Focus on Cancer

Springer
London
Berlin
Heidelberg
New York
Barcelona
Budapest
Hong Kong
Milan
Paris
Santa Clara
Singapore
Tokyo

Also available in this series:

Evaluation of Cancer Screening
J. Chamberlain and S. Moss (Eds)
ISBN 3-540-19957-8

Cancer: Palliative Care
R. Dunlop
ISBN 3-540-19974-8

Maurice L. Slevin and Teresa Tate (Eds)

Cancer: How Worthwhile is Non-Curative Treatment?

With 16 Figures

Springer

Maurice L. Slevin, MB, ChB, MD, FRCP
Teresa Tate, FRCP, FRCR

Department of Medical Oncology, St Bartholomew's Hospital, West Smithfield, London EC1A 7BE, UK

ISBN 3-540-76083-0 Springer-Verlag Berlin Heidelberg New York

British Library Cataloguing in Publication Data
Cancer: how worthwhile is non-curative treatment?. -
(Focus on cancer)
1. Cancer - Palliative treatment
I. Slevin, Maurice II. Tate, Anne Teresa
616.9'94'06
ISBN 3540760830

Library of Congress Cataloging-in-Publication Data
Cancer: how worthwhile is non-curative treatment? / M.L. Slevin and T. Tate (eds.).
p. cm. - (Focus on cancer)
Includes bibliographical references and index.
ISBN 3-540-76083-0 (pbk. : alk. paper)
1. Cancer-Palliative treatment. I. Slevin, Maurice L. II. Tate, T. (Teresa) III. Series.
[DNLM: 1. Neoplasms-therapy. 2. Palliative Care. 3. Quality of Life. QZ 266 C21438 1997]
RC271.P33C36 1997
616.99'4-dc21
DNLM/DLC 97-18096
for Library of Congress CIP

Typeset by Wilmaset Ltd, Birkenhead, Wirral
Printed at the Athenæum Press Ltd., Gateshead, Tyne & Wear
28/3830-543210 Printed on acid-free paper

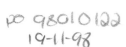

Series Editor's Foreword

Cancer is a major issue in the provision of health care. It is estimated that one in four people in developed countries are likely to develop it at some time. As longevity steadily increases, the incidence of malignant disease is expected to rise further. Important advances in the control of cancer have taken place and curative treatment has improved, notably in some of the rarer tumours, particularly in children. Advances in the more common cancers have been less marked, although adjunctive systemic treatment and population screening are lowering mortality from the most prevalent cancer - carcinoma of the breast. Despite this progress, complete control of malignant disease is still a long way off. However, our understanding of the molecular biology of cancer has increased enormously in recent years and the application of this knowledge holds considerable promise for developing new therapeutic strategies. As for prevention, the cause of most cancers is still poorly understood although it is clear that tobacco avoidance would prevent most lung cancers and several others.

Cancer is studied at many different levels: molecular and cellular biology, pathology in patients (particularly clinical trials), and prevention and populations (epidemiology). The psychosocial problems caused to patients and their families are being increasingly recognized and subjected to systematic study. Workers in the field, therefore, range from basic scientists to epidemiologists, from hospital specialists to community support teams. Each needs to have at least some knowledge of the role the others play. However, to bring all together in a single educational forum is impractical. Nevertheless, this ideal underlies the ethos of this series. Cancer issues are well served by a burgeoning literature of learned journals, newsletters, student textbooks and specialized monographs. Less available are concise overviews of general aspects for the busy oncologist and equally to those many professionals who are involved in the subject but are not specialists in it. Springer-Verlag's Focus on Cancer series has been designed to meet this information need. Each issue is devoted to a well-defined theme such as basic science and clinical application, diagnostic methods (including clinical appraisal of new technology), treatment, complications of cancer and psychosocial problems. The reader will judge whether this aim has been achieved and I will be pleased to receive comments and suggestions, including further topics for coverage in this series.

April, 1995 R.D. Rubens
United Medical and Dental Schools
Guy's and St Thomas's Hospitals, London

Preface

Many advances have taken place in the treatment of cancer over the past 25 years and treatment continues to improve year by year. However, more than 50% of all patients with cancer are still treated knowing that cure is not feasible or, at least, a very remote possibility. The therapeutic intent for these patients must be the prolongation of good quality life and, if this is not possible, optimising the quality of the remaining time.

The non-curative treatment of cancer may involve surgery, radiotherapy, chemotherapy and hormone therapies, physical and psychosocial symptom management, all used in varying combinations depending on the individual situation. When these treatments are proposed for patients in whom cure is not possible, there may be great concern that the morbidity associated, particularly with the anti-cancer therapies, will outweigh the benefits that the patient may receive. This concern often results in failure to refer the patient for a specialist oncological opinion. In fact, recent research increasingly indicates that achieving optimal tumour control by active treatment of the cancer can maximise the quality of life. The benefits of a reduction in symptoms from the cancer itself outweigh any toxicity to the therapy.

There nevertheless remains considerable confusion and uncertainty among doctors treating cancer patients as to how to balance the potential benefits and toxicities when considering the active treatment of non-curable cancer. Even the terminology is confused. The conventional understanding of "palliative treatment" is of that given in the last months of life, with the intention of relieving symptoms related to the cancer, but with the implicit proviso that anti-cancer treatments are not included or are specifically confined to controlling symptoms, for example, radiotherapy for bone pain. It would in many ways be helpful if a different term could be used to describe the treatment of patients whose tumours are managed with active but non-curative intent by surgery, radiotherapy or chemotherapy. A hunt through the thesaurus does not provide many easy alternatives, the best probably being "ameliorative", which is cumbersome and unfamiliar but which might, with persistence, come into common usage.

This book brings together in a single volume the current state-of-the-art in the non-curative, but active treatment of cancer. The chapters have been written by leading experts in their fields and, as far as possible, are evidence based. There are, however, many aspects of the difficult topic for which hard data does not exist. The authors then suggest logical approaches for various situations and problems. We hope that this book stimulates and contributes to the debate on this very important topic, and that it will help clinicians in the practical management of their patients.

M. L. Slevin and T. Tate

Contents

Section 1. Non-Curative Surgery

Section 2. Non-Curative Radiotherapy

Section 3. Non-Curative Chemotherapy

Contributors

Dr S.J. Arnott
Consultant Radiotherapist
St Bartholomew's Hospital
West Smithfield
London EC1A 7BE

Dr R. Barton
Academic Unit of Radiotherapy and Oncology
The Royal Marsden NHS Trust
Downs Road
Sutton
Surrey SM2 5PT

Dr P.R. Blake
Consultant Clinical Oncologist
The Royal Marsden NHS Trust
Fulham Road
London SW3 6JJ

Professor N.M. Bleehen
Department of Clinical Oncology
Addenbrooke's Hospital
Hills Road
Cambridge CB2 2QQ

Dr D.J. Boote
Department of Clinical Oncology
Addenbrooke's Hospital
Hills Road
Cambridge CB2 2QQ

Dr Michael Brada
Academic Unit of Radiotherapy and Oncology
The Royal Marsden NHS Trust
Downs Road
Sutton
Surrey SM2 5PT

Dr L. Brazil
Academic Unit of Radiotherapy and Oncology
The Royal Marsden NHS Trust
Downs Road
Sutton
Surrey SM2 5PT

Mr Robin Crawford
St Bartholomew's Hospital
West Smithfield
London EC1A 7BE

Dr M.H. Cullen
Consultant Medical Oncologist
Birmingham Oncology Centre
Queen Elizabeth Hospital
Edgbaston
Birmingham B15 2TH

Dr D. Cunningham
Consultant Medical Oncologist
CRC Section of Medicine
The Royal Marsden NHS Trust
Downs Road
Sutton
Surrey SM2 5PT

Mr John W.L. Fielding
Surgical Oncology Unit
Queen Elizabeth Hospital
Edgbaston
Birmingham B15 2TH

Mr Peter Goldstraw
Consultant Thoracic Surgeon
Royal Brompton Hospital
Sydney Street
London SW3 6NP

Dr M.E. Gore
Consultant Cancer Physician
The Royal Marsden NHS Trust
Fulham Road
London SW3 6JJ

Dr F. Anthony Greco
Medical Director
Centennial Medical Center
The Sarah Cannon Cancer Center
250 25th Avenue North
Suite 412, The Atrium
Nashville
TN 37203, USA

Dr John D. Hainsworth
Centennial Medical Center
The Sarah Cannon Cancer Center
250 25th Avenue North
Suite 412, The Atrium
Nashville
TN 37203, USA

Mr Jonathan D. Harrison
Surgical Oncology Unit
Queen Elizabeth Hospital
Edgbaston
Birmingham B15 2TH

Mr W.F. Hendry
Consultant Urologist
St Bartholomew's Hospital
West Smithfield
London EC1A 7BE

Dr P.J. Hoskin
Marie Curie Research Wing for Oncology
Mount Vernon Centre for Cancer Treatment
Mount Vernon Hospital
Rickmansworth Road
Northwood
Middlesex HA6 2RN

Dr A. Jones
Consultant Medical Oncologist
Department of Clinical Oncology
The Royal Free Hospital
Pond Street
London NW3 2QG

Dr R.C.F. Leonard
Consultant & Honorary Senior Lecturer
Department of Clinical Oncology
The University of Edinburgh
Western General Hospital
Edinburgh EH4 2XU

Dr C.M. McLean
Department of Clinical Oncology
The University of Edinburgh
Western General Hospital
Edinburgh EH4 2XU

Dr G. Middleton
CRC Section of Medicine
The Royal Marsden NHS Trust
Downs Road
Sutton
Surrey SM2 5PT

Mr R.J. Nicholls
Consultant Surgeon
Academic Institute
Northwick Park and St Mark's Hospitals
Northwick Park
Watford Road
Harrow
Middlesex HA1 3UJ

Mr Ugo Pastorino
Royal Brompton Hospital
Sydney Street
London SW3 6NP

Mr D.G. Porter
The National Hospital for Nervous Diseases
Queen Square
London WC1N 3BG

Dr M.E.B. Powell
Marie Curie Research Wing for Oncology
Mount Vernon Centre for Cancer Treatment
Mount Vernon Hospital
Rickmansworth Road
Northwood
Middlesex HA6 2RN

Dr J.A. Prendiville
The Royal Marsden NHS Trust
Fulham Road
London SW3 6JJ

Dr Gillian M. Sadler
Senior Registrar
Meyerstein Institute of Oncology
The Middlesex Hospital
Mortimer Street
London W1

Dr D.J. Sebag-Montefiore
Yorkshire Regional Centre for Cancer Treatment
Cookridge Hospital
Hospital Lane
Leeds LS16 6QB

Mr John H. Shepherd
Consultant Gynaecologist
St Bartholomew's Hospital
West Smithfield
London EC1A 7BE

Professor D.G.T. Thomas
The National Hospital for Nervous Diseases
Queen Square
London WC1N 3BG

Dr Jeffrey S. Tobias
Clinical Director Cancer Services
Meyerstein Institute of Oncology
The Middlesex Hospital
Mortimer Street
London W1

Mr S.J. Watson
Department of General Surgery
Sir Charles Gardiner Hospital
Verdun Street
Nedlands
Western Australia WA6009
Australia

Section 1

Non-Curative Surgery

1 – Non-Curative Surgery for Upper Gastrointestinal Malignancy

Jonathan D. Harrison and John W.L. Fielding

Introduction

The surgical management of upper gastrointestinal malignancy is commonly "non-curative" or "palliative", since the majority of patients present with advanced stage disease and local or distant failure occurs fairly frequently even in patients receiving potentially curative resections. The objective of surgery is thus moving toward providing *stage appropriate* treatment, with the intention of maximizing survival and allowing an optimum quality of life.

The selection of patients for radical or palliative surgery depends on a number of factors which are assessed by staging investigations which may be preoperative in the case of radiological assessments or perioperative in the case of frozen section lymph node assessments. These factors are:

1. The primary tumour.
2. Lymph node metastases.
3. Distant metastases.
4. Histology.
5. Lack of safe and effective therapy for advanced disease.

Other factors involved in the intention to treat the cancer are the general condition and age of the patient, although age is not as significant a barrier to curative surgery as it once was, with patients now being assessed according to their merits.

Oesophageal Carcinoma

Surgery

Oesophageal cancer is a lesion that is commonly advanced at presentation and thus not curable. Patients with stage I disease are considered to be surgically curable, but unfortunately these patients comprise less than 10% of patients in hospital series [1]. The corollary of this is that the majority of operations for oesophageal cancer are non-curative.

The resectability rate of oesophageal tumours depends upon the stage of the lesion and the technical experience and expertise of the operating surgeon. Resectability rates have generally increased over the last three decades and in many studies are now around 50–60% [2].

The majority of surgeons resect and replace in one session, the choice of a two- or three-phase procedure usually being based on the level of the tumour in the oesophagus. The most commonly used reconstruction conduit is the mobilized gastric fundus and although some surgeons report the same mortality rates with either stomach or colon interposition [3], some have found the latter procedure to have a higher mortality rate [4].

Operative mortality rates have fallen significantly in the last 30 years. In the 20-year period 1957–76 the mortality for the "occasional" resectionist ($\leqslant$ 3 per year) was 39.4% and 21.6% for the "frequent" resectionist ($\geqslant$ 6 per year) [5]. Mortality has since fallen by between 5% and 10%, particularly in the last decade [2, 4, 6–9].

The overall 5-year survival rate after surgical resection is around 20% as compared to the overall survival of 5% at 5 years [2]. The only patients who have a higher survival rate than this are the selected group of patients undergoing an *en bloc* radical resection [10]. Surgical resection is thus of benefit in terms of patient survival, and although it is infrequently curative because of the advanced stage of the disease, the quality of palliation in terms of swallowing is superior in the majority of patients. The place of palliative bypass surgery for irresectable tumours is more contentious, since the same swallowing advantages accrue from these procedures, but at the expense of what many surgeons consider to be an unacceptable morbidity and mortality rate [10–13].

As many patients are elderly and have complicating serious medical conditions which preclude major resection, endoscopic therapy has become the mainstay of treatment for this group. The endoscopic approach includes dilatation, insertion of prostheses, alcohol injection, photodynamic therapy (PDT) and thermal destruction with Bicap probes or lasers.

Laser Therapy

Laser irradiation can be used either directly or indirectly in the therapy of gastric cancer. When used directly (usually using a Neodymium: Yttrium Aluminium Garnet (Nd:YAG) source), the laser can vaporize obstructing exphytic tissue at the cardia, with satisfactory resolution of dysphagia in the majority of cases. The potential advantage of this method over intubation is that the patient should be able to take a more normal diet, provided that the obstructing lesion is less than around 4 cm [14]. The main disadvantage is that multiple treatments are often necessary [15–18]. In the initial stages of development this form of therapy was a "non-contact" technique, but recently new ceramic probes have been developed which allow contact photocoagulation. This allows a greater degree of control, and also lower levels of power are required for the same effect, making the requisite laser equipment simpler and cheaper [19].

Photodynamic Therapy

Laser irradiation may be employed in an indirect capacity in PDT. This form of treatment uses a photosensitizing agent coupled with laser radiation of a specific wavelength to destroy tumour tissue. The photosensitizing agent most commonly used is haematoporphyrin derivative (HpD), which is produced by treating haematoporphyrin with acetic and sulphuric acid [20]. HpD is administered 72 h prior to treatment, as the agent is retained in malignant tissue for longer periods than normal tissue [21]. HpD has a strong absorption peak at 630 nm and so for this application an argon dye laser is used, so that red light of wavelength 630 nm is produced by use of the dye Rhodamine B.

Electron microscopy has shown that therapy results in mitochondrial damage, dilatation of the rough endoplasmic reticulum and alteration of the nuclear membrane.

The cytotoxic effect is thought to be mediated by the production of singlet oxygen within the malignant cells [22]. In Japan, over 1600 patients with gastric carcinoma have been treated with endoscopic laser therapy [23], including a group of patients with early gastric cancer. The advantage of this form of treatment is that multiple treatments can be safely performed with a low complication rate.

Intubation

The endoscopic insertion of a rigid plastic tube across a neoplastic stricture has become an accepted approach to the palliation of oesophageal malignancy [24, 25]. The disease is commonly advanced, often with distant metastases, and the patients are usually malnourished. The complication rate of the tube insertion, which requires a dilatation of up to 54F, is thus often high and the survival in this group of patients is limited. The advantage of this form of palliation is that the treatment is usually the only intervention required unless there is tube blockage or migration. The main disadvantage of intubation is that the quality of swallowing is limited and reflux symptoms are common.

Ethanol-Induced Tumour Necrosis

A number of studies have shown that effective palliation of malignant dysphagia can be achieved by the direct injection of absolute alcohol or polidocanol into the tumour. This results in necrosis of the tumour and as a result of this an increase in the diameter of the lumen, which has the effect of improving dysphagia scores [26, 27].

Bipolar Diathermy Tumour Probes

The BICAP™ (ACMI, Connecticut, USA) multipolar endoscopic diathermy probe is another method of palliating malignant dysphagia. Its olive-shaped ceramic probe tip has three pairs of longitudinal electrodes of alternate polarity which results in heat generation when an electric current is applied. The probes come in a range of sizes to suit the diameter of the tumour and they have a central channel for a guidewire. Studies have shown the BICAP probe to be similar in efficacy to the Nd:YAG laser at improving dysphagia scores over similar periods of time [28–30].

The major flaw with these local endoscopic treatments (dilatation, laser, alcohol injection and BICAP) is that the improvement in dysphagia scores is temporary and the therapies usually need to be repeated a variable number of times before the patient's death.

Conclusion

Oesophageal cancer is a challenging disease to treat, since the majority of patients present with advanced disease and recurrence even after aggressive surgical treatment is common. Nevertheless, if surgical resection is possible, it gives the most satisfactory outcome in terms of disease-free survival and quality of life.

Gastric Cancer

Gastric carcinoma remains the fourth commonest cause of cancer mortality in England and Wales and despite a modest reduction in the incidence of gastric cancer this century, it still accounts for approximately 10 000 deaths annually. The overall 5-year survival rate remains static at around 5% in England and Wales [31]. The principal reason for this poor prognosis is that the stage at presentation is stage III or IV in the majority of cases [32]. This means that although surgery has been possible in an increasing proportion of these patients in the last 20 years, the possibility of cure is limited by the spread of the disease and the object of treatment has thus been palliation.

The changing pattern of site in gastric cancer also makes the choice of palliation more difficult, with an increase in the proportion of patients with proximal tumours in the last two decades [33]. This provides a dilemma, since many surgeons now feel that total gastrectomy is not an appropriate means of palliation in patients with advanced disease given the high morbidity and mortality rates associated with this procedure and the length of recovery time after it compared to the likely survival time in such patients.

Because of the greater potential for spread of the diffuse type of tumour, some authors have suggested that wider margins (> 6 cm) need to be taken to be sure of adequate clearance. This approach often leads to the routine performance of total gastrectomy for diffuse-type tumours [34].

Surgery

There has been a steady increase in the tumour resectability rate reported in various series. Mine and colleagues [45] showed an increase from 22% in 1907–16 to 55% in 1950–59 in the rate of resection.

Gall and Hermanek [34] reported an increase from 60.8% to 75.9% over two consecutive 5-year periods, which was mainly due to an increase in the number of non-curative resections. While tumour stage clearly is the major determinant of resectability, the surgeons' approach is also important, as illustrated by the resectability rates reported in a co-operative study [35], in which seven centres reported resection rates varying between 37% and 73%, with similar laparotomy rates over the same time period. This effect was also seen in the West Midlands over the 25-year period 1957–81. During this time, 42.5% of 31 567 patients reported to the Cancer Registry had an "open and close" laparotomy with no attempt at surgical palliation and only 29.2% of these patients had a resection. The policy of not attempting to resect gastric cancers prevalent 20 years ago is particularly seen with increasing patient age: only 21.5% of patients aged 50–59 years were offered no treatment compared to 51.6% of patients aged 70–79 years [36].

There is no doubt that if a tumour is resectable then the prognosis is considerably superior to the group whose tumours are irresectable [35, 37–40], although this is clearly stage dependent, rather than the operation being a prognostic indicator *per se*. Surgeons must ensure an adequate clearance above and below the primary tumour, since it has been demonstrated that the presence of tumour at either resection margin has a marked negative effect upon survival [32].

The effect of surgeons as a prognostic factor is also seen in their ability to conclude gastric resections safely with a low operative mortality rate. It has been shown that operative mortality falls with increasing experience and frequent performance of partial gastrectomy [36].

In Japan, and to a lesser extent in Europe until recently, there has been increasing enthusiasm for the use of extended radical lymphadenectomy to effect a cure in gastric carcinoma, since the prognosis has not been improved by less radical surgery. The gastric region lymph nodes are customarily divided into four groups defined by the General Rules of the Japanese Research Society for Gastric Cancer [41] (Table 1.1).

Operations to remove groups of nodes *en bloc* with the stomach are termed "Dn" procedures, such that "D" should exceed the number of the group of lymph nodes affected by disease, in order to completely excise the local disease [42]. The degree of lymph node involvement is known to have a significant effect upon prognosis [43, 44], although not as an independent variable, since lymph node spread is dependent upon the degree of infiltration of the primary tumour through the gastric wall [45, 46]. This has stimulated surgical efforts to remove the next group of nodes to the one that is involved in each patient, such that D > n. Evidence for the efficacy of this approach comes from studies showing a steady decline in hospital mortality rates and a steady increase in the 5-year survival of patients treated by radical lymphadenectomy, which is only seen in the node-positive patients. Nakajima and Kajitani [46] showed a steady increase in the 5-year survival of 5415 patients treated between 1946 and 1973, which they attribute to the aggressive approach to lymph node surgery. Although many of the gastrectomies in Japanese series are done with curative intent, it is clear that many of the patients have involvement of lymph nodes and a significant proportion of these patients will die from recurrent disease.

Table 1.1 Classification of lymph node groups in gastric cancer

Group 1	Involvement of perigastric lymph nodes within 3 cm of the primary tumour
Group 2	Involvement of perigastric lymph nodes more than 3 cm from the primary tumour, including those along the left gastric, common hepatic, splenic and coeliac arteries.
Group 3	Involvement of retropancreatic, para-aortic or diaphragmatic nodes
Group 4	Involvement of nodes more distant than group 3

Nevertheless, it is evident from the literature that very satisfactory palliation is achieved in this group of patients in whom a near-normal quality of life can be expected, with 5-year survival in the region of 30% [42, 45–47].

There have also been a number of studies in the literature examining the relative merits of palliative resection in patients with advanced disease. The data in the literature are difficult to interpret as most of the studies are retrospective and there is almost certainly a significant degree of selection bias which is impossible to quantify. Despite this, it would seem that there are advantages to be gained from palliative partial gastric resection compared to lesser procedures such as gastroenterostomy or laparotomy and no procedure. These advantages are seen in terms of a lower hospital mortality rate, prolonged survival and a superior quality of life [48–53].

Conclusion

It is clear that since gastric carcinoma most commonly presents at an advanced stage when there is no hope of cure, the most important advances that can be made in the Western world, as in Japan, are in changing the natural history of the disease by early diagnosis, and in developing safe and effective forms of palliation for patients with advanced disease, but in the meantime surgical palliation will remain the mainstay of management for gastric carcinoma.

Liver

Palliative Surgery for Primary Hepatocellular Cancer

Hepatocellular carcinoma (HCC) accounts for more than 1 million deaths a year worldwide and even quite small untreated tumours have a poor prognosis, with only <13% of patients alive at 3 years [54]. Many patients with HCC will have chronic hepatic damage due to hepatitis B or C, and cirrhosis in more than three-quarters makes surgery hazardous. In advanced cases, only palliative treatment is possible with chemotherapy. Tumour irradiation, alcohol injection or cryotherapy are current options being explored. Transarterial catheter embolization has also been advocated and 1-year survival of 50–78% has been reported [55, 56]. Complete hepatic tumour resection offers the only realistic prospect of cure, and a contentious area at present is whether a hepatic resection should be partial or total, followed by hepatic transplantation.

In the absence of cirrhosis, resection is the treatment of choice and can be undertaken with a low morbidity and hospital mortality of 3–15%. Five-year survival is high in tumours less than 2 cm in size, although this falls to between 20% and 37% when the tumour size exceeds 5 cm [57]. Nevertheless, this still represents significant palliation in these survivors, with an expectation of a normal quality of life in these non-cirrhotic survivors.

Extended hepatic resections of HCC tumours with major vascular invasion have been reported and results may be improved by preoperative chemotherapy. Complete hepatectomy followed by transplantation will be reserved for those relatively few non-cirrhotic patients with all major compartments of the liver involved by cancer, yet staging indicating that disease is still confined to the liver.

The surgical approach in cirrhotic patients is less clearly defined. Resection rates are low with advancing or decompensating liver disease (Child's B/C categories), with the significant risks of haemorrhage, infection and liver decompensation.

Resection in Child's B/C cirrhosis is usually confined to tumours situated peripherally, less than 5 cm in size, which can be removed by non-anatomical or segmental resection, maximizing the residual liver mass. In this situation mortality rates below 10% are reported, yet it is important that an adequate tumour clearance margin of at least 1 cm is achieved if local tumour recurrence is to be avoided.

The ultimate patient survival depends not only on the likelihood of tumour recurrence, but also the underlying stability of the liver cirrhosis. Progression of the underlying liver cirrhosis means that less than 30% of Child's B/C cases will avoid complications of variceal haemorrhage or hepatic decompensation. In the long term, as many patients succumb due to progression of cirrhosis as to recurrent tumour and 5-year survival rates are low (0–23%) [58, 59]. Larger tumours or those more centrally situated may be irresectable because of inadequate hepatic reserve, and even with modern surgical technique mortality rises. Nagasue et al. [59] report a 3-year survival of only 16% in Child's B/C cirrhotic patients under 60 years old with tumours less than 5 cm in size or in patients with multicentric HCC nodules. It is concluded that such patients should be considered for transplantation.

The high rate of recurrence which marked the early disappointing results of transplantation was often due to the advanced tumour stage, with residual tumour in coeliac nodes in a high proportion of patients. Less than 20% of such patients survived longer than 2 years. However, Ringe et al. clearly showed that when coeliac lymph nodes did not contain tumour, then nearly 50% of all patients survived more than 3 years after transplantation [60].

The European Liver Transplantation Registry now reports over 40% 3-year patient survival in transplantation for HCC, although this figure includes "incidental" tumours [61]. An attempt to address the issue of residual lymph node disease led to a radical hepatic excision and *en bloc* clearance of the coeliac lymph nodes and adjacent tissue prior to transplantation, the so-called "cluster" operation [62]. These complex procedures were largely abandoned when it became clear that 2-year survival was less than 20% in patients whose coeliac lymph nodes contained tumour [63]. In those patients with negative lymph nodes and therefore in whom such a radical procedure was performed, the 2-year survival was more than 70%, not significantly different from patients undergoing "simpler" hepatic transplantation [64]. Following this early experience of transplantation for HCC, meticulous cancer staging is now undertaken in patients with Child's B/C category cirrhosis.

The progression of cirrhosis in conditions such as haemochromatosis, chronic active hepatitis, primary biliary cirrhosis or alcoholic liver disease means that the risk of hepatic decompensation is significant. The uncertain prognosis of the underlying parenchymal liver disease combined with concern about recurrent or metachronous HCC, especially if inadequate tumour clearance occurs, has led to a reappraisal of the benefits of complete hepatic resection and transplantation [65].

With the improvements in immunosuppression and modification of the surgical techniques involved in hepatic transplantation, the majority of elective patients can now be grafted safely with low mobidity – a mean hospital stay of less than 20 days and in-hospital mortality of less than 8%.

In cirrhotic patients with comparable tumour staging, a recent analysis showed a 5-year survival of 35.6% following complete hepatic resection and transplantation compared to no survivors in patients who had a partial hepatic resection [64]. Clearly complete hepatic excision and transplantation of the liver will not be appropriate for all cirrhotic patients and requires careful assessment, especially when alcoholic cirrhosis is the underlying disease. Against its benefits must of course be balanced its significant cost, the need for lifelong immunosuppression and the relative shortage of donor organs. Also, hepatitis B may recur in the grafted liver even in spite of hyperimmune globulin. The option of transplantation of the liver is clearly not appropriate for elderly patients with concomitant major disease. However, in a patient under 60 years old with underlying cirrhosis, a large central tumour or multi-focal disease will be considered.

Elsewhere, for patients with HCC and cirrhosis, increasingly, management protocols will include the complete range of options, both surgical and oncological, adding complete hepatic excision and transplantation to the standard technique of partial hepatic excision. Only by combining the screening of patients and the earlier diagnosis of HCC with a wider range of complementary surgical options will the prognosis of this dreadful condition be improved.

Secondary Adenocarcinoma

Approximately 25% of patients undergoing resection for a colonic or rectal carcinoma have hepatic metastases and a further 25% have "occult" metastases which progress and may or may not present clinically before the death of the patient [66]. Until the last two to three decades the presence of liver metastases was generally regarded as an untreatable terminal event. More recently it has been increasingly recognized that a proportion of patients may be considered for a hepatic resection to remove metastases from colorectal cancers.

The problem in evaluating the degree of palliation achieved by major hepatic resection is that the natural history of hepatic metastases is variable, with median survival ranging from 9 months in patients with widespread bilobar disease to 21 months for patients with solitary metastases [67]. This makes comparing the tumour load in different patients an inexact science, although improvements in cross-sectional imaging techniques have improved the accuracy of such comparisons.

Detection of Metastases

While the educated surgical hand has been the "gold standard" in the detection of liver metastases for many years, there have been a number of developments which have increased our ability to identify these lesions at an earlier phase in their natural history. Non-invasive techniques with a resolution of around 5 mm include external ultrasound, computed tomographic (CT) and magnetic resonance (MR) imaging. All of these techniques are more sensitive than palpation alone for small lesions deep in the hepatic parenchyma. Complementary to these investigations is intraoperative ultrasound scanning, which can achieve higher resolution by use of higher frequency probes in direct contact with the liver [68, 69]. Another method of detecting lesions which remain occult to all current imaging techniques is by using the hepatic perfusion index. This relies on the phenomenon by which hepatic metastases derive the majority of their blood supply early in their development and this is manifested as an increase in the arterial blood flow relative to the portal venous flow in the relevant part of the liver. This can be detected either by a radiopharmaceutical method [70] or more recently by a combination of colour Doppler imaging with an injection of galactose microparticles [71]. Scintigraphic detection of metastases from carcinoid tumours may also be detected using radiolabelled octreotide [72].

Prognostic Factors

Early reports on hepatic resection for metastatic liver disease concentrated on resection of small lesions with good results, which prompted the consideration of larger lesions for surgical management [73]. There is now considerable experience of such resections in many centres, which has allowed an analysis of the most important clinical indices in the prognosis of patients with liver metastases. While such major surgery can now be routinely performed with mortality rates of around 5% [74–79], it is clear that certain factors result in a poor prognosis which is not significantly different from unresected patients with a similar tumour load [78].

One of the most important determinants which have come out of many univariate and multivariate analyses is tumour load, with patients having less than four discrete metastases enjoying a significantly better prognosis than patients with four or more lesions. Other important negative prognostic factors are resection margins less than 10 mm from the tumour, the presence of extrahepatic metastases, synchronous tumours, satellite metastases and non-anatomical resections [80–86]. Many authors have found that the stage of the primary does not have an effect on survival after hepatic resection for metastases, which seems counter-intuitive. Other authors have found a significant effect, with Dukes' stage C tumours having a median survival of 27 months compared to 123 months for stage B tumours in the Sloan-Kettering Memorial Hospital series [87, 88].

Advances in hepatic surgery have allowed repeat resections of lesions which have recurred in 10–20% of cases after an initial resection due either to residual disease or progression of occult metastases. This approach has been combined with resection of localized extrahepatic lesions such as pulmonary metastases, with good disease-free palliation in this highly selected group of patients [89–93].

The techniques of liver transplantation have also been applied to this area, with surgeons performing extracorporeal "bench resections" after perfusing the liver with preservation solution and then reimplanting the remaining liver for lesions that are deemed to be inoperable by conventional techniques [94].

While the majority of studies have been into palliative surgery for colorectal metastases, there has also been some interest and also some encouraging results for the treatment of selected patients with metastases from gastric cancer, with similar survival figures to colorectal metastatic disease [95].

It seems clear from the many series in the literature that while this form of surgery is rarely curative, it can result in significant palliation with a good quality of life in 25–30% of a selected group of around 20% of patients with metastases at 5 years.

Metastatic Neuroendocrine Tumours

When gastroenteropancreatic carcinomas metastasize to the liver the clinical manifestation of the lesion depends on the cell type involved, one of the commonest of which is the serotonin-secreting carcinoid tumour. These metastatic lesions are most commonly treatable medically by means of the somatostatin analogue octreotide, interferon or chemo-embolization of the tumour [96–98], but there is a small group of patients with symptoms which are uncontrollable by medical means and who have surgically resectable lesions who may benefit from surgical debulking of the liver disease [99–102].

If there is major hepatic involvement, uncontrollable symptoms and clear evidence of disease limited to the liver, then complete hepatic excision followed by orthotopic liver transplantation may be considered in a small group of selected patients [103].

Cryotherapy

There are a number of ways in which the bulk of a liver tumour which is inoperable according to conventional criteria may be reduced, such as cryotherapy or interstitial laser irradiation. Hepatic cryotherapy for neoplastic disease has been under evaluation for some time and it has been shown to be a safe technique which may be used alone or in combination with regional chemotherapy [104–107]. Promising results have been shown in terms of tumour destruction, as evidenced by sharp falls in serum carcinoembryonic antigen (CEA) levels [108], and survival data from 33 patients having hepatic cryotherapy for colorectal metastases have recently been published showing an advantage for those patients with a major fall in CEA level [109].

Regional Chemotherapy

It is appropriate to mention regional cytotoxic perfusion in this section since the infusion equipment is implanted at a major laparotomy and the technique is complementary to other forms of surgical management including resection and cryotherapy.

The implantation of catheters into either the portal vein or the hepatic artery, usually by placing a cannula into the gastroduodenal artery, has been practised for the last three decades and a number of uncontrolled studies with disparate cytotoxic agents have shown some promising results, with increases in the objective response rate to around 60% with a combination of 5-fluorouracil (5-FU) and folinic acid, which is approximately double the response rate seen with the same agents given systematically. Operative mortality is very low (usually less than 1%) but morbidity is relatively high, particularly in the series using fluorodeoxyuridine (FUDR) which is commonly associated with an irreversible sclerosing cholangitis. This does not seem to be a problem in the studies using 5-FU, which is associated with little toxicity when given intra-arterially [110–113].

Cholangiocellular Carcinoma

It is generally appreciated that cholangiocarcinomata, particularly those at the hepatic hilum, are difficult to manage due to their anatomical location and opinion has been expressed to doubt that the lesion is surgically curable. Despite this view it seems clear that a radical resection in a patient with clear margins and uninvolved lymph nodes gives the best chance of a cure or at least prolonged palliation with a good quality of life [114–116]. The patients in most surgical series with the longest survival are those who have had a radical resection, with histologically uninvolved margins and nodes, although it has to be conceded that there are few long-term survivors.

Resection

The resectability rate in many series has increased steadily over the last 20 years with the development of surgical techniques and technology [117]. The resectability rate in many series is 10–30% [115, 117, 118]. The importance of excising segment I in addition to the tumour is being increasingly recognised, since this may be invaded by tumour in a significant proportion of cases [119]. Removal of the lesion by either radical partial resection or total hepatic excision and replacement was possible in 33% of the patients in this series and the majority of these resections (12/14) took place after 1987.

Transplantation

The role of orthotopic liver transplantation (OLT) in the management of cholangiocarcinoma is the cause of some controversy, although many units have moved away from an active policy of transplanting for this indication, even though it is not an uncommon incidental finding in patients having an OLT for sclerosing cholangitis (SC) [120]. This group with incidental tumours has a much better prognosis than those having an OLT for known malignancy, but significantly worse than the patients with SC without a cholangiocarcinoma [120, 121]. Similar disappointing results have been seen in other studies for patients transplanted for known cholangiocarcinoma, with early recurrence and median survival of around 1 year [122–124].

It may be that the lsions that are most suitable for treatment by hepatic excison and OLT are those which are demonstrably intrahepatic with no extrahepatic disease, as opposed to previous recommendations [117, 123] to transplant patients with the most advanced tumours, which are probably more likely to have metastasized to lymph nodes and are thus incurable even by total hepatectomy.

Palliative Procedures

The optimal management for patients with irresectable disease is another area of controversy. Many surgeons will argue that a surgical approach such as the segment III–IV duct bypass popularized by Bismuth and Corlette [125] gives the patient an uninterrupted period of good health before the terminal stages of the disease, while the longer endoscopically placed stents required to decompress hilar lesions often result in one or more subsequent admissions for stent changes, with the resulting ill-health associated with cholangitis before and after the procedure [117]. The advent of the wallstent with its wider lumen [126] may tip the balance in favour of non-surgical biliary decompression, but objective evidence for this contention is currently lacking. The optimal management of the irresectable cholangiocarcinoma awaits confirmation by clinical trial.

Adjuvant Therapy

Due to the comparative rarity of this condition it has proved difficult to recruit sufficient numbers of patients to trials of adjuvant drug or radiation treatment. Radiation may be administered either by external beam [127, 128] using ^{192}Iridium brachytherapy [129, 130] or by ^{131}Iodine-labelled anti-CEA antibody with chemotherapy [131]. Response rates have been variable and a significant effect on survival has yet to be demonstrated.

Radical resection can give prolonged palliation and possibly a cure, particularly in patients who have negative lymph nodes. OLT gives satisfactory results when the tumour has not metastasized to extrahepatic lymph nodes, but is probably not indicated as a treatment for advanced cholangiocarcinoma until better methods of excluding extrahepatic disease are developed. Prolonged survival is seen in a proportion of patients receiving both endoscopic and surgical palliation.

Pancreatic Cancer

Adenocarcinoma of the pancreas is the fifth commonest cause of cancer mortality in England and Wales and the incidence of the disease in the Western world has been increasing in the last three decades [132]. It has a marked tendency to present with advanced stage disease such that curative surgery is rarely possible, and even when macroscopic disease clearance has been achieved it is not uncommon for the patient to succumb to local disease recurrence.

Nevertheless, there is still a very important role for surgery in the management of the majority of patients with pancreatic cancer for whom the disease has progressed beyond the stage of resectability. The principal conditions in which non-curative surgery may be of value are in the relief of obstruction to the common bile duct or gastric outlet, the palliation of chronic pain and, as mortality rates have fallen in the last two decades, some surgeons are recommending palliative resection in patients who clearly have residual disease at the time of surgery [133, 134].

Resectability

The resectability of pancreatic cancers has increased over the last 20 years from 10% to around 20%. The incidence of palliative surgical bypass has also increased steadily from 45% to nearly 60%, while the number of patients having a laparotomy only has fallen by about 5% to around 20% [135].

The decision to offer the patient a resection depends upon the philosophy of the physician or surgeon making the initial assessment of the tumour. Some clinicians are prepared to accept apparent inoperability on imaging and simply relieve jaundice with endoscopically or radiologically placed endoprostheses. Many surgeons with an interest in pancreatic surgery contend that cross-sectional imaging modalities such as CT or MRI, even when combined with angiography, are not sufficiently sensitive to categorically rule that a patient is inoperable and the only certain method of deciding operability is by trial dissection. If, after this dissection, the patient's tumour is deemed irresectable, then the opportunity exists for a surgical biliary diversion which has the advantage of a low complication rate compared to endoscopically placed endoprostheses, which commonly block after 3–6 months, requiring replacement and causing a period of recurrent jaundice and ill-health during the limited period before the patients' terminal decline.

Survival after Resection

Postoperative survival has improved steadily over the last 20 years, with the mean survival time increasing from 12 to 17 months over successive decades from 1970. Studies over the last 20 years have shown a longer survival time for patients having a resection than for those having a palliative bypass, but if the lesion is irresectable then a biliary bypass results in a significantly longer survival (3 versus 6 months) than a laparotomy alone [135].

Although selection bias must play a part in these statistics, the fact that resection can now be performed with a similar or even lower mortality rate as a palliative bypass means that all patients who are fit for such surgery should be staged by CT scanning, angiography to exclude arterial or portal venous encasement and probably laparoscopy, which has a higher sensitivity for peritoneal spread than radiological imaging.

Patients with periampullary or small (< 5 cm) pancreatic head lesions who have no evidence of peritoneal or hepatic metastases and no evidence of vascular involvement should be considered for an exploration with a view to resection if possible and a palliative bypass if resection is inappropriate. The choice of resectional procedure is usually of the pancreatic head, with an end-to-end or end-to-side pancreatojejunostomy, since total pancreatectomy results in a higher mortality rate [136] and brittle diabetes mellitus in a proportion of patients. Mortality has been decreasing steadily for major pancreatic resections, with most series in the last decade reporting mortality rates of less than 10% even for patients over 70 years old [136–138], or in patients having combined resections of the pancreatic head and portal vein [139]. Significant series have also been published where no hospital deaths have occurred after major resection [133].

The position of the lesion in the pancreas is highly significant, since it is uncommon for lesions in the body or tail of the pancreas to be resectable as they are free to invade widely before causing symptoms, unless they are discovered incidentally. These tumours are rarely resectable and appropriate palliative biliary or gastric bypass surgery and pain-relieving techniques are usually the only appropriate measures in these patients [136].

Biliary Drainage

The type of biliary drainage employed to palliate the jaundice caused by pancreatic malignancy is still the subject of controversy. There is no doubt that if a patient has unequivocal evidence of metastatic disease, then a minimally invasive method of stent insertion is appropriate, by either endoscopic or percutaneous routes.

If, however, there is no metastatic disease and the patient is fit for major surgery, then the situation is less clear, as palliative surgery has the considerable advantage of rarely requiring multiple readmissions for recurrent jaundice or cholangitis which is often the case with the smaller diameter plastic stents, while having the significant disadvantage of a higher mortality rate compared with endoprosthesis insertion. Studies examining the role of these two techniques have found endoprosthesis insertion to be a valuable alternative to surgical bypass with advantages and disadvantages for each. The endoscopic route seems to be superior for the insertion of plastic prostheses compared to the percutaneous route [140–142]. This advantage may also be negated by the advent of the much wider diameter afforded by the wallstent, which seem to block less frequently than the 10 French gauge stents [126].

The type of surgical biliary bypass used most commonly is the cholecystojejunostomy, although the data from studies comparing the results from this procedure and choledochojejunostomy suggest that the latter procedure may be performed with similar rates of morbidity and mortality, but a considerably lower rate of recurrent jaundice. This is presumed to be due to the common phenomenon of the cystic duct joining the common bile duct (CBD) parallel with the gall bladder, but entering the CBD much lower down, so allowing the tumour to involve this junction more easily. Other popular structures used for biliary bypass are the stomach or the duodenum. Theoretical problems with these techniques are biliary gastritis and blockage due to direct tumour extension respectively.

Gastric Bypass

It is not proven whether the stomach should be bypassed selectively or as a routine in patients who are already having a biliary bypass. Proponents of routine gastroenterostomy cite the group of around 20% of patients who develop gastric outlet obstruction after a surgical biliary diversion alone, and also the very high mortality rate of these patients undergoing a gastroenterostomy. It has also been demonstrated that the addition of gastroenterostomy has no effect on operative mortality [135].

There is, however, a higher incidence of upper gastrointestinal bleeding if gastroenterostomy is added to a biliary diversion [143, 144]. Also, in patients with a lesion to the left of the pancreatic head in whom duodenal obstruction is less likely, or in patients with a limited prognosis and a small primary tumour, the addition of the gastroenterostomy is probably inappropriate, so each patient must be taken on their merits.

Pain Relief

This is a very important area in pancreatic cancer, since neoplastic involvement of the rich nervous plexus around the coeliac axis results in a very severe constant pain. This may be achieved by percutaneous means, but if the patient is having palliative surgery for biliary or gastric obstruction, then a chemical ablation of the coeliac plexus by absolute alcohol or oily phenol can be worth while in a significant number of patients [145]. This procedure can be recommended in any patient in whom pain is a significant feature.

Another novel approach recently described for the relief of pancreatic pain is to divide the splanchnic nerves in the chest thorascopically, with good effect in one patient [146].

Conclusion

Pancreatic cancer remains a disease with a very limited prognosis, despite improvements in resectability and surgical safety. There seems little doubt that good palliation is achieved even in the patients who are operated upon for cure, but who subsequently die of recurrent disease.

Surgical biliary bypass allows the majority of patients receiving this form of palliation less risk of recurrent jaundice and cholangitis compared to endoprostheses, although it seems likely that the new generation of wider lumen stents may lessen this advantage. Gastric bypass relieves distressing symptoms of gastric outlet obstruction and simultaneous chemical splanchnicectomy can relieve the severe pain of coeliac plexus invasion where pain is a feature.

References

1. Moghissi K (1992) Surgical resection for stage I cancer of the oesophagus and cardia. Br J Surg 79:935–937.
2. Muller J, Erasmi H, Stelzner M, Zieren U, Pichlmaier H (1990) Surgical therapy of oesophageal carcinoma. Br J Surg 77:845–857.
3. Bernstein JM, Juler GL (1980) Colon interposition versus esophagogastrostomy for esophageal carcinoma. Am Surg 46(4):216–222.
4. Schattenkerk M, Obertop H, Mud H, Eijkenboom W, Andel Jv, Houten Hv (1987) Survival after resection for carcinoma of the oesophagus. Br J Surg 74:165–168.
5. Matthews H, Powell D, McConkey C (1986) Effect of surgical expertise on the results of resection for oesophageal carcinoma. Br J Surg 73:621–623.
6. Galandiuk S, Hermann R, Gassman J, Cosgrove D (1986) Cancer of the esophagus: the Cleveland Clinic experience. Ann Surg 203:101–108.
7. Giuli R, Gignoux M (1980) Treatment of carcinoma of the esophagus: retrospective study of 2400 patients. Ann Surg 192(1):44–53.
8. Launois B, Paul J, Lygidakis N, Campion J, Malledant Y, Grossetti D et al. (1983) Results of the surgical treatment of carcinoma of the oesophagus. Surg Gynecol Obstet 156:753–760.

9. Nishi M, Hiramatsu Y, Hatano T, Yamamoto M (1988) Pulmonary complications after subtotal oesophagectomy. Br J Surg 75:527–530.
10. Skinner DB, Little AG, Ferguson MK, Soriano A, Staszak VM (1986) Selection of operation for esophageal cancer based on staging. Ann Surg 204(4):391–401.
11. Collard JM, Otte JB, Reynaert M, Fiasse R, Kestens PJ (1991) Feasibility and effectiveness of en bloc resection of the esophagus for esophageal cancer. Results of a prospective study. Int Surg 76(4):209–213.
12. Holting T, Friedl P. Schraube N, Fritz P, Schlag P, Herfarth C (1991) Palliation of esophageal cancer – operative resection versus laser and afterloading therapy. Surg Endosc 5(1):4–8.
13. Segalin A, Little AG, Ruol A, Ferguson MK, Bardini R, Norberto L et al. (1989) Surgical and endoscopic palliation of esophageal carcinoma. Ann Thorac Surg 48(2):267–271.
14. Alderson D, Wright P (1990) Laser recanalization versus endoscopic intubation in the palliation of malignant dysphagia. Br J Surg 77:1151–1153.
15. Krasner N, Beard J (1984) Laser irradiation of tumours of the oesophagus and gastric cardia. Br Med J 288:829.
16. Swain C, Bown S, Edwards D, Kirkham J, Salmon P, Clark A (1984) Laser recanalisation of obstructing foregut cancer. Br J Surg 71:112–115.
17. Mellow M, Pinkas H (1985) Endoscopic laser therapy for malignancies affecting the esophagus and gastroesophageal junction. Arch Intern Med 145:1443–1448.
18. Fleischer D, Sivak M (1985) Endoscopic Nd:YAG laser therapy as palliation for esophagogastric cancer. Gastroenterology 89:827–831.
19. Koyama S, Ozaki A, Iwasaki Y, Sakita T, Osuga T, Watanabe A et al. (1986) Randomized controlled study of postoperative adjuvant immunochemotherapy with Nocardia rubra cell wall skeleton (N-CWS) and Tegafur for gastric carcinoma. Cancer Immunol Immunother 22(2):148–154.
20. Hayata Y, Kato H, Okitsu H, Kawaguchi M, Konaka C (1985) Photodynamic therapy with haematoprophyrin derivative in cancer of the upper gastrointestinal tract. Semin Surg Oncol. 1:1–11.
21. Douglass H, Nara H, Weishaupt K, Boyle D, Sugerman M, Halpern E et al. (1983) Intra-abdominal applications of haematoporphyrin photoradiation therapy. Adv Exp Med Biol 160:15–21.
22. Tatsuta M, Yamamoto R, Yamamura H, Iishi H, Noguchi S, M MI, et al. (1984) Photodynamic effects of exposure to hematoporphyrin derivatives and dye-laser radiation on human gastric adenocarcinoma cells. JNCI 73(1):59–63.
23. Ito Y, Kasugai T (1987) Use of endoscopic laser in gastroenterology. Ann Acad Med 16:290–293.
24. Atkinson M, Ferguson R (1977) Fibreoptic endoscopic palliative intubation of inoperable oesophago-gastric neoplasm. Br Med J 1:266–277.
25. Jager FDH, Bartelsman J, Tytgat G (1987) Palliative treatment of obstructing gastric malignancy by endoscopic positioning of a plastic prosthesis. Gastroenterology 77:1008–1014.
26. Spiller R, Misiewicz J (1987) Ethanol-induced tumour necrosis for palliation of malignant dysphagia. Lancet 2:792.
27. Nwokolo C, Payne-James J, Silk D, Loft D (1994) Palliation of malignant dysphagia by ethanol induced tumour necrosis. Gut 35:299–303.
28. Fleischer D (1987) A comparison of endoscopic laser therapy and BICAP tumor probe therapy for esophageal cancer. Am J Gastroenterol 82(7):608–612.
29. Jensen DM, Machicado G, Randall G, Tung LA, English ZS (1988) Comparison of low-power YAG laser and BICAP tumor probe for palliation of esophageal cancer strictures. Gastroenterology 94(6):1263–1270.
30. Johnston JH, Fleischer D, Petrini J, Nord HJ (1987) Palliative bipolar electrocoagulation therapy of obstructing esophageal cancer. Gastrointest Endosc 33(5):349–353.
31. Surveys OPCS (1974–85) Mortality statistics. HMSO, London.

32. Fielding J, Roginski C, Ellis D, Jones B, Powell J, Waterhouse J et al. (1984) Clinicopathological staging of gastric cancer. Br J Surg 71:677–680.
33. Allum W, Roginski C, Fielding J, Jones B, Ellis D, Waterhouse J et al. (1986) Adenocarcinoma of the cardia: a 10 year regional review. World J Surg 10:462–467.
34. Gall F, Hermanek P (1985) New aspects in the surgical treatment of gastric carcinoma – a comparative study of 1636 patients operated on between 1969 and 1982. Eur J Surg Oncol 11:219–225.
35. Lundh G, Burn J, Kolig G, Richard C, Thomson J, Eik Pv et al. (1974) A co-operative international study of gastric cancer. Ann R Coll Surg Engl 54:219–228.
36. Fielding J, Powell J, Allum W, Waterhouse J, McConkey C (1989) Cancer of the stomach. Macmillan Press, London.
37. Borch K, Hammarstrom E, Liedberg G (1982) Gastric cancer: diagnosis and prognosis in clinical routine. Acta Chir Scand 148:517–523.
38. Brookes V, Waterhouse J, Powell D (1965) Carcinoma of the stomach: a 10 year survey of results and of factors affecting prognosis. Br Med J II:1577–1583.
39. Sjostedt S, Pieper R (1986) Gastric cancer: factors influencing long term survival and postoperative mortality. Acta Chir Scand 530:25–29.
40. Swynnerton B, Truelove S (1952) Carcinoma of the stomach. Br Med J I:287–293.
41. Murakami T (JRSGC) (1973) The general rules for the gastric cancer study in surgery. Jpn J Surg 3(1):61–71.
42. Kodama Y, Sugimachi K, Soejima K, Matsusaka T, Inokuchi K (1981) Evaluation of extensive lymph node dissection for carcinoma of the stomach. World J Surg 5:241–248.
43. Hawley P, Westerholm P, Morson B (1970) Pathology and prognosis of carcinoma of the stomach. Br J Surg 57:877–883.
44. Hermanek P (1986). Prognostic factors in stomach cancer surgery. Eur J Surg Oncol 12:241–246.
45. Mine M, Majima S, Harada M, Etani S (1970) End results of gastrectomy for gastric cancer: effect of extensive lymph node dissection. Surgery 68:753–758.
46. Nakajima T, Kajitani T (1981) Surgical treatment of gastric cancer with special reference to lymph node dissection. In: Friedman M, Ogawa M, Kisner D (eds) Diagnosis and treatment of upper gastrointestinal tumours. Excerpta Medica, Amsterdam, pp 207–225.
47. Soga J, Kobayashi K, Saito J, Fujimachi M, Muto T (1979) The role of lymphadenectomy in curative surgery for gastric cancer. World J Surg 3:701–708.
48. Buchholtz T, Welch C, Malt R (1978) Clinical correlates of resectability and survival in gastric carcinoma. Ann Surg 188:711–715.
49. Choi T, Koo J, Wong J, Ong G (1982) Survival after surgery for advanced carcinoma of the stomach other than cardia. Am J Surg 143:748–750.
50. Dupont J, Lee J, Burton G, Cohn I (1978) Adenocarcinoma of the stomach: review of 1497 cases. Cancer 41:941–947.
51. Ekbom G, Gleysteen J (1980) Gastric malignancy: resection for palliation. Surgery 88(4):476–481.
52. Hallissey M, Allum W, Roginski C, Fielding J (1988) Palliative surgery for gastric cancer. Cancer 62:440–444.
53. Haugstvedt T, Viste A, Eide GE, Soreide O (1989) The survival benefit of resection in patients with advanced stomach cancer: the Norwegian multicenter experience. Norwegian stomach cancer trial. World J Surg 13(5):617–621.
54. Ezaki T (1992) Hepatocellular carcinoma. Br Med J 304:196–197.
55. Yamada K, Kishi K, Sonomura T, Tsuda M, Nomura S, Satoh M (1990) Transcatheter arterial embolization in unresectable hepatocellular carcinoma. Cardiovasc Intervent Radiol 13:135–139.
56. Dusheiko G, Hobbs K, Dick R, Burroughs A (1992) Treatment of small hepatocellular carcinomas. Lancet 340:285–288.

57. Yamasaki S, Makuuchi M, Hasegawa H (1991) Results of hepatectomy for hepatocellular carcinoma at the National Cancer Center Hospital. HPB Surg 3(3):235–249.
58. Liver Cancer Study Group of Japan (1990) Primary liver cancer in Japan. Ann Surg 211:277–287.
59. Nagasue N, Kohno H, Chang Y-C, Taniura H, Yamanoi A, Uchida M et al. (1993) Liver resection for hepatocellular carcinoma: results of 229 consecutive patients during 11 years. Ann Surg 217(4):375–384.
60. Ringe B, Pichlmayr R, Wittekind C, Tusch G (1991) Surgical treatment of hepatocellular carcinoma: experience with liver resection and transplantation in 198 patients. World J Surg 15:270–285.
61. European liver transplant registry – 1992 update.
62. Starzl T, Todo S, Tzakis A, Podesta L, Mieles L, Demetris A et al. (1989) Abdominal organ cluster transplantation for the treatment of upper abdominal malignancies. Ann Surg 210(3):374–386.
63. Tzakis A, Todo S, Madariaga J, Tzoracoeleftherakis E, Fung J, Starzl T (1991) Upper-abdominal exenteration in transplantation for extensive malignancies of the upper abdomen – an update. Transplantation 51(3):727–728.
64. Iwatsuki S, Starzl Y, Sheahan D, Yokoyama I, Demetris A, Todo S et al. (1991) Hepatic resection versus transplantation for hepatocellular carcinoma Ann Surg 214:221–229.
65. Bismuth H, Chiche L, Adam R, Castaing D (1993) Surgical treatment of hepatocellular carcinoma in cirrhosis: liver resection or transplantation. Trans Proc 25(1):1066–1067.
66. Finlay I, McArdle C (1986) Occult hepatic metastases in colorectal carcinoma. Br J Surg 73:732–735.
67. Wagner J, Adson M, Heerden Jv, Adson M, Ilstrup D (1984) The natural history of hepatic metastases from colorectal cancer. Ann Surg 199:502–507.
68. Machi J, Isomoto H, Kurohiji T, Shirouzu K, Yameshita Y, Kakegawa T et al. (1986) Detection of unrecognised liver metastases from colorectal cancers by routine use of operative ultrasonography. Dis Colon Rectum 29:405–409.
69. Olsen AK (1990) Intraoperative ultrasonography and the detection of liver metastases in patients with colorectal cancer. Br J Surg 77(9):998–999.
70. Leveson S, Wiggins P, Giles G et al. (1985) Deranged blood flow patterns in the detection of liver metastases. Br J Surg 72:128–130.
71. Leen E, Angerson W, Warren H, O'Gorman P, Moule B, Carter E et al. (1994) Improved sensitivity of colour Doppler flow imaging of colorectal hepatic metastases using galactose microparticles: a preliminary report. Br J Surg 81:252–254.
72. Ahlman H, Wangberg B, Tisell L, Nilsson O, Forsell-Aronsson E (1994) Clinical efficacy of octreotide scintigraphy in patients with midgut carcinoid tumours and evaluation of intra-operative scintillation detection. Br J Surg 81:1144–1149.
73. Adson M, Heerden JV (1980) Major hepatic resection for metastatic colorectal cancer. Ann Surg 191:576–581.
74. Nims T (1984) Resection of the liver for metastatic cancer. Surg Gynecol Obstet 158:46–48.
75. Gennari L, Doci R, Bozzetti F, Bignami P (1986) Surgical treatment of hepatic metastases from colorectal cancer. Ann Surg 203:49–54.
76. Hanks J, Meyers W, Filston H, Killenberg P, Jones R (1980) Surgical resection for benign and malignant disease. Ann Surg 191:584–590.
77. Iwatsuki S, Shaw B, Starzl T (1983) Experience with 150 liver resections. Ann Surg 197:247–253.
78. Scheele J, Stangl R, Altendorf-Hofmann A (1990) Hepatic metastases from colorectal carcinoma: impact of surgical resection on the natural history. Br J Surg 77:1241–1246.
79. Savage A, Malt R (1991) Elective and emergency hepatic resection: determinants of operative mortality and morbidity. Ann Surg 214:689–695.

80. August D, Sugarbaker P, Ottow R, Gianola F, Schneider P (1986) Hepatic resection for colorectal metastases. Ann Surg 201:210–218.
81. Cady B, McDermott W (1986) Major hepatic resection for metachronous metastases from colon cancer. Ann Surg 201:204–209.
82. Ekberg H, Tranberg K-G, Anderson R, Lundstedt C, Hagerstrand I, Ranstam J et al. (1986) Determinants of survival in liver resection for colorectal secondaries. Br J Surg 73:727–731.
83. Savage A, Malt R (1992) Survival after hepatic resection for malignant tumours. Br J Surg 79:1095–1101.
84. Sugihara K, Hojo K, Moriya Y, Yamasaki S, Kosuge T, Takayama T (1993) Pattern of recurrence after hepatic resection for colorectal metastases. Br J Surg 80:1032–1035.
85. Scheele J, Stangl R, Altendorf-Hofmann A, Gall F (1991) Indicators of prognosis after hepatic resection for colorectal secondaries. Surgery 110:13–29.
86. Tomas-de la Vega JE, Donahue E, Doolas A, Roseman D, Straus A, Bonomi P et al. (1984) A ten year experience with hepatic resection. Surg Gynecol Obstet 159:223–228.
87. Fortner J (1984) Multivariate analysis of a personal series of 247 consecutive patients with liver metastases from colorectal cancer. Ann Surg 199:306–316.
88. Butler J, Attiyeh F, Daly J (1986) Hepatic resection for metastases of the colon and rectum. Surg Gynecol Obstet 162:109–113.
89. Lange J, Leese T, Castaing D, Bismuth H (1989) Repeat hepatectomy for recurrent malignant tumours of the liver. Surg Gynecol Obstet 169:119–126.
90. Griffith K, Sugarbaker P, Chang A (1990) Repeat hepatic resections for colorectal metastases. Surgery 106:106–116.
91. Bozzetti F, Bignami P, Montalto F, Doci R, Gennari L (1992) Repeated hepatic resection for recurrent metastases from colorectal cancer. Br J Surg 79:146–148.
92. Nakamura S, Yokoi Y, Suzuki S, Baba S, Muro H (1992) Results of extensive surgery for liver metastases in colorectal carcinoma. Br J Surg 79:35–38.
93. Que F, Nagorney D (1994) Resection of "recurrent" colorectal metastases to the liver. Br J Surg 81:255–258.
94. Yanaga K, Kishikawa K, Shimada M, Kakizoe S, Higashi H, Nishizaki T et al. (1993) Extracorporeal hepatic resection for previously unresectable neoplasms. Surgery 113:637–643.
95. Ochiai T, Sasako M, Mizuno S, Konoshita T, Takayama T, Kosuge T et al. (1994) Hepatic resection for metastatic tumours from gastric cancer: analysis of prognostic factors. Br J Surg 81: 1175–1178.
96. Hanssen LE, Schrumpf E, Kolbenstvedt AN, Tausjo J, Dolva LO (1989) Treatment of malignant metastatic midgut carcinoid tumours with recombinant human alpha2b interferon with or without prior hepatic artery embolization. Scand J Gastroenterol 24(7):787–795.
97. Hajarizadeh H, Ivancev K, Mueller CR, Fletcher WS, Woltering EA (1992) Effective palliative treatment of metastatic carcinoid tumours with intra-arterial chemotherapy-chemoembolization combined with octreotide acetate. Am J Surg 163(5):479–483.
98. Odurny A, Birch SJ (1985) Hepatic arterial embolisation in patients with metastatic carcinoid tumours. Clin Radiol 36(6):597–602.
99. Stephen JL, Grahame SD (1972) Treatment of the carcinoid syndrome by local removal of hepatic metastases. Proc R Soc Med 65(5):444–445.
100. McEntee G, Nagorney K, Kvols L, Moertel C, Grant C (1990) Cytoreductive hepatic surgery for neuroendocrine tumours. Surgery 108:1091–1096.
101. Soreide O, Berstad T, Bakka A, Schrumpf E, Hanssen LE, Engh V et al. (1992) Surgical treatment as a principle in patients with advanced abdominal carcinoid tumors. Surgery 111(1):48–54.
102. Basson MD, Ahlman H, Wangberg B, Modlin IM (1993) Biology and management of the midgut carcinoid. Am J Surg 165(2):288–297.
103. Alsina AE, Bartus S, Hull D, Rosson R, Schweizer RT (1990) Liver transplant for metastatic neuroendocrine tumor. J Clin Gastroenterol 12(5):533–537.

104. Charnley RM, Doran J, Morris DL (1989) Cryotherapy for liver metastases: a new approach. Br J Surg 76(10):1040–1041.
105. Morris D, Horton M, Dilley A, Warlters A, Clingan P (1993) Treatment of hepatic metastases by cryotherapy and regional cytotoxic perfusion. Gut 34:1156–1157.
106. Ravikumar T, Kane R, Cady B, Jenkins R, Clouse M, Steele G (1987) Hepatic cryosurgery with intraoperative ultrasound monitoring for metastatic colon carcinoma. Arch Surg 122:403–409.
107. Ravikumar T, Kane R, Cady B, Jenkins R, Clouse M, Steele G (1991) A 5-year study of cryosurgery in the treatment of liver tumours. Arch Surg 126:1520–1524.
108. Charnley R, Thomas M, Morris D (1991) Effect of hepatic cryotherapy on serum CEA concentration in patients with multiple inoperable hepatic metastases from colorectal cancer. Aust NZ J Surg 61(1):55–58.
109. Preketes AP, King J, Caplehorn JR, Clingan PR, Ross WB, Morris DL (1994) CEA reduction after cryotherapy for liver metastases from colon cancer predicts survival. Aust NZ J Surg 64(9):612–614.
110. Fortner J, Silva J, Cox E, Golbey R, Gallowitz H, Maclean B (1984) Multivariate analysis of a personal series of 247 consecutive patients with liver metastases from colorectal cancer. II Treatment by intrahepatic chemotherapy. Ann Surg 199:317–324.
111. Goldberg JA, Kerr DJ, Wilmott N, McKillop JH, McArdle CS (1990) Regional chemotherapy for colorectal liver metastases: a phase II evaluation of targeted hepatic arterial 5-fluorouracil for colorectal liver metastases. Br J Surg 77(11):1238–1240.
112. Grage T, Vassilopoulos P, Shingleton W, Elias E, Aust J, Moss S (1979) Results of a prospective randomised study of hepatic artery infusion with 5-fluorouracil versus intravenous 5-fluorouracil in patients with hepatic metastases from colorectal cancer: A Central Oncology Group study. Surgery 86:550–555.
113. Kemeny MM, Goldberg D, Beatty JD, Blayney D, Browning S, Doroshow J et al. (1986) Results of a prospective randomized trial of continuous regional chemotherapy and hepatic resection as treatment of hepatic metastases from colorectal primaries. Cancer 57(3):492–498.
114. Pinson C, Rossi R (1988) Extended right hepatic lobectomy, left hepatic lobectomy and skeletonization resection for proximal bile duct cancer. World J Surg 12:52–59.
115. Hadjis NS, Blenkharn JI, Alexander N, Benjamin IS, Blumgart LH (1990) Outcome of radical surgery in hilar cholangiocarcinoma. Surgery 107(6):597–604.
116. Stain SC, Baer HU, Dennison AR, Blumgart LH (1992) Current management of hilar cholangiocarcinoma. Surg Gynecol Obstet 175(6):579–588.
117. Bismuth H, Castaing D, Traynor O (1988) Resection or palliation: priority of surgery in the treatment of hilar cancer. World J Surg 12:39–47.
118. Reding R, Buard J-L, Lebeau G, Launois B (1991) Surgical management of 552 carcinomas of the extrahepatic bile ducts (gallbladder and periampullary tumours excluded). Ann Surg 213(3):236–241.
119. Tashiro S, Tsuji T, Kanemitsu K, Kamimoto Y, Hiraoka T, Miyauchi Y (1993) Prolongation of survival for carcinoma at the bile duct confluence. Surgery 113:270–278.
120. Abu-Elmagd K, Selby R, Iwatsuki S, Fung J, Tzakis A, Todo S et al. (1993) Cholangiocarcinoma and sclerosing cholangitis: clinical characteristics and effect on survival after liver transplantation. Transplant Proc 25(1):1124–1125.
121. Iwatsuki S, Gordon R, Shaw B, Starzl T (1985) Role of liver transplantation in cancer therapy. Ann Surg 202(4):401–408.
122. O'Grady J, Polson R, Rolles K, Calne R, Williams R (1988) Liver transplantation for malignant disease. Ann Surg 207(4):373–379.
123. Pichlmayr R, Ringe B, Lauchart W, Bechstein W, Gubernatis G, Wagner E (1988) Radical resection and liver grafting as the two main components of surgical strategy in the treatment of proximal bile duct cancer. World J Surg 12:68–77.

124. Olthoff KM, Millis JM, Rosove MH, Goldstein LI, Ramming KP, Busuttil RW (1990) Is liver transplantation justified for the treatment of hepatic malignancies? Arch Surg 125(10):1261–1266.
125. Bismuth H, Corlette M (1975) Intrahepatic cholangioenteric anastomosis in carcinoma of the hilus of the liver. Surg Gynecol Obstet 140:170–178.
126. Adam A, Chetty N, Roddie M, Yeung E, Benjamin IS (1991) Self-expandable stainless steel endoprostheses for treatment of malignant bile duct obstruction. Am J Roentgenol 156(2):321–325.
127. Shiina T, Mikuriya S, Uno T, Toita T, Serizawa S, Itami J et al. (1992) Radiotherapy of cholangiocarcinoma: the roles for primary and adjuvant therapies. Cancer Chemother Pharmacol 31(suppl)115–118.
128. Flickinger J, Epstein A, Iwatsuki S, Carr B, Starzl T (1991) Radiation therapy for primary carcinoma of the extrahepatic biliary system. An analysis of 63 cases. Cancer 68:289–294.
129. Karani J, Fletcher M, Brinkley D, Dawson JL, Williams R, Nunnerley H (1985) Internal biliary drainage and local radiotherapy with iridium-192 wire in treatment of hilar cholangiocarcinoma. Clin Radiol 36(6):603–606.
130. Levitt MD, Laurence BH, Cameron F, Klemp PF (1988) Transpapillary iridium-192 wire in the treatment of malignant bile duct obstruction. Gut 29(2):149–152.
131. Stillwagon GB, Order SE, Haulk T, Herpst J, Ettinger DS, Fishman EK et al. (1991) Variable low dose rate irradiation (131I-anti-CEA) and integrated low dose chemotherapy in the treatment of nonresectable primary intrahepatic cholangiocarcinoma. Int J Radiat Oncol Biol Phys 21(6):1601–1605.
132. OPCS. (1975–85) Mortality statistics. HMSO, London.
133. Trede M, Schwall G, Saeger H-D (1990) Survival after pancreatoduodenectomy: 118 consecutive resections without an operative mortality. Ann Surg 211(4):447–458.
134. Klinkenbijl J, Jeekel J, Schmitz P, Rombout P, Nix G, Bruining H et al. (1993) Carcinoma of the pancreas and periampullary region: palliation versus cure. Br J Surg 80:1575–1578.
135. Watanapa P, Williamson R (1992) Surgical palliation for pancreatic cancer: developments during the past two decades. Br J Surg 79:8–20.
136. Baumel H, Huguier M, Manderscheid J, Fabre J, Houry S, Fagot H (1994) Results of resection for cancer of the exocrine pancreas: a study from the French Association of Surgery. Br J Surg 81:102–107.
137. Kairaluoma M, Kiviniemi H, Stahlberg M (1987) Pancreatic resection for carcinoma of the pancreas and the periampullary region in patients over 70 years of age. Br J Surg 74:116–118.
138. Spencer M, Sarr M, Nagorney D (1990) Radical pancreatectomy for pancreatic cancer in the elderly: Is it safe and justified? Ann Surg 212:140–143.
139. Takahashi S, Ogata Y, Tsuzuki T (1994) Combined resection of the pancreas and portal vein for pancreatic cancer. Br J Surg 81:1190–1193.
140. Bornman P, Harries-Jones E, Tobias R, VanStiegmann G, Terblanche J (1986) Prospective controlled trial of transhepatic biliary endoprosthesis versus bypass surgery for incurable carcinoma of head of pancreas. Lancet I:69–71.
141. Speer A, Cotton P, Russell R, Mason R, Hatfield A, Leung J et al. (1987) Randomized trial of endoscopic versus percutaneous stent insertion in malignant obstructive jaundice. Lancet II:57–62.
142. Andersen J, Sorensen S, Kruse A, Rokkjaer M, Matzen P (1989) Randomised trial of endoscopic endoprosthesis versus operative bypass in malignant obstructive jaundice. Gut 30:1132–1135.
143. Schantz S, Schickler W, Evans T, Coffey R (1984) Palliative gastroenterostomy for pancreatic cancer. Am J Surg 147:793–796.
144. Jacobs P, vanderSluis H, Wobbes T (1989) Role of gastroenterostomy in the palliative surgical treatment of pancreatic cancer. J Surg Oncol 42:145–149.

145. Gardner A, Solomou G (1984) Relief of pain of unresectable carcinoma of pancreas by chemical splanchnicectomy during laparotomy. Ann R Coll Surg Engl 66:409–411.
146. Worsey J, Ferson P, Keenan R, Julian T, Landrenau R (1993) Thoracoscopic pancreatic denervation for pain control in irresectable pancreatic cancer. Br J Surg 80:1051–1052.

2 – Non-Curative Surgery for Cancer of the Large Bowel

S.J. Watson and R.J. Nicholls*

Introduction

In England and Wales, approximately 24 000 patients present each year with colorectal adenocarcinoma [1]. In the USA there are 157 000 new cases annually [2]. The main treatment modality is surgical, but due to the insidious nature of the disease and the lack of a suitable screening tool, only about 50–82% [1, 3–8] have surgery undertaken with curative intent. This leaves a very large number of patients with colorectal cancer who require palliation of symptoms.

The main principle of palliative surgery is to relieve symptoms by the least traumatic operation possible. In this chapter, palliative surgery is taken to mean surgery aimed at local disease or its effects and is not directed at metastases alone. The factors in planning palliative surgery include the following considerations:

1. Palliative surgery has a higher morbidity and mortality compared with curative surgery.
2. Patients have a short life expectancy.
3. It is likely that other treatment modalities will be used in management (radiotherapy, chemotherapy).

Natural History of Unresected Primary Disease

In a review of 422 cases of colorectal cancer from 1883–1922, the average duration of survival from onset of illness ranged from 16 to 26 months [9]. Survival was less in younger patients (less than 35 years of age), in men and in colon cancer. Only patients who had no surgery or non-resection surgery were included, but positive histology was not always obtained.

In 1936, Daland and Welch reported 100 cases of untreated rectal cancers [10]. The median age was 59 years. The median survival was 14 months from the onset of symptoms. In only 35 of these, however, was the diagnosis confirmed by biopsy or at autopsy. In another 84 patients from the same report, survival was unchanged by colostomy formation alone (median 14 months survival from symptoms) [10].

* Mr S.J. Watson is supported by the Robert Luff Foundation.

A review in 1964 from the Mayo Clinic [11] reported 440 cases of colorectal cancer untreated or undergoing non-resection surgery. The average survival was 10.1 months from diagnosis, with symptoms noted an average of 8.5 prior to diagnosis [11]. The longest survivals were seen in women, well-differentiated tumours and tumours with local invasion (mean survival with tumour invasion to local organs was 14.7 months vs. 9 months with hepatic metastases) [11]. Unlike an earlier study [9], age had no influence on survival.

Specific survival times in patients with distant metastases and advanced local disease who do not have resection of the primary tumour will be discussed later.

Assessment of Palliative Surgery

The value of palliative surgery is difficult to assess. There are little control data on untreated colorectal cancer. There are no randomized, prospective trials that assess the palliative effects of surgery, radiotherapy or other treatment modalities. It is apparent from published reports that patients with more extensive disease tend to undergo less radical procedures.

Comparison of reports in the literature is difficult due to differences in the definition of palliative intent. Surgery can be classified as palliative because of advanced local disease, regional and distant metastases or a combination of these. There are obvious differences between these groups, but they are all classed as palliative. Patients with significant co-morbid conditions may undergo palliative treatment despite presenting with potentially resectable disease.

On review of the literature, it is apparent that in most circumstances little attempt is made to quantitate palliation objectively. In some situations, a subjective judgement is made by the clinician. Where palliation has been scored, relief of symptoms such as pain, bleeding, diarrhoea, tenesmus and constipation have been recorded. A measure of performance status (Karnovsky Index) has been used in some reports.

Mortality and Morbidity Following Palliative Resection in Primary Colorectal Cancer

Surgical resection of advanced colorectal cancer must be accomplished with a low mortality and acceptable morbidity if it is to be used for palliative therapy. Mortality rates following palliative resection in colorectal cancer range from 1% to 11.7% (Table 2.1) Mortality is greater in patients having non-resection surgery who generally have more advanced disease. The data show that in selected patients palliative colonic resection, anterior resection, Hartmann's resection and abdominoperineal excision can be performed with acceptable mortality.

Morbidity is more difficult to measure, with definitions that vary between authors. Generally, morbidity following palliative resection is high, with rates up to 50% reported [12–14], but this depends on the definition of morbidity and the procedure performed. Major palliative procedures such as pelvic exenteration and sacral resection report morbidity rates up to 100% [15–18].

Patients who are not resected also experience significant morbidity. In 103 patients with advanced rectal cancer, Longo et al. [19] reported 35% morbidity in patients who did not have resection compared to 26% in patients having anterior resection or abdominoperineal excision.

Table 2.1 Mortality and morbidity in resection and non-resection surgery in palliative colorectal cancer

Reference	n	Age (years)	Operation	Mortality (%)	Morbidity (%)
Rectal tumours					
Longo [19]	68	61*	AR and APER	4.3	26
	35	66.9*	Not resection	3	34
Bordos [14]	34	61.5	APER	2.9	50
Moran [7]	95	68.9	AR, APER, HR	1	18
	17		Colostomy	0	
	13		Local procedure		
Johnson [4]	239	n.a.	Resection	11.7	
	61		Colostomy	4.9	
	38		Laparotomy	5.3	
Colorectal tumours					
Makela [199]	66	65*	Resection	5	24
	17		Enterostomy	24	29
	6		Bypass	0	17
	7		Laparotomy	14	14
Joffe [12]	81		Resection	10	50
Takaki [13]	78	64.8	Resection	6.4	43.5
Bacon [21]	25		Colostomy	24	
			Laparotomy	12	
Boey [200]	72		Bypass, resection, laparotomy, colostomy	17	
Stearns [20]	57	n.a.	Resection	3.5	
	54		Colostomy	5.5	
Welch [201]	241		Resection	10.8	
	132		Non-resection	26.5	
Wanebo [23]	175		Resection	10	
	15		Non-resection	7	

Age median unless otherwise stated (* mean)

Survival Following Palliative Surgery for Primary Colorectal Cancer

There are no randomized studies, but survival appears to be prolonged in patients who have resection compared to non-resection or no surgery (Table 2.2). However, this improvement may be due to selection of patients with less advanced disease for palliative resection. Tumour burden from more advanced disease may account for reported differences in survival following resection of the primary tumour. The effect of tumour burden can be seen in the reduced survival in patients with substantial tumour replacement of the liver (Table 2.3) and with reduced survival in patients with distant metastases compared with locoregional spread (Table 2.4).

Besides massive liver replacement, age over 75 years and a history of cardiovascular disease are reported as adverse risk factors [12].

Palliation of Symptoms in Advanced Primary Colorectal Cancer

Mortality, morbidity and survival rates can be measured, but assessment of palliation is far more difficult. This difficulty is reflected in the relative paucity of reports which address the question of palliation of symptoms.

Table 2.2 Median or mean survival in resection and non-resection palliative colorectal and rectal surgery in primary tumours

Reference	*n*	Surgery	Median survival (months)
Colorectal cancer			
Makela et al. [45]	66	Resection	15
	30	No resection	7
Joffe [12]	81	Resection	9
Moran et al. [73]	95	Resection	14.8
	13	Local excision	14.7
	17	Colostomy alone	6.4
Silverman et al. [47]	1248	Resection	10.5
	519	No resection	2.8
Pestana et al. [11]	269	Resection	13.0 (mean)
	137	Bypass/colostomy	6.3 (mean)
	177	Laparotomy alone	6.2 (mean)
Takaki et al. [3]	78	Resection	9.1
Cady et al. [161]	203	AP resection	14.1 (mean)
	38	Resection	12.3 (mean)
	15	Bypass	4.1 (mean)
	13	Laparotomy only	3.3 (mean)
Rectal cancer			
Bussey [202]	511	Resection	17*
	171	No resection	7*
Longo [19]	68	Resection	16
	35	No resection	5
Johnson [4]	239	Resection	14
	100	No resection	6
Bordos [14]	34	APER	58% alive at 1 year
	18	No resection	26% alive at 1 year
Moran [7]	95	Resection	14.8
	17	No resection	6.4
Silverman et al. [47]	463	Resection	10.7
	414	No resection	5.0

Table 2.3 Tumour volume and survival in hepatic metastases from colorectal cancer

Reference	*n*	Liver replacement	Median survival (months)
Bengtsson [28]	155	< 25%	6.2
		25–50%	5.5
		> 75%	3.4
Johnson [4]	12	Solitary metastasis	18
	6	Multiple, one lobe	7
	33	Multiple, both lobes	8
Joffe [12]	7	{Solitary metastasis / Multiple, one lobe}	16.5*
	24	Multiple, both lobes	8.5*
Finan [203]	90	< 20%	16.4
		20–80%	5.6
Wood [30]	15	Solitary metastasis	16.7
	11	Multiple, one lobe	10.6
	87	Multiple, both lobes	3.1

Survival median unless otherwise stated (* mean).

Table 2.4 Median survival in rectal cancer; increased tumour load where there is local and distant metastases reduces survival (From Longo et al. [19])

Extent of disease	n	Median (months)
Local invasion	30	15
Local metastases	18	14
Distant metastases	55	8
Total	103	11.6

What symptoms do patients with incurable colorectal cancer present with? There is no suitable screening programme for sporadic colorectal cancer and most patients will present with local tumour symptoms. A few will have symptoms from disseminated disease alone. Local tumour effects include bleeding, anaemia, pain, obstruction and perforation, and symptoms due to disseminated disease are weight loss, malaise, jaundice, ascites, pain and mass effects upon other organs.

Stearns and Binkley [20] reported complete relief of symptoms in 34 of 57 patients undergoing palliative resection for colorectal cancer. The median duration of complete relief of symptoms was 10 months (range 3–72 months), with a median duration of survival of 16 months. Symptomatic relief depended on whether the incurable nature of the cancer was due to local, regional or distant disease. Palliation was complete in 4 of 12 patients where local tumour could not be resected compared with 30 of 43 patients with regional or distant metastases [20].

Bacon and Martin [21] report that 68.5% of selected patients with advanced colorectal cancer were able to return to work or usual activity after resection, but this was not the case if the patients did not have the primary tumour resected. However, few details are given regarding case selection or assessment of palliation.

Local tumour clearance is important in a palliative resection, especially in the pelvis. Several groups have reported control of local perineal symptoms with palliative anterior resection and abdominoperineal excision [14, 19, 21, 22]. Bordos et al. [14] performed palliative abdominoperineal resection in 34 patients. Fifty-eight per cent were alive at 12 months with successful palliation of symptoms in 76%. Colostomy alone produced poor palliation (Table 2.5).

There are concerns about the safety of a palliative anterior resection, but few reports specifically address this point. A clinical anastomotic leak follows palliative anterior resection in 1.5–3% of cases [7, 19]. Obstruction requiring surgery following anterior resection occurs in only 1.5–4% [7, 19]. Symptomatic pelvic recurrence occurs in 10% following a palliative anterior resection [23]. On the basis of these reports it appears that, where possible, anterior resection should be performed. There is no reported incontinence after a palliative anterior

Table 2.5 Palliation of symptoms following abdominoperineal excision (From Bordos et al. [14])

Procedure	n	Survivors at 1 year (%)	Pelvic symptoms at 1 year (%)
Curative APER	102	95	7
Palliative APER	34	58	24
Other palliative procedures	18	26	100

resection; however, in curative low anterior resections a colonic pouch may improve function [24]. This is an important consideration in a palliative low anterior resection where the patient does not have a prolonged period for adaptation to a neorectum.

Common Clinical Situations in Palliative Colorectal Cancer

Patients may present with primary or recurrent colorectal cancer and be classified as palliative for a variety of reasons. These situations are reviewed, and by drawing on reports in the literature and on personal experience, recommendations are made on a surgical approach. Reports in the literature are often fragmented and incomplete. Some of the clinical situations are overlapping with, for example, multiple metastases to different sites.

Initial Presentation

Pathology

Resectable Local Disease but with Metastases

Metastases may be regional, distant or both and diagnosed by preoperative investigations or found at operation. The relative frequency of metastases is different in rectal and colonic cancer due to differences in venous drainage. Necropsy data have shown that rectal cancers metastasize less often to the liver (62% vs. 76%) and more often to the lungs (64% vs. 48%) and skeleton (19% vs. 11%) [25].

Hepatic Metastases in Primary Colorectal Cancer

Liver metastases are found at laparotomy in 15–20% of cases, but another 25–30% will develop liver metastases that are not clinically evident at the primary operation [26, 27]. The natural history of untreated liver secondaries from colorectal cancer shows that mean survival is just 6–9 months (Table 2.6). However, survival is probably related to the extent of tumour replacement (Table 2.3) [28–31], tumour doubling time and the biological characteristics of the tumour.

The greater the sensitivity in detection of liver metastases, the smaller the tumour volume and the longer a patient will survive after palliative surgery. This lead time may be important in considering reported results from resection of hepatic metastases [32]. The mean age of overt hepatic metastases detectable at surgery is 3.7 years, whereas the mean age of occult metastases seen only on computed tomography (CT) is 2.3 years [33].

Intraoperative ultrasound (IOUS) is the most sensitive method of detecting hepatic secondaries. Clark et al. [34] found that IOUS showed 25–35% additional lesions compared with preoperative ultrasound and CT. Parker et al. [35] prospectively compared intraoperative palpation, IOUS and preoperative CT scanning in detecting hepatic metastases from a number of types of primaries.

Table 2.6 Survival in colorectal cancer with liver metastases: resection and non-resection of the primary tumour

Reference	*n*	Proven metastases	Survival (months)	
			Non-resection	Resection
Silverman [47]	636 Colonic	No	2.6	10
Silverman [47]	305 Rectal	No	4.7	10.4
Stearns [20]	22	No	–	18*
Baden [204]	105	No		10
Bacon [21]	50	Yes	6.5*	15.1*
Oxley [205]	86	No	8% alive at 12 months	36% alive at 12 months
Nielson [206]	103 Colonic	Yes	5	12.3
Nielsen [207]	59 Rectal	No	7*	24*
Jaffe [39]	177	No	1.2 biopsy 3.4 stoma	5.7
Swinton [208]	41	No	–	7
Cady [209]	269	No	3*	14*
Wood [30]	113	No		6.6
Abrams [210]	58	Yes	2	7
Johnson [4]	265	No	3 biopsy 10 stoma	13

Survival is median except where indicated (*mean).

Intraoperative ultrasound detected 98% and finger palpation 91% [35]. Others have also found IOUS more sensitive than finger palpation [36].

Although new contrast agents allow preoperative CT scanning to detect lesions as small as 0.5 cm [37], with an accuracy of 61–77% [35], IOUS has resolution thresholds of 3–5 mm, even in the left lobe of the liver [36, 38].

Increased sensitivity of scanning methods for hepatic secondaries will mean some patients that are now classified as curative will be palliative. These patients are not symptomatic and may not become so for months or years. Therefore, with greater sensitivity in detecting hepatic lesions that are unlikely to have a clinical impact for some time, a complete resection of the local tumour is required even if screening tests declare the operation to be palliative.

Reported rates of survival following resection and non-resection surgery for primary colorectal cancer in the presence of liver metastases are shown in Table 2.6. Older reports rely on less sensitive screening methods than are now available.

Survival is related to the degree of tumour replacement, presence of ascites and jaundice and abnormal biochemistry. Figure 2.1 (*overleaf*) shows that improved median survival in palliative resection in the presence of liver metastases is due to case selection. Most of the patients with ascites had a laparotomy or diversion without resection [39].

Bengsston et al. [28] showed that abnormal alkaline phosphatase is associated with reduced survival in 155 patients with liver metastases from a median of 6.2 months to 2.8 months. Abnormal liver function tests are indicators of advanced disease and are a poor prognostic indicator [29, 30, 39–41].

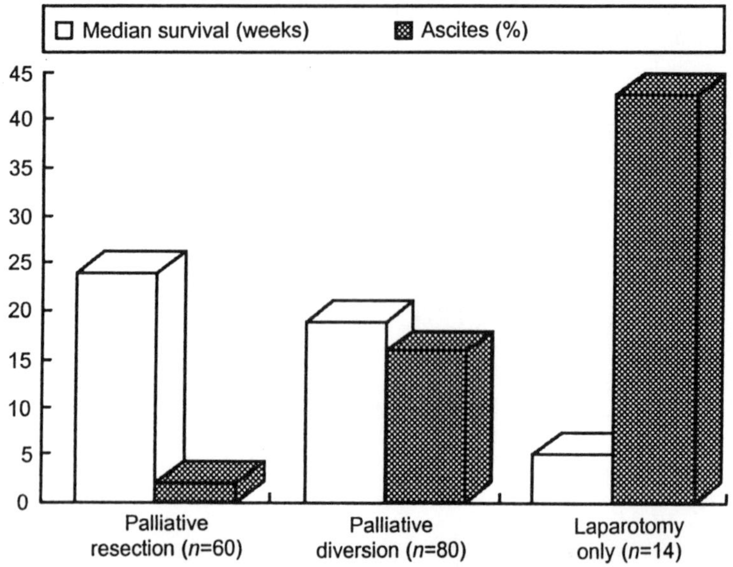

Fig. 2.1 Survival after resection, diversion or laparotomy alone in patients with colorectal cancer and known hepatic metastases, with or without ascites. Palliative resection was performed in patients without ascites and non resection surgery in patients with ascites. Survival is probably related to ascites rather than resection. The degree of liver replacement by tumour was similar in each group. (From Jaffe et al [39])

Recommendation Resection of the primary colorectal cancer in the presence of liver secondaries is indicated in selected cases when the extent of tumour replacement of the liver is not too extensive, and ascites and jaundice are absent. The patient can successfully be palliated for many months.

Lung Metastases in Primary Colorectal Cancer

After the liver, the lungs are the most common site of metastases from colorectal adenocarcinoma. This supports the cascade theory of tumour dissemination [25, 42, 43]. About 10% of patients with colorectal cancer will develop detectable pulmonary metastases during the course of their disease and in 90% this will be part of generalized disease [44].

The incidence of pulmonary metastases, like liver secondaries, is a function of the screening test. In primary colorectal cancer, lung metastases are present on chest roentgenograms in about 5–15% [45–47]. Compared with CT, plain chest roentgenograms miss occult pulmonary metastases in 10–15% of patients [48]. Necropsy series show pulmonary metastases in 64% of rectal and 48% of colonic adenocarcinomas [25].

In the presence of asymptomatic pulmonary metastases, survival of up to 18 months may be seen in selected patients having a resection of the primary tumour [20, 21, 46] (Table 2.7).

Recommendation The detection of isolated asymptomatic lung metastases should not alter surgical management of the primary tumour. Lung metastases as part of

Table 2.7 Survival in resection and non-resection of the primary tumour in the presence of lung metastases only

Reference	Resection	Survival (months)	Non-resection	Survival (months)
Silverman [47]	119 (colon)	16.4*	41	3.8*
Silverman [47]	52 (rectum)	12.3*	27	6.7*
Modlin and Walker [46]	2	18†	20	8.7†
Stearns and Binkley [20]	3	13.6†	4	9.5
Bacon and Martin [21]	3	14.3†	5	8.4†

* Median.
† Mean.

widespread disease may influence management, but this will depend on the total tumour load, in particular evidence of ascites and liver failure.

Peritoneal Metastases in Primary Colorectal Cancer

Minor local involvement of the peritoneum can be removed *en bloc* with the primary colorectal tumour. This forms part of the description of adjacent organ involvement and is discussed below.

Diffuse peritoneal carcinomatosis is more difficult to manage and, unless associated with ascites or obstruction, is difficult to predict preoperatively [49]. The main mode of presentation of peritoneal carcinomatosis is intestinal obstruction [50]. Poor prognosis indicators associated with peritoneal carcinomatosis in colorectal carcinoma are ascites and lung metastases [51]. The presence of ascites is associated with a median survival in colorectal malignancies of 4 months [52]. Compared with ascites from gynaecological malignancies, the protein concentration of ascitic fluid in gastrointestinal malignancies is lower and associated with a reduced survival. The critical ascitic/serum protein ratio is 0.4, below which survival is reduced [52].

Recommendation In the presence of ascites, palliative surgery should be the minimum needed to relieve immediate symptoms.

Bone Metastases in Primary Colorectal Cancer

Symptomatic bone secondaries from colorectal cancer are rare [53–56]. In primary colorectal cancer, asymptomatic isolated bone metastases are detected in 0.6–1.8% [47, 54, 57] and 4–6% of patients have bone metastases as part of generalized disease [54, 57]. Necropsy data show metastatic disease in 0.96–19.4% of patients with a diagnosis of colorectal cancer [25, 42, 58–60].

Bone scans show that asymptomatic skeletal involvement in colorectal cancer is common. The actual incidence depends on technique and is 33–61% [54, 57, 61–65].

Lindeman et al. [66] have conducted a prospective study using an immunocytochemical assay for epithelial cytokeratin protein CK 18 in curative colorectal resection. The presence of the CK 18 marker in the bone marrow was an independent prognostic factor, with a 71% 5-year survival in negative scans vs. a 32% 5-year survival in positive scans [66]. A positive scan should not alter the approach to the primary colorectal tumour, but should indicate the need for systemic therapy.

There may be an interval of up to 3 years after a positive scan, with bone secondaries presenting 21 to 34 months after curative resection of a colorectal tumour [53, 54, 56]. Mean survival after diagnosis of bone secondaries is 6–13 months [53, 54].

Symptomatic bone metastasis at the time of diagnosis of a primary colorectal cancer is a poor prognostic indicator. This is because it is likely that there will be generalized disease with a high tumour burden.

Recommendation A positive bone scan in an asymptomatic patient with a primary colorectal cancer should not alter the management of the primary tumour. A positive bone scan may be present in up to two-thirds of patients, possibly indicate the need for systemic therapy and may not become symptomatic for up to 3 years.

Unresectable Local Disease with or without Metastases in Primary Colorectal Cancer

Thus far, it has been assumed that the local tumour is resectable. Resection should follow the usual oncological guidelines, unless there is overwhelming tumour burden as indicated by extensive liver replacement, ascites, deranged liver biochemistry or multiple distant metastases. There are other palliative situations where the local tumour appears to be unresectable with or without evidence of distant disease.

Locally Invasive Tumour without Evidence of Metastases

Staging of distant metastases has been discussed. The accurate preoperative staging of a primary colorectal tumour is more difficult. Endoluminal ultrasound is more accurate in staging rectal tumours than CT [67]. Contrast agents, helical CT and magnetic resonance imaging using an intrarectal coil may increase the sensitivity and accuracy of these imaging techniques.

Unless there is a clinical suspicion of a fixed pelvic rectal carcinoma, preoperative staging of the local tumour is not routinely performed. At operation, unresectable intra-abdominal malignant disease may be found. It is impossible clinically to differentiate tumour from inflammatory adhesions. Cutting across malignant adhesions, either deliberately for a frozen section or unintentionally, renders the operation palliative. Table 2.8 shows the result of

Table 2.8 Failure to excise an adherent colorectal tumour *en bloc* increases recurrence and reduces survival (From Hunter et al. [68])

	No adherence (177)	Tumour adherence to another organ (41)		*p* value
Operation	Colectomy	*En bloc* (28)	Separation (13)	
5-year survival	55%	61%	23%	0.03
Recurrence	33%	36%	77%	0.02
Local recurrence	11%	18%	69%	0.002

failure to remove a tumour *en bloc*. Local recurrence increases from 18% to 69% and 5-year survival falls from 61% to 23% [68].

Large bulky primary tumours display a non-metastasizing behaviour, as described by Spratt [69]. These invade locally in a manner similar to basal cell carcinoma of the skin. Excision of such a tumour *en bloc* is associated with good survival [68, 70, 71].

Recommendation Therefore, when there is no evidence of metastases, even large tumours that may be deemed palliative by some are potentially curative. Preoperative radiotherapy has an important place in this clinical situation. *En bloc* excision should include involved contiguous structures. The difficulty is when adhesions involve vital structures. Although there are reports of pelvic exenteration as a palliative procedure [72], extensive procedures such as total pelvic exenteration and sacropelvic resection are justified only if performed with curative intent. This is despite falling mortality rates from 30% [73] to 0% to 20% in recent decades. The morbidity rates from total pelvic exenteration and sacropelvic resection are 50–100% [15–17, 71, 73–83].

Locally Invasive Tumour with Evidence of Metastases

As discussed, a large bulky tumour with apparent malignant adhesions should be resected if possible. However, the presence of definite distant metastases calls for an individual patient assessment. There are no specific data to assist judgement. It is reasonable to remove a locally invasive tumour *en bloc* when massive tumour burden is not present and a major exenteration is not required. Palliative abdominoperineal resection has a mortality rate of 2.9% [14]. Surgical excision, if possible, offers good palliation. External beam radiotherapy alone after subtotal excision of a rectal tumour does not alter survival or recurrence [84, 85].

Clinical Presentation

Obstruction, perforation and intraoperative spillage are associated with increased recurrence and decreased survival. These are palliative situations.

Obstruction

Large bowel obstruction is usually due to occlusion of the lumen from the primary colorectal tumour, and small bowel obstruction is more commonly due to extramural obstruction from peritoneal carcinomatosis.

Primary Obstruction

Obstruction is the presenting feature in 7–29% of cases [86–89]. Large bowel obstruction can be diagnosed on plain or contrast radiographs, clinically or at laparotomy. The methods of classification can affect the reported incidence of obstruction in primary colorectal cancer. For instance, in 44 patients demonstrating a complete retrograde blockage to barium, only 22 had clinical evidence of antegrade obstruction [90]. The site of obstruction is more commonly found in the colon than the rectum (24% vs. 4% [91]), and occurs in almost half of all splenic flexure tumours [87, 92–94].

Survival in obstructed colorectal cancer is less than in elective cases. Obstructive symptoms reduce 5-year survival from 38% to 19% [95]. Reduced survival in obstructed cases may be due to age [96] and advanced tumour stage [86, 97–100], although this is disputed [87].

In 42–50% of obstructed colorectal cancer, the disease is deemed incurable at presentation [86, 88, 91]. Distant metastases are said to be present in 25% [91], which is probably an underestimate. Preoperative and perioperative staging investigations are not usually performed in emergency presentations of colorectal cancer and we have already seen that palpation of the liver is not as sensitive as IOUS.

Patients with obstruction are more likely to have an advanced tumour stage and may have decreased survival stage for stage. The surgical alternatives are a two- or three-stage resection, primary resection with anastomosis (with or without on-table antegrade lavage), resection with colostomy or bypass or colostomy alone. The range in mortality rates is 6–60% (Table 2.9).

A staged resection has the disadvantage of formation of a stoma which has morbidity and may never be closed. On an intention-to-treat basis, there is no significant difference between primary resection and staged resection in either the in-hospital mortality rate (19% vs. 22%) or age-adjusted 5-year survival (29% vs. 31%) [87]. In this study of 713 patients with obstruction, hospital stay was shorter in the primary resection group (20 days vs. 40 days) and there was no difference in intra-abdominal sepsis or chest complications [87].

Right-sided lesions are generally managed now with resection and primary anastomosis. The situation relating to left-sided obstruction is less clear. A randomized study of 55 patients with acute left-sided obstruction [101] showed no difference in mortality (20–25%), morbidity or survival between a three-stage procedure with an initial stoma and a two-stage procedure with an initial Hartmann's operation. Four of the 20 survivors in the Hartmann's group did not have stoma closure.

In left-sided obstruction, resection and primary anastomosis the leak rate is 6% in elective and 18% in obstructed cases [87]. On-table lavage reduces the clinical leak rate to 5–10% [102]. A 10-year review of 130 cases with left-sided

Table 2.9 Mortality and survival in *palliative* emergency colorectal surgery for large bowel obstruction

Reference	*n*	Surgery	Mortality (%)
Kyllonen [91]	140	Resection	32 colonic 22 rectal
Phillips [87]	713	Resection	22
Dutton [212]	69	Curative resection	13
Runkel [115]	28	Resection	14
	29	No resection	29
Serpell [213]	49	Resection	6
		No resection	7
Gandrup [96]	59	Resection	49
Sjodahl [103]	27	Resection	30
Irvin [98]	27	Resection	59

obstruction reported no deaths in five patients with primary resection and anastomosis [96].

Although reported in 5–15% [88, 103], obstruction in rectal cancer is less common than colonic cancer. Differences in classification in some series see results from rectosigmoid obstruction considered in the same grouping as rectal tumours.

In addition to anterior resection, Hartmann's resection or abdominoperineal excision, obstruction from a rectal cancer can be dealt with via an endo-anal approach. The alternatives are local excision, electrocoagulation, cryotherapy and laser therapy (see below).

Recommendation Due to advanced stage at presentation and poor prognosis even within the same stage, obstructed tumours have a poor prognosis. Although not palliative by our earlier definition, the treatment of obstructed and perforated tumours can be considered at least "partially" palliative. Although traditionally treated with staged procedures, primary resection has become more widely used in obstructed colonic tumours. A primary resection has the same mortality as a staged resection on an intention-to-treat basis. Immediate anastomosis (perhaps with on-table lavage) is preferred, but there are no prospective studies. Patient and surgeon variables may dictate what procedure is performed.

Small Bowel Obstruction

Many of the reports relating to malignant small bowel obstruction do not make a clear distinction between primary and recurrent colorectal disease. Malignant tumours are responsible for 9–16% of all small bowel obstruction, with the colon and rectum the most common primary tumours [104–107]. When colorectal metastases are the cause of small bowel obstruction, median survival is 2–7 months [104, 105, 108], with a worse prognosis if ascites is present [51].

The alternatives are surgical excision of the obstructing tumour(s) or conservative treatment. Surgical mortality is 12–46% and is adversely affected by age, advanced disease and malnutrition [50, 104, 109]. Morbidity in a single report was 22%, although 10% had an enterocutaneous fistula [104].

Conservative management with nasogastric suction is not beneficial [109–112] and increases the risk of gangrene [110]. In selected patients the use of a long decompression jejunostomy tube may be helpful [113].

Recommendation Compared with pancreatic, genitourinary or gastric cancers, small bowel obstruction from a colorectal malignancy has a better prognosis [51]. However, in the presence of ascites, surgery is advised with caution.

Perforation

Intraoperative perforation has a worse prognosis than a spontaneous perforation. The 5-year survival in 111 curative resections with a spontaneous perforation was 44% compared with 32% following intraoperative perforation [114].

Table 2.10 Survival in intraoperative tumour spillage (From Slanetz [114])

	Dukes' category	n	5-year survival (%)
Perforation into cancer:			
colon	A	1	0
	B	6	20
	C	10	11
rectum	A	2	100
	B	22	17
	C	26	4.3
Perforation away from the cancer:			
colon	A	1	100
	B	17	29
	C	18	24
rectum	A	15	80
	B	30	38
	C	26	48

Perforated Bowel on Presentation

Three to 8% of colorectal cancers present with perforation [115]. In contrast to obstructed tumours, the relative risk for perforation increases from the left to the right colon [115].

As for obstructed tumour, a perforated tumour is at high risk of recurrence. Recurrence rates following perforation range from 28% to 51% [116–118]. Life expectancy in perforation is less than elective surgery for the same tumour stage [119].

The surgical options for perforation are similar to obstruction. Defunctioning colostomy alone in perforation is not advised. The mortality of a staged resection in perforation of the left colon is 27–73% and with primary resection mortality is 8–30% [115].

Perforation of the Bowel during Mobilization

Perforation of the tumour site carries a far graver prognosis than if perforation is distant to the tumour. The site (colon or rectum) and stage of the tumour affects survival (Table 2.10). In 1174 curative resections [114], inadvertent perforation resulted in 5-year survival falling from 63% to 23% in colon cancer and from 54% to 33% in rectal cancer. There was a four-fold increase in postoperative mortality when the cancer was disrupted during resection [114].

Subsequent Presentation

Pathology

Local Recurrence with and without Metastases

Median survival in patients with recurrent colorectal cancer is 5 months without treatment and 21 months after resection [120]. There are conflicting reports on the relative value of resection and non-resection surgery, radiotherapy and chemotherapy [121].

Relief of symptoms with external beam radiotherapy is 33–90% [122–124]. However, duration of response with radiotherapy is short-lived and long-term symptom-free survival is rare [125–128].

The pattern of recurrence after colonic and rectal cancer resection differs. In colonic cancer, local recurrences occur with distant and especially hepatic metastases [129, 130]. Local rectal cancer recurrence has less widesprad dissemination [131–133]. In patients who develop recurrence following curative surgery for rectal or sigmoid cancer, 30–50% of such recurrence is confined to the pelvis [132, 134, 135]. Forty-five per cent die an average of 7–9 months later because of isolated pelvic recurrence [132, 134, 135].

Most cases of recurrent colorectal cancers are palliative. Preoperative assessment may identify a few that are potentially resectable. Assessment of pelvic recurrence is difficult, especially following radiotherapy or abdominoperineal excision. Computed tomography and magnetic resonance imaging demonstrate soft-tissue masses but lack tissue specificity [136]. Positron emission tomography after intravenous injection of 18F-fluorodeoxyglucose may help in differentiating recurrent tumour from scar tissue [137].

Reoperation rate for cure is 10–65% [121, 138–140], although the overall chance of cure in a patient with locally recurrent colorectal cancer is low. Philipshen et al. [141] state that "despite consideration of re-resection wherever possible", 89% of patients with pelvic recurrence died and just 3.8% were free of disease.

Operative mortality in palliative resection is higher in recurrent compared with primary colorectal cancer. Makela et al. [121] report a mortality of 21.7% after palliative resection. Morbidity was 42%, 60% and 60% for resection, bypass and enterostomy procedures, respectively [121].

In patients with apparently local recurrence only, complete resection with negative microscopic margins has a median survival of 59 months [142]. A wide *en bloc* excision of local tumour recurrence has a 5-year survival of 15–49% [142–144].

Recommendation Local recurrence often reflects tumour dissemination and the prognosis is generally poor. However, a few patients may benefit from a salvage resection.

Obstruction

The important point here is not to assume tumour recurrence as the cause of obstruction in a patient previously resected for curative colorectal cancer. Obstruction after curative resection for colorectal cancer is not due to tumour recurrence in 25–41% and surgery produces long-term survival in 40% [109, 145]. When obstruction is due to tumour recurrence, operative mortality is 27%, with a median survival of 2 months. The prognosis is also bleak where a patient undergoes a primary palliative procedure and re-presents with obstruction.

Weiss et al. [110] use a "performance grading system" to try to predict survival in patients with obstruction (Table 2.11). Patients who are obviously terminally ill, too weak to get out of bed and often with visceral metastases have little hope of benefiting from surgery.

Table 2.11 Survival in patients with previous diagnosis of colon cancer presenting with bowel obstruction (from Weiss et al [110])

Performance status*	n	Mean survival (months)
0–1	19	12.4
2–3	13	6.0
4	2	0.38

* Performance grades:
0: Fully active, no restriction to daily activity.
1: Ambulatory and performs light work.
2: Ambulatory and self-caring but no work activities.
3: Limited self-care. Confined to bed or chair more than 50% of waking hours.
4: No self-care. Confined to bed or chair.

Recommendation If a patient presents with small bowel obstruction after a curative excision of a colorectal tumour, laparotomy should be performed if obstruction persists after 3–4 days of nasogastric suction.

Ascites

Re-presentation with ascites after excision of a colorectal tumour is a grave prognostic sign. Many of these patients will present with obstruction as part of peritoneal carcinomatosis (see above). The presence of ascites with obstruction after resection of a tumour reduces survival. In patients with symptomatic tense ascites alone, percutaneous draining with concomitant albumin replacement and spironolactone is probably the best that can be offered. Systematic peritoneal shunting confers no advantage over this approach.

Surgical Options

Stoma Alone

In patients with ascites and massive liver deposits, survival is measured in weeks or days rather than months. In these patients a resection should only be performed where there is low morbidity. In obstructed cases, a well-constructed stoma or a bypass procedure can offer good short-term palliation.

In patients with palliative primary colorectal cancer, we have already seen that survival of many months is possible. In this situation, resection of the primary is preferable to a stoma alone.

In recurrent cancer, salvage surgery is usually more extensive, especially in the pelvis. Although, generally performed with curative intent, results are not good in the long term (see above).

The surgical options for resection in primary palliative rectal cancer are local excision, a Hartmann's procedure, anterior resection and abdominoperineal excision. In obstructed or perforated colonic cancer, the resection options are staged or primary resection with or without immediate anastomosis (see above).

Anterior resection, Hartmann's procedure and abdominoperineal excision have already been discussed.

Local Procedures

Local procedures may be used as palliative treatment in advanced disease or where the condition of the patient prevents the usual method of surgical excision. Except where the tumour is removed as a full-thickness local procedure, there is difficulty in comparing local procedures as the tumour cannot be pathologically staged.

Local Excision

A palliative local excision avoids a stoma and can be performed under regional anaesthesia. Moran et al. [7] report 13 cases of peranal local resection in a group of 108 undergoing palliative resection. There was no morbidity or mortality after local excision and none of the patients died of pelvic disease. One did have symptoms of pelvic recurrence. The authors did not describe the method of selection for operation, the operative technique or tumour pathology. Control of disease may require repeated attempts at excision [146, 147] and it may be impossible to excise the tumour completely [147]. Local excision can be combined with radiotherapy and chemotherapy in curative cases, but there are no reports of this technique in palliative cases.

The reported techniques of local excision of rectal cancer are disc excision [148], a trans-sphincteric excision [149], endoscopic transanal excision using a urological resectoscope [147, 150, 151] and transanal endoscopic microsurgery [152].

Graham et al. [153] reported palliative submucous excision [154] in just a few patients. Although pathological details are not given, these cases were probably deemed palliative due to co-morbidity, as submucous resection is not suitable for a locally advanced tumour.

One of the difficulties in recommending local excision is the lack of a suitable sensitive and specific preoperative technique to identify local pelvic nodal spread.

In palliative rectal cancer due to extreme age and associated co-morbid conditions, local excision may be a worthwhile alternative to anterior resection and abdominoperineal excision. However, in patients with colorectal cancer aged 70 and over, there is no significant difference in mortality (9% vs. 5%) or morbidity (18% vs. 17%) in resection of advanced and localized disease [155]. However, there were more rectal tumours in the localized tumour group than the advanced group (61% vs. 18%) which may account for the good results in the advanced group. Compared with colonic tumours, surgery for advanced rectal tumours is usually associated with higher mortality and morbidity.

Laser Therapy

Laser treatment may be by contact or non-contact photoablation (coagulation necrosis or vaporization with immediate destruction) or by photodynamic therapy. The role of photodynamic therapy in palliative colorectal cancer requires further study [156].

The Nd:YAG laser is a deep coagulator with a depth of injury of 4 mm. It is

Table 2.12 Laser therapy* in palliative colorectal cancer with obstruction and bleeding

Reference	n	Relief of symptoms (%)		Morbidity (%)
		Obstruction	Bleeding	
Mathus [164]	156	83	93	13
Escudero [214]	25	67	100	0
Brunetaud [162]	161	88		3
Spinelli [215]	227	93	100	3

* Nd:YAF laser used as coagulation at low power of 80 W.

especially suited for endoscopic use due to a flexible delivery system. The indications for laser treatment in advanced colorectal cancer are palliation of local symptoms or relief of obstruction as the sole therapy or to enable patient preparation prior to definitive surgery. Laser therapy is effective in the treatment of bleeding and the relief of obstruction (Table 2.12). However, pain, tenesmus [157, 158] and incontinence [157] are not well palliated. In addition, surgery is required after poor laser palliation for large lesions, lesions located near the anus [159] and long, circumferential strictures [160] at the rectosigmoid junction [159]. Bright et al. [161] found that 12 of 18 patients with tumours > 5 cm required surgery after failed laser treatment.

In obstruction, recanalization of the lumen with laser is not always associated with relief. Mellow [159] employed criteria from Brunetaud [162] and found that in 18 of 20 patients successfully recanalized with laser, only 14 had a qualitative success.

Morbidity of laser treatment is zero to 13% [163–165]. Perforation, rectovaginal fistula, stenosis and bleeding are the main complications. Some authors [162] feel that repeated coagulation with the laser at a lower power is safer than vaporization at high power. However, one of the drawbacks of laser therapy is that repeated treatment is required. Usually laser treatment is once or twice a week until the treatment goal is attained. Treatment is then repeated at monthly intervals.

Radiotherapy reduces the frequency and dose of laser treatment, albeit at an increased risk of stricture formation [166].

The financial benefits of laser therapy in patients with obstruction and bleeding are a shorter hospital and intensive care stay [159]. In this report [159], the capital expenses of laser treatment were not taken into account. Laser can potentially treat more proximal lesions than other local methods.

A word of caution on laser treatment comes from Forde [167], who urges careful selection of patients because patients may "... survive longer than anticipated only to succumb to long term complications of laser ablation such as stenosis and then require a colostomy. ..."

Comparison with Other Methods of Palliation

There are no randomized studies that compare laser with other methods of palliation. In a retrospective study of 79 patients from a single centre, there was little difference in mortality or morbidity in patients treated with laser, a transanal procedure or abdominoperineal or anterior resection [165]. There were no differences between the groups in patient wellbeing after surgery.

Another group reviewed their experience with palliative resection or laser therapy in 46 patients with distant metastases or co-morbid conditions that prevented a radical procedure [159]. Of 21 treated with laser, three suffered bleeding or a perirectal abscess and two required surgery later for obstruction. In the 35 treated with a surgical procedure, 19 suffered complications with five requiring reoperation [159].

Electrocoagulation Treatment

Electrocoagulation treatment of rectal cancer has been reported with varying results in a small number of series [168–172]. There are difficulties with bleeding, poor palliation with surgical intervention required and frequent and often prolonged treatment sessions. In a mixture of patients where electrocoagulation was performed with both curative and palliative intent, postoperative bleeding occurred in 22% and perforation in 2.5% [170].

Although some claim a "boiling" technique with lower energy to be more effective [168], the limitation of electrocoagulation to the distal 10 cm of rectum and the option of laser therapy renders electrocoagulation treatment an unappealing method, to be used sparingly as a palliative measure [169].

Endoscopic Transanal Resection

The operative technique is similar to transurethral resection of the prostate or bladder tumour. Resection is performed with a deep cutting loop. The tumour is removed piecemeal, perforation of the bowel may result and for this reason the procedure should be limited to rectal tumours below the peritoneal reflection. Results show poor relief of symptoms, with a mortality rate of 12% [150]. There is little to recommend this method.

Cryosurgery

Cryosurgery uses liquid nitrogen delivering a temperature of up to −195°C at the tip of the probe. Due to dangers of perforation, cryotherapy cannot be applied above 10–12 cm from the anal verge. Treatment must be applied repeatedly and patients are at risk of mucous discharge for up to 6 weeks, as is seen after cryosurgery for haemorrhoids [173].

Palliation for bleeding and pain is not good, with no change in symptoms in over 50% of 112 patients [174]. In this series, morbidity was 17% [174].

Palliative Colorectal Surgery in the Elderly

One of the factors that influences the clinician in the difficult decision to resect in a palliative case is the chronological and biological age of the patient. Colorectal tumours are frequently seen in the elderly. The overall lifetime risk of developing colorectal cancer is 1:20; the incidence in persons younger than 65 years is 19 per 100 000 but rises to 337 per 100 000 in persons older than 65 [175].

In colonic cancer, age alone should not alter the surgical decision in cases of obstruction, perforation or local disease control [155, 176, 177]. However, in rectal cancer there is a higher morbidity and mortality with co-morbid factors becoming more significant [178–181]. In the presence of distant metastases, local excision of a rectal malignancy may be more appropriate than a pelvic dissection. However, abdominoperineal resection may be necessary to control the debilitating effects of advanced pelvic disease [180].

Most of the above figures relate to elderly patients over 65, 70 or 75 years. However, in patients over 80 years of age, surgery for palliative colorectal cancer is probably not indicated [182].

Palliative Laparoscopic Surgery

There may well be a place for this technique in palliative resection of large bowel cancer [183], but no results have been reported.

Anal Cancer

Anal Canal Tumours

Generally, abdominoperineal excision is reserved for salvage treatment following persistent or recurrent local disease. In a review of 16 studies involving 636 patients treated with multimodality therapy for anal canal cancer, Beck et al. [184] found persistent tumour present in 14%. Careful follow-up with core biopsies is required to recognize persisting tumour. Salvage abdominoperineal excision in cases of persisting tumour prevents another relapse in 70–90% of cases [185–187], although long-term cure with salvage abdominoperineal excision is reported in only 29–50% [188, 189]. Salvage therapy with additional chemotherapy and radiotherapy produced disappointing results in a recent report [189] and colostomy alone had no benefit.

Median survival is 1 month in patients with untreated distant metastases compared with 11 months and 12 months with mitomycin C + 5-FU and cisplatin + 5-FU respectively [190]. In view of this poor prognosis in patients with combined local and distant recurrence, salvage abdominoperineal excision for the local recurrence should be combined with chemotherapy to treat the distant metastases.

Malignant Melanoma

Presenting features from an anorectal melanoma are usually bleeding, a mass, pain or sometimes an incidental finding on pathological examination of haemorrhoidectomy specimens [191, 192]. Abdominoperineal resection, inguinal or pelvic lymphadenectomy do not increase survival whether metastases are present or not [192–194]. Local excision of the primary tumour offers the best palliation with low mortality.

Local recurrence is more common after a local excision than after abdominoperineal excision [191–194]. However, local recurrence is usually associated with disseminated disease and a median survival of just 2 months [193, 194].

In such an uncommon condition, recommendations are based on a small number of cases. However, local excision is supported as the treatment for primary anorectal malignant melanoma [191, 194–198]. Abdominoperineal excision in anorectal malignant melanoma should be reserved for bulky primary tumours or local recurrence when indicated.

Conclusions

In primary and recurrent colorectal cancer, palliation is a common consideration. Curative surgery for primary colorectal cancer is possible in only 50–82% of cases. In the remainder, resection of the primary tumour offers the best method of palliation. Local recurrence after curative surgery for colorectal cancer occurs in 2.6–32%, but curative resection of this recurrence is usually not possible due to disseminated disease.

The difficulty lies in selecting patients who will benefit from palliative resection of the primary or recurrent tumour. Review of the literature shows that in cases with asymptomatic metastases of the liver, lung and bone, resection of the primary tumour is entirely justified. Where there is extensive tumour involvement of the liver or other evidence of advanced disease demonstrated by jaundice or ascites, or symptomatic bone secondaries, the benefits of palliative surgery are less clear. The possible symptomatic benefit from resectional surgery in recurrent disease must be balanced against high mortality and morbidity of extensive procedures.

Factors such as age and the presence of associated medical conditions also influence mortality and survival. Furthermore, it is not easy to quantify the tumour load and the decision on palliative surgery is often a result of subjective assessment by the surgeon. Although mortality rates and survival figures can be recorded, assessment of palliation of symptoms is more difficult.

Local resection, resection with anastomosis and abdominoperineal resection of palliative rectal cancers can be performed with acceptable mortality and morbidity. Although pelvic symptoms are palliated by major resection such as pelvic exenteration and sacropelvic exenteration, the high morbidity and mortality combined with the economics of such surgery means that this approach should be used only with curative intent.

References

1. Slaney G. Results of treatment of carcinoma of the colon and rectum. In: Irvine WT, eds. Modern trends in surgery. London: Butterworths. 1971: 69–89.
2. Boring CC, Squires TS, Tong T. Ca-a cancer journal for clinicians. Cancer Statistics 1991; 41: 19-36.
3. Brown SC, Abraham JS, Walsh S, Sykes PA. Risk factors and operative mortality in surgery for colorectal cancer. Ann R Coll Surg Engl 1991; 73: 269–72.
4. Johnson WR, McDermott FT, Pihl E, Milne BJ, Price AB, Hughes ESR. Palliative operative management in rectal carcinoma. Dis Colon Rectum 1981; 24: 606–609.
5. Lockhart-Mummery HE, Ritchie JK, Hawley PR. The results of surgical treatment for

carcinoma of the rectum at St Mark's Hospital from 1948 to 1972. Br J Surg 1976; 63: 673–677.
6. McArdle CS, Hole D, Hansell D, Blumgart LH, Wood CB. Prospective study of colorectal cancer in the West of Scotland: 10 year follow up. Br J Surg 1990; 77: 280–282.
7. Moran MR, Rothenberger DA, Lahr CJ, Buls JG, Goldberg SM. Palliation for rectal cancer. Resection? Anastomosis? Arch Surg 1987; 122: 640–643.
8. Phillips RKS, Hittinger R, Blesovsky L, Fry JS, Fielding LP. Local recurrence following "curative" surgery for large bowel cancer: I. The overall picture. Br J Surg 1984; 71: 12-16.
9. Lazarus-Barlow WS, Leeming JH. The natural duration of cancer. Br Med J 1924; 2: 266.
10. Daland EM, Welch CE, Nathanson I. One hundred untreated cancers of the rectum. New England J Med 1936; 214: 451–456.
11. Pestana C, Reitemeier RJ, Moertel CG, Judd ES, Dockerty MB. The natural history of carcinoma of the colon and rectum. Am J Surg 1964; 108: 826–829.
12. Joffe J, Gordon PH. Palliative resection for colorectal cancer. Dis Colon Rectum 1981; 24: 355–360.
13. Takaki HS, Ujiki GT, Shields TS. Palliative resections in the treatment of primary colorectal cancer. Am J Surg 1977; 133: 548–550.
14. Bordos DC, Baker RR, Cameron JL. An evaluation of palliative abdominoperineal resection for carcinoma of the rectum. Surg Gynecol Obstet 1974; 139: 731–733.
15. Sardi A, Bolton JS, Hicks TC, Skenderis BS. Total pelvic exenteration with or without sacral resection in patients with recurrent colorectal cancer. South Med J 1994; 87: 363–369.
16. Pearlman NW, Donohue RE, Stiegman GV et al. Pelvic and sacropelvic exenteration for locally advanced or recurrent anorectal cancer. Arch Surg 1987; 122: 537–540.
17. Hafner GH, Herrera L, Petrelli NJ. Morbidity and mortality after pelvic exenteration for colorectal adenocarcinoma. Ann Surg 1992; 215: 63–67.
18. Wanebo H, Gaker D, Whitehill R, Morgan R, Constable W. Pelvic recurrence of rectal cancer. Options for curative resection. Ann Surg 1987; 205: 482–495.
19. Longo WE, Ballantyne GH, Bilchik AJ, Modlin IM. Advanced rectal cancer: What is the best palliation? Dis Colon Rectum 1988; 31:
20. Stearns MWJ, Binkley GE. Palliative surgery for cancer of the rectum and colon. Cancer 1954; 7: 1016–1019.
21. Bacon HE, Martin PV. The rationale of palliative resection for primary cancer of the colon and rectum complicated by liver and lung metastases. Dis Colon Rectum 1964; 7: 211–217.
22. Martin RG, Soriano SJ, Clark LR, White EC. Abdominoperineal resection as palliation for advanced rectal cancer. Cancer Bull 1966; 2: 28–32.
23. Wanebo HJ, Semoglou C, Attiyeh F, Stearns MJJ. Surgical management of patients with primary operable colorectal cancer and synchronous liver metastases. Am J Surg 1978; 135: 81–85.
24. Parc R, Tiret E, Frileux P, Moszkowski E, Loygue J. Resection and colo-anal anastomosis with colonic reservoir for rectal carcinoma. Br J Surg 1986; 73: 139–141.
25. Berge T, Ekelund G, Mellner C, Pihl B, Weinckert A. Carcinoma of the colon and rectum in a defined population. Acta Chir Scand 1973; 438 (Suppl.): 45–49.
26. Steele GJ, Posner MR. Adjuvant treatment of colorectal adenocarcinoma. Curr Probl Cancer 1993; 17: 223–69.
27. Finlay IG, McArdle CS. Occult hepatic metastases in colorectal cancer. Br J Surg 1986; 73: 732–735.
28. Bengtsson G, Carlsson G, Hafstrom L, Jonsson P. Natural history of patients with untreated liver metastases from colorectal cancer. Am J Surg 1981; 141: 586–589.
29. Bengmark S, Hafstrom L. The natural history of primary and secondary malignant tumours of the liver. Cancer 1969; 23: 198–202.

30. Wood CB, Gillis CR, Blumgart LH. A retrospective study of the natural history of patients with liver metastases from colorectal cancer. Clin Oncol 1976; 2: 285–288.
31. Steele G, Ravikumar TS. Resection of hepatic metastases from colorectal cancer. Ann Surg 1989; 210: 127–138.
32. Silen W. Hepatic resection for metastases from colorectal cancer is of dubious value. Arch Surg 1989; 124: 1021–1022.
33. Finlay IG, Meek D, Brunton F, McArdle CS. Growth rate of hepatic metastases in colorectal carcinoma. Br J Surg 1988; 75: 641–644.
34. Clarke MP, Kane RA, Steele GJ, Hamilton ES, Ravikumar TS et al. Prospective comparison of preoperative imaging and intraoperative ultrasonography in the decison of liver tumors. Surgery 1989; 106: 849–855.
35. Parker GA, Lawrence WJ, Horsley JS, Neifeld JP, Cook D et al. Intraoperative ultrasound of the liver affects operative decision making. Ann Surg 1989; 209: 569–577.
36. Steele G Jr., Ravikumar TS, Benotti PN. New surgical treatments for recurrent colorectal cancer. Cancer 1990; 65: 723–30.
37. Hughes K, Scheele J, Sugarbaker PH. Surgery for colorectal cancer metastatic to the liver. Surg Clin North Am 1989; 69: 339–359.
38. Carlsson U, Lasson A, Ekelund G. Recurrence rates after curative surgery for rectal carcinoma with special reference to their accuracy. Dis Colon Rectum 1987; 30: 431–434.
39. Jaffe BM, Donegan WL, Watson F, Spratt JSJ. Factors influencing survival in patients with untreated hepatic metastases. Surg Gynecol Obstet 1968; 127: 1–11.
40. Lahr CJ, Scong S-J, Cloud G et al. A multifactorial analysis of progniostic factors in patients with liver metastases from colorectal carcinoma. J Clin Oncol 1983; 1: 720–723.
41. Goslin R, Steele GJ, Zamcheck N et al. Factors influencing survival in patients with hepatic metastases from adenocarcinoma of the colon and rectum. Dis Colon Rectum 1982; 25:
42. Weiss L, Grundmann E, Thorhorst J, Harveit F, Moberg I et al. Haematognous metastatic patterns in colonic carcinoma: an analysis of 1541 necropsies. J Pathol 1986; 150: 195–202.
43. Weiss L, Voit A, Lane WW. Metastatic patterns in patients with carcinomas of the lower esophagus and upper rectum. Invasion and Metastasis 1984; 4: 47–60.
44. McCormack PM. Resected pulmonary metastases from colorectal cancer. Dis Colon Rectum 1979; 22: 553–556.
45. Dionne L. The pattern of blood borne metastasis from carcinoma of the rectum. Cancer 1965; 18: 775.
46. Modlin J, Walker HS. Palliative resections in cancer of the colon and rectum. Cancer 1949; 2: 767–776.
47. Silverman DT, Murray JL, Smart CR, Brown CC, Myers MH. Estimated median survival times of patients with colorectal cancer based on experience with 9,745 patients. Am J Surg 1977; 133: 289–97.
48. Steele GJ, Osteen RT, Wilson RE et al. Patterns of failure after surgical cure of large liver tumours. Am J Surg 1984; 147:
49. Nelson RC, Chezmar JL, Hoel MJ, Buck DR, Sugarbaker PH. Peritoneal carcinomatosis: preoperative CT with intraperitoneal contrast material. Radiology 1992; 182: 133–138.
50. Annest LS, Jolly PC. The result of surgical treatment of bowel obstruction caused by peritoneal carcinomatosis. Am Surg 1979; 45: 718–721.
51. Chu DZ, Lang NP, Thompson C, Osteen PK, Westbrook KC. Peritoneal carcinomatosis in nongynecologic malignancy. A prospective study of prognostic factors. Cancer 1989; 63: 364–7.
52. Garrison RN, Karlin LD, Galloway RH, Houser LS. Malignant ascites: Clinical and experimental observations. Ann Surg 1986; 203: 644–651.

53. Besbeas S, Stearns MW. Osseous metastases from carcinoma of the colon and rectum. Dis Colon Rectum 1978; 21: 266.
54. Bonnheim DC, Petrelli NJ, Herrera L, Walsh D, Mittleman A. Osseous metastases from colorectal cancer. Am J Surg 1986; 151: 457–459.
55. Hoehn JL, Ousley JL, Avecilla CS. Occult carcinoma of the colon and rectum manifesting as osseous metastasis. Dis Colon Rectum 1979; 129–132.
56. Talbot RW, Irvine B, Jass JR, Dowd GS, Northover JM. Bone metastases in carcinoma of the rectum: a clinical and pathological review. Eur J Surg Oncol 1989; 15: 449–452.
57. Bonfanti G, Bozzetti F, Doci R, Baticci F, Marolda R et al. Results of extended surgery for cancer of the rectum and sigmoid. Br J Surg 1982; 69: 305–307.
58. Swinton NW, Legg MA, Lewis FG. Metastasis of cancer of the rectum and sigmoid flexure. Dis Colon Rectum 1964; 7: 273–277.
59. Hindo WA, Soleimani PK, Miller WA et al. Patterns of recurrent and metastatic carcinoma of the colon and rectum treated with radiation. Dis Colon Rectum 1972; 15: 436.
60. Buirge RE. Carcinoma of the large intestine: Review of four hundred and sixteen autopsy reports. Arch Surg 1941; 42: 801.
61. Antoniades J, Croll MN, Walner RJ, Brady LW. Bone scanning in carcinoma of the colon and rectum. Dis Colon Rectum 1976; 19: 139–143.
62. Nabi HA, Doerr RJ. Radiolabeled monoclonal antibody imaging (immunoscintaigraphy) of colorectal cancers: current status and future perspectives. Am J Surg 1992; 163: 448–456.
63. Shirazi PH, Rayundu GVS, Fordham EW. 18F bone scanning: Review of indications and results of 1500 scans. Radiology 1974; 112: 361–368.
64. Tofe AJ, Francis MD, Harvey WJ. Correlation of neoplasms with incidence and localization of skeletal metastases: An analysis of 1355 diphosphonate bone scans. J Nucl Med 1975; 16: 986–989.
65. Vider M, Maruyama Y, Navarez R. Significance of the vertebral venous (Batson's) plexus in metastatic spread in colorectal cancer. Cancer 1977; 40: 67–71.
66. Lindemann F, Schlimok G, Dirschedl P, Witte J, Riethmuller G. Prognostic significance of micrometastatic tumour cells in bone marrow of colorectal cancer. Lancet 1992; 340: 685–689.
67. Rifkin MD, Ehelich SM, Marks G. Staging of rectal carcinoma: Prospective comparison of endorectal US and CT. Radiology 1989; 170: 319.
68. Hunter JA, Ryan JJ, Schultz P. En bloc resection of colon cancer adherent to other organs. Am J Surg 1987; 154: 67–71.
69. Spratt JS, Watson FR, Pratt JL. Characteristics of variants of colorectal cancer that do not metastasize to lymph nodes. Dis Col Rectum 1970; 13: 243–246.
70. McGlone TP, Bernie WA, Elliot DW. Survival following extended resection for extracolonic invasion by colon cancer. Arch Surg 1982; 117: 595–599.
71. Butcher HR, Spjut HJ. An evaluation of pelvic extenteration for advanced carcinoma of the lower colon. Cancer 1959; 12: 681–687.
72. Deckers P, Olsson C, Williams LF, Mozden PJ. Pelvic exenteration as palliation of malignant disease. Am J Surg 1976; 131: 509–515.
73. Brunschwig A. Complete excision of pelvic viscera for advanced carcinoma. Cancer 1948; 1: 177–183.
74. Eckhauser FE, Lindenauer SM, Morley GW. Pelvic exenteration for advanced rectal carcinoma. Am J Surg 1979; 138: 411–414.
75. Boey J, Wong J, Ong GB. Pelvic exenteration for locally advanced colorectal carcinoma. Ann Surg 1982; 195: 513–8.
76. Bricker HR, Butcher EM. Results of the radical surgical treatment of advanced pelvic cancer. Ann Surg 1967; 166: 428.
77. Kiselow M, Butcher HR, Bricker EM. Results of the radical surgical treatment of advanced pelvic cancer. Ann Surg 1967; 166: 428–436.

78. Ledesma EJ, Bruno S, Mittelman A. Total pelvic exenteration colorectal disease: a twenty year experience. Ann Surg 1981; 194: 701–703.
79. Lindsey WF, Wood DK, Briele HA, Greager JA, Walker MJ et al. Pelvic exenteration. J Surg Oncol 1985; 30: 231–234.
80. Lopez MJ, Kraybill WG, Downey RS et al. Exenterative surgery for locally advanced rectosigmoid cancers: is it worthwhile? Surgery 1987; 102: 644–651.
81. Takagi H, Morimoto T, Yasue M et al. Total pelvic exenteration for advanced carcinoma of the lower colon. J Surg Oncol 1985; 28: 59–62.
82. Williams LFJ, Huddleston CB, Sawyers JL, Potts JR, Sharp KW, McDougal SW. Is total pelvic exenteration reasonable primary treatment for rectal carcinoma? Ann Surg 1988; 207: 670–678.
83. Yeung RS, Moffat FL, Falk RE. Pelvic exenteration for recurrent and extensive primary colorectal adenocarcinoma. Cancer 1993; 72: 1853–8.
84. Ghossein NA, Samala EC, Alpert S, DeLuca FR, Ragins H et al. Elective post-operative radiotherapy after incomplete resection of colorectal cancer. Dis Colon Rectum 1981; 24: 252–256.
85. Schild SE, Martenson JA, Gunderson LL et al. Long-term survival and patterns of failure after postoperative radiation therapy for subtotally resected rectal adenocarcinoma. Int J Radiat Oncol Biol Phys 1989; 16: 459.
86. Ohman U. Prognosis in patients with obstructing colorectal carcinoma. Am J Surg 1982; 143: 742–747.
87. Phillips RKS, Hittinger R, Fry JS, Fielding LP. Malignant large bowel obstruction. Br J Surg 1985; 72: 296–302.
88. Umpleby HC, Williamson RCN. Survival in acute obstructing colorectal carcinoma. Dis Colon Rectum 1984; 27: 299–304.
89. Fielding LP, Wells BW. Survival after primary and after staged resection for large bowel obstruction caused by cancer. Br J Surg 1974; 61: 16–18.
90. Faulconer HT, Ferguson JA, Van Zwalenburg BR. The surgical influence of complete retrograde obstruction of the colon. Dis Colon Rectum 1971; 14: 428.
91. Kyllonen LE. Obstruction and perforation complicating colorectal carcinoma. An epidemiologic and clinical study with special reference to incidence and survival. Acta Chir Scand 1987; 153: 607–14.
92. Levien DH, Gibbons S, Begos D, Byrne DW. Survival after resection of carcinoma of the splenic flexure. Dis Colon Rectum 1991; 34: 401–403.
93. Steffen C, Bokey EL, Chapuis PH. Carcinoma of the splenic flexure. Dis Colon Rectum 1987; 30: 872–874.
94. Waldron RP, Donovan IA. Mortality in patients with obstructing colorectal cancer. Ann R Coll Surg Engl 1986; 68: 219–221.
95. Chapuis PH, Dent OF, Fisher R, Newland RC, Pheils MT et al. A multivariate analysis of clinical and pathological variables in prognosis after resection of large bowel cancer. Br J Surg 1985; 72: 698–702.
96. Gandrup P, Lund L, Balslev I. Surgical treatment of acute malignant large bowel obstruction. Eur J Surg 1992; 158: 427–30.
97. Garcia-Valdecasas JC, Llovera JM, deLacy AM, Reverter JC, Grande L et al. Obstructing colorectal carcinomas: Prospective study. Dis Colon Rect 1991; 34: 759–762.
98. Irvin TT, Greaney MG. The treatment of colonic cancer presenting with intestinal obstruction. Br J Surg 1977; 64: 741–744.
99. Ragland JJ, Londe AM, Spratt JS. Correlation of the prognosis of obstructing colorectal carcinoma with clinincal and pathological variables. Am J Surg 1971; 121: 552.
100. Schein CJ, Gemming RH. The prognosis of obstructing left colonic cancers. Dis Colon Rectum 1981; 24: 454–455.
101. Kronborg O. The missing randomized trial of two surgical treatments for acute

obstruction due to carcinoma of the left colon and rectum. Int J Colorect Dis 1986; 1: 162–166.
102. Glass RL, Smith LE, Cochran RC. Subtotal colectomy for obstructing carcinoma of the left colon. Am J Surg 1983; 145: 335.
103. Sjodahl R, Franzen T, Nystrom P. Primary versus staged resection for acute obsructing colorectal carcinoma. Br J Surg 1992; 79: 685–688.
104. Aranha GV, Folk FA, Greenlee HB. Surgical palliation of small bowel obstruction due to metastatic carcinoma. Am Surg 1981; 47: 99–102.
105. Glass RL, LeDuc RJ. Small intestinal obstruction from peritoneal carcinomatosis. Am J Surg 1973; 125: 316–317.
106. Davis SE, Sperlings L. Obstruction of the small intestine. Arch Surg 1969; 99: 424–426.
107. Sise JG, Crichlow RW. Obstruction due to malignant tumours. Semin Oncol 1978; 5: 213.
108. Aabo K, Pedusen H, Bach F, Knudsen J. Surgical management of intestinal obstruction in the late course of malignant disease. Acta Chir Scand 1984; 150: 173–176.
109. Ketchman AS, Hoye RC, Pilch YH, Morton DL. Delayed intestinal obstruction following treatment for cancer. Cancer 1970; 25: 406–410.
110. Weiss SM, Skibber JM, Rosato FE. Bowel obstruction in cancer patients: performance status as a predictor of survival. J Surg Oncol 1984; 25: 15–17.
111. Osteen RT, Guyton S, Steele G, Wilson RE. Malignant intestinal obstruction. Surgery 1980; 87: 611–615.
112. Baines M, Oliver DJ, Carter RL. Medical management of intestinal obstruction in patients ith advanced malignant disease. Lancet 1985; 2(8462): 990–993.
113. McCarthy JD. A strategy for intestinal obstruction of peritoneal carcinomatosis. Arch Surg 1986; 121: 1081–1082.
114. Slanetz CAJ. The effect of inadvertent intraoperative perforation on survival and recurrence in colorectal cancer. Dis Colon Rectum 1984; 27: 792–7.
115. Runkel NS, Schlag P, Schwarz V, Herfarth C. Outcome after emergency surgery for cancer of the large intestine. Br J Surg 1991; 78: 183–8.
116. Phillips RKS, Hittinger R, Blesovsky L, Fry JS, Fielding LP. Local recurrence following 'curative' surgery for large bowel cancer: II. The rectum and rectosigmoid. Br J Surg 1984; 71: 17–20.
117. Wiggers T, Arends JW, Volovics A. Regression analysis of prognostic factors in colorectal cancer after curative resection. Dis Colon Rectum 1988; 31: 33–41.
118. Zirngibl H, Husemann B, Hermanek P. Intraoperative spillage of tumour cells in surgery for colorectal cancer. Dis Colon Rectum 1990; 33: 610–614.
119. Willet C, Tepper JE, Cohen A, Orlow E, Welch C. Obstructive and perforative colonic cancer: patterns of failure. J Clin Oncol 1985; 3: 379–384.
120. Polk HCJ, Spratt JSJ. Recurrent colorectal carcinoma: Detection, treatment and other considerations. Surgery 1971; 69: 9–23.
121. Makela J, Haukipuro K, Laitinen S, Kairaluoma MI. Surgical treatment of recurrent colorectal cancer. Five-year follow-up. Arch Surg 1989; 124: 1029–32.
122. Whitely HW, Stearns MWJ, Leaming RH, Deddish MR. Palliative radiation therapy in patients with cancer of the colon and rectum. Cancer 1970; 25: 343.
123. Nordman E, Gronroos M, Aho AJ, Numminen S. Inoperable and recurrent carcinoma of the rectum and rectosigmoid: aspects of radiation treatment and prognosis. Ann Chir Gynae 1977; 66: 265–268.
124. Arnott SJ. Colorectal cancer: Radiotherapy. Recent results. Cancer Res 1982; 83: 113–125.
125. Pacini P, Cionini L, Pirtoli L, Ciatto S, Tucci E, Sebaste L. Symptomatic recurrences of carcinoma of the rectum and sigmoid. Dis Colon Rectum 1986; 29: 865–868.
126. Overgaard M, Overgaard J, Sell A. Dose-response relationship for radiation therapy of recurrent, residual and primarily inoperable colorectal cancer. Radiother Oncol 1984; 1: 217.

127. Dobrowosky W, Schmid AP. Radiotherapy of presacral recurrence following radical surgery or rectal carcinoma. Dis Colon Rectum 1985; 28: 917–919.
128. James RD, Johnson RJ, Eddleston B, Zheng GL, Jones JM. Prognostic factors in locally recurrent rectal carcinoma treated by radiotherapy. Br J Surg 1983; 70: 469–472.
129. Malcolm AW, Perencevich NP, Olson RM, Hanley JA, Chaffey JT, Wilson RE. Analysis of recurrence of patterns following curative resection for carcinoma of the colon and rectum. Surg Gynecol Obstet 1981; 152: 131.
130. Russell AH, Tong D, Dawson LE, Wisbeck W. Adenocarcinoma of the proximal colon. Sites of initial dissemination and patterns of recurrence following surgery alone. Cancer 1984; 53: 360–367.
131. Rao AR, Kagan AR, Chan PM, Gilbert HA, Nussbaum H, Hintz BL. Patterns of recurrence following curative resection alone for adenocarcinoma of the rectum and sigmoid colon. Cancer 1981; 48: 1492–1495.
132. Cass AW, Pfaff FA, Million RR. Patterns of recurrence following surgery alone for adenocarcinoma of the colon and rectum. Cancer 1976; 37: 2861.
133. Patel SC, Tovee EB, Langer B. Twenty-five years' experience with radical surgical treatment of carcinoma of the extraperitoneal rectum. Surgery 1977; 82: 460–465.
134. Gilbertsen VA. Improving the prognosis for patients with intestinal cancer. Surg Gynecol Obstet 1967; 124: 1253.
135. Olson RM, Perencevich NP, Malcolm AW, Chaffey JT, Wilson RE. Patterns of recurrence following curative resection of adenocarcinoma of the colon and rectum. Cancer 1980; 45: 2969–2974.
136. Thompson WM, Trenkner SW. Staging colorectal carcinoma. Radiologic Clinics N Am 1994; 32: 25–37.
137. Schlag P, Lehner B, Strauss G. Scar or recurrent cancer. Arch Surg 1989; 124: 197.
138. Schiessel R, Wunderlich M, Herbst F. Local recurrence of colorectal cancer: effect of early detection and aggressive surgery. Br J Surg 1986; 73: 242–244.
139. Stipa S, Nicolanti V, Botti C, Cosimelli M, Mannella E et al. Local recurrence after curative resection for colorectal cancer: frequency, risk factors and treatment. J Surg Oncol Suppl 1991; 2: 155–60.
140. Quentmeier A, Schlag P, Smok M, Herfarth C. Re-operation for recurrent colorectal cancer: the importance of early diagnosis for resectability and survival. European J Surg Oncol 1990; 16: 319–325.
141. Pilipshen SJ, Heilweil M, Quan SHQ, Sternberg SS, Enker WE. Patterns of pelvic recurrence following definitive resections of rectal cancer. Cancer 1984; 53: 1354–1362.
142. Vassilopoulos PP, Yoon JM, Ledesma EJ. Treatment of recurrence of adenocarcinoma of the colon and rectum at the anastomotic site. Surg Gynecol Obstet 1981; 152: 777–780.
143. Welch JP, Donaldson GA. Detection and treatment of recurrent cancer of the colon and rectum. Am J Surg 1978; 135: 505–11.
144. Bacon HE, Berkley JL. The rationale of re-resection for recurrent cancer of the colon and rectum. Dis Colon Rectum 1959; 2: 549.
145. Spears H, Petrelli NJ, Herrera L, Mittelman A. Treatment of bowel obstruction after operation for colorectal cancer. Am J Surg 1988; 155: 383–386.
146. Whiteway J, Nicholls RJ, Morson BC. The role of surgical local excision in the treatment of rectal cancer. Br J Surg 1985; 72: 694–697.
147. Savage AP, Reece-Smith H, Faber RG. Survival after peranal and abdominoperineal resection for rectal carcinoma. Br J Surg 1994; 81: 1482–1484.
148. Parks AG, Nicholls RJ. Per-anal endo-rectal operative techniques. In: Todd IP , Fielding LP, eds. Operative Surgery. Colon, Rectum and Anus . 4 th. London and Boston: Butterworths. 1983: 316–216.
149. Mason AY. In: Todd IP, eds. Operative surgery. Colon, Rectum and Anus . 3rd. London and Boston: Butterworth. 1978: 178–181.

150. Berry AR, Souter RG, Campbell WB, Mortensen NJM. Endoscopic transanal resection of rectal tumours - a preliminary report of its use. Br J Surg 1990; 77: 134–137.
151. Dickinson AJ, Savage AP, Mortensen NJM, Kettlewell MGW. Long-term survival after endoscopic transanal resection of rectal tumours. Br J Surg 1993; 80: 1401–1404.
152. Buess G, Mentges B, Manncke K, Starlinger M, Becker H. Technique and results of transanal endoscopic microsurgery in early rectal cancer. Am J Surg 1992; 163: 63–70.
153. Graham RA, Atkins MB, Karp DD, Wazer DE, Hackford AW. Local excision of rectal carcinoma. Dis Colon Rectum 1994; 37: 308–312.
154. Parks AG, Stuart AE. The management of villous adenomas of the large bowel. Br J Surg 1973; 60: 688–695.
155. Fitzgerald SD, Longo WE, Daniel GL, Vernava A3. Advanced colorectal neoplasia in the high-risk elderly patient: is surgical resection justified? Dis Colon Rectum 1993; 36: 161–6.
156. Barr H, Bown SG, Krasner N, Boulos PB. Photodynamic therapy for colorectal disease. Int J Colorect Dis 1989; 4: 15–19.
157. McGowan I, Barr H, Krasner N. Palliative laser therapy for inoperable rectal cancer–does it work? A prospective study of quality of life. Cancer 1989; 63: 967–9.
158. Birnbaum PL, Mercer CD. Laser fulguration for palliation of rectal tumours. Can J Surg 1990; 33: 299–301.
159. Mellow MH. Endoscopic laser therapy in colorectal cancer. Int J Colorectal Dis 1989; 4: 12–14.
160. Van CE, Boonen A, Geboes K, Coremans G, Hiele M et al. Risk factors which determine the long term outcome of Neodymium-YAG laser palliation of colorectal carcinoma. Int J Colorectal Dis 1989; 4: 9–11.
161. Bright N, Hale P, Mason R. Poor palliation of colorectal malignancy with the neodymium yttrium-aluminium-garnet laser. Br J Surg 1992; 79: 308–9.
162. Brunetaud JM, Maunoury V, Cochelard D, Cortot A, Paris JC. Laser palliation for rectosigmoid cancers. Int J Colorectal Dis 1989; 4: 6–8.
163. Eckhauser ML. Laser therapy of gastrointestinal tumors. World J Surg 1992; 16: 1054–9.
164. Mathus VE, Tytgat GN. Analysis of failures and complications of neodymium: YAG laser photocoagulation in gastrointestinal tract tumors. A retrospective survey of 18 years' experience. Endoscopy 1990; 22: 17–23.
165. Tacke W, Paech S, kruis w, Stuetzer H, Mueller JM et al. Comparison between endoscopic laser and different surgical treatments for palliation of advanced rectal cancer. Dis Colon Rectum 1993; 36: 377.
166. Sargeant IR, Tobias JS, Blackman G, Thorpe S, Bown SG. Radiation enhancement of laser palliation for advanced rectal and rectosigmoid cancer: a pilot study. Gut 1993; 34: 958–62.
167. Forde KA. Therapeutic colonoscopy. World J Surg 1992; 16: 1048–53.
168. Hoekstra HJ, Verschueren RCJ, Oldhoff J, van der Ploeg E. Palliative and curative electrocoagulation for rectal cancer: experience and results. Cancer 1985; 55: 210–213.
169. Hughes EPJ, Veidenheimer MC, Corman ML, Coller JA. Electrocoagulation of rectal cancer. Dis Colon Rectum 1982; 25: 215–218.
170. Madden JL, Kandalaft S. Clinical evaluation of electrocoagulation in the treatment of cancer of the rectum. Am J Surg 1971; 122: 347–352.
171. Ramsey WH. Treatment of inoperable cancer of the rectum by fulguration. 1962; 114–117.
172. Strauss AA, Strauss SF, Crawford RA, Strauss HA. Surgical diathermy of carcinoma of the rectum: Its clinical end results. JAMA 1935; 104: 1480.
173. Smith LE, Goodreau JJ, Fouty WJ. Operative haemorrhoidectomy versus cryodestruction. Dis Colon Rectum 1978; 22: 10–16.
174. Heberer G, Denecke H, Demmel N, Wirsching R. Local procedures in the management of rectal cancer. World J Surg 1987; 11: 499–503.

175. DeCosse JJ, Ptiolias GJ, Jacobson JS. Colorectal cancer, detection treatment and rehabilitation. CA Cancer J Clin 1994; 44: 27–42.
176. Gwin JL, Hoffman JP, Eisenberg BL. Surgical management of nonhepatic intraabdominal recurrence of carcinoma of the colon. Dis Colon Rect 1993; 36: 540–544.
177. Nogueras JJ, Jagelman BG. Principles of surgical resection: influences of surgical technique on treatment outcome. Surg Clin North Am 1993; 73:
178. Ota DM, Skibber J, Rich TA. Anderson Cancer Center experience with local excision and multimodularity therapy for rectal cancer. Surg Oncol Clin North Am 1992; 1: 147–152.
179. Staniunas RJ, Schoetz DJ. Extended resection for carcinoma of colon and rectum. Surg Clin North Am 1993; 73: 117–29.
180. Summers GE, Medenhall WM, Copeland EMI. Update on the University of Florida experience with local excision and postoperative radiation for the treatment of early rectal cancer. Surg Oncol Clinic North Am 1992; 1: 125–130.
181. Enker WE, Paty PB, Minsky BD, Cohen AM. Restorative or preservation operations in the treatment of rectal cancer. Surg Oncol Clin North Am 1992; 1: 117–129.
182. Lewis AAM, Khoury GA. Resection for colorectal cancer in the very old: are the risks too high? BMJ 1988; 296: 459–461.
183. O'Rourke NA, Heald RJ. Laparoscopic surgery for colorectal cancer. Br J Surg 1993; 80: 1229–1330.
184. Beck DE. Anal neoplasms. In: Beck DE , Welling DG, eds. Patient care in colorectal cancer . Boston: Little, Brown & Co. 1991:
185. Tanum G, Tveit K, Karlsen KO, Hauer JM. Chemotherapy and radiation therapy for anal carcinoma. Survival and late morbidity. Cancer 1991; 67: 2462–6.
186. Cummings BJ. Treatment of primary epidermoid carcinoma of the anus. Int J Colorect Dis 1987; 2: 107–112.
187. Nigro ND. Multidisciniplary treatment of carcinoma of the anus. World J Surg 1987; 11: 449.
188. Zelnick RS, Haas PA, Ajlouni M et al. Results of abdominoperineal resections for failures after combination chemotherapy and radiation therapy for anal canal cancers. Dis Colon Rectum 1992; 35: 574–578.
189. Longo WE, Vernava AM, Wade TP, Coplin MA, Virgo KS, Johnson FE. Recurrent squamous cell carcinoma of the anal canal. Predictors of initial treatment failure and results of salvage. Ann Surg 1994; 220: 40–49.
190. Tanum G. Treatment of relapsing anal carcinoma. Acta Oncol 1993; 32: 33–5.
191. Cooper PH, Mills SE, Allen MSJ. Malignant melanoma of the anus: report of 12 patients and analysis of 255 additional cases. Dis Colon Rectum 1982; 25: 693–703.
192. Brady MS, Kavolius JP, Quan SH. Anorectal melanoma. A 64-year experience at Memorial Sloan-Kettering Cancer Center. Dis Colon Rectum 1995; 38: 146–51.
193. Goldman S, Glimelius B, Pahlman L. Anorectal malignant melanoma in Sweden. Dis Colon Rectum 1990; 33: 874–877.
194. Ross M, Pezzi C, Pezzi T, Meurer D, Hickey R, Balch C. Patterns of failure in anorectal melanoma. Arch Surg 1990; 125: 313–316.
195. Morson BC, Volkstadt H. Malignant melanoma of the anal canal. J Clin Pathol 1963; 16: 126–132.
196. Pack GT, Oropeza RA. A comparative study of melanoma and epidermoid carcinoma of the anal canal: a review of 20 melanomas and 29 epidermoid carcinomas. Dis Colon Rectum 1967; 10: 161–176.
197. Siegal B, Cohen D, Jacob E. Surgical treatment of anorectal melanoma. Am J Surg 1983; 146: 336–338.
198. Ward MWN, Romano G, Nicholls RJ. The surgical treatment of anorectal malignant melanoma. Br J Surg 1986; 73: 68–69.
199. Makela J, Haukipuro K, Laitinen S, Kairaluoma MI. Palliative operations for colorectal cancer. Dis Colon Rectum 1990; 33: 846–50.

200. Boey J, Choi TK, Wong J et al. Carcinoma of the colon and rectum with liver involvement. Surg Gynecol Obstet 1981; 153: 864–868.
201. Welch JP, Donaldson GA. Recent experience in the management of cancer of the colon and rectum. Am J Surg 1974; 127: 258–266.
202. Bussey HJ. The survival rate of patients with advanced rectal cancer. Proc R Soc Med 1969; 62: 1221–1223.
203. Finan PJ, Marshall RJ, Cooper EH, Giles GR. Factors affecting survival in patients presenting with synchronous hepatic metastases from colorectal cancer. Br J Surg 1985; 72: 373–377.
204. Baden H, Anderson B. Survival of patients with untreated liver metastases from coloectal cancer. Scand J Gastroenterol 1975; 10: 221–223.
205. Oxley EM, Ellis H. Prognosis of carcinoma of the large bowel in the presence of liver metastases. Br J Surg 1969; 56: 149–152.
206. Nielsen J, Balslev I, Jensen HE. Carcinoma of the colon with liver metastases: operative indications and prognosis. Acta Chir Scand 1971; 137: 463–465.
207. Nielsen J, Balsev J, Fenger HJ, Jensen HE, Kragelund E. Carcinoma of the rectum with liver metastases. Acta Chir Scand 1973; 139: 479–481.
208. Swinton NW, Samann S, Rosenthal D. Cancer of the rectum and sigmoid. Surg Clin N Am 1967; 47: 657–662.
209. Cady B, Monson DO, Swinton NWS. Survival of patients after colonic resection for carcinoma with simultaneous liver metastases. Surg Gynecol Obstet 1970; 131: 697–700.
210. Abrams MS, Lerner HJ. Survival of patients at Pennsylvannia Hospital with hepatic metastases from carcinoma of the colon and rectum. Dis Colon Rectum 1971; 12: 431–434.
211. Appelqvist P, Silvo J, Salmela L, Kostiainen S. On the treatment and prognosis of malignant ascites: Is the survival time determined when abdominal paracentesis is needed? J Surg Oncol 1982; 20: 238–242.
212. Dutton JW, Hreno A, Hampson LG. Mortality and prognosis of obstructing carcinoma of thelarge bowel. Am J Surg 1976; 131: 36–41.
213. Serpell J W., McDemott FT, Katrivessis H, Hughes ES. Obstructing carcinomas of the colon. Br J Surg 1989; 76: 965–969.
214. Escudero-Fabre A, Sack J. Endoscopic laser therapy for neoplastic lesions of the colorectum. Am J Surg 1992; 163: 260–2.
215. Spinelli P, Dal-Fante M, Mancini A. Current role of laser and photodynamic therapy in gastrointestinal tumors and analysis of a 10-year experience. Semin Surg Oncol 1992; 8: 204–13.

3 – Non-Curative Surgery for Gynaecological Malignancy

John H. Shepherd and Robin Crawford

Introduction

Worldwide, gynaecological malignancies continue to be the most common group of cancers affecting women. In the underdeveloped world, cervical cancer is more common than breast cancer, with the majority of cases presenting at an advanced stage. In the Western world, breast cancer is the commonest tumour, with cervical cancer the fourth most frequent in the UK [1]. It is a salutary fact that, despite the huge financial support for research into the causes of and treatments for cancer, it would appear that the incidence and the mortality of this disease in the developed world may even be increasing [2]. This may be due to increased longevity which will lead to an increase in the incidence of cancer, but also due to improved diagnosis and data recording. Although clinicians may doubt the accuracy of the cancer registry statistics [3], which document over 90% of cancer-related deaths, it can be seen that modern treatment is contributing little to an overall reduction in these mortality figures [4]. However, this rather depressing observation does not mean that the enormous progress made over the last 50 years has been in vain. When one considers the present quality of life of these dying women in the palliative setting, it is obvious that both treatment and management have been improved vastly.

Surgery still plays a lead role, both in terms of diagnosis and treatment, for potentially curable early stage and for palliation of advanced stage cases. Gynaecological oncologists must use their knowledge of the natural history of the disease to assess their patients in a sympathetic and constructive manner.

There are four areas for surgery in advanced gynaecological malignancy:

1. The initial assessment and diagnosis of the disease.
2. The local control of the disease process.
3. The control of symptomatic discharge, haemorrhage and pain.
4. Reconstruction and rehabilitation.

It is important when dealing within a palliative setting that clear objectives of any particular treatment are established. All doctors aim to cure their patients, but in gynaecological cancer 50% of patients will probably still die despite the best efforts. Therefore, a realistic approach to the patients' management and especially surgery must be taken.

Breast Cancer

This is the most common female malignancy in the Western world and the commonest cause of death in the 35–55-year age group. In the UK, 25 000 cases occur annually, with over 15 000 deaths. Approximately one in five of all cases present in an advanced stage, with little chance of cure even when treated aggressively. Early stage disease has an over 50% change of relapse, with metastatic disease even up to 20 years later, despite apparent complete remission. Breast cancer is one of the few tumours that has such a potential for late recurrence.

Local Control

The original Halstead radical mastectomy was described almost 90 years ago to deal with fungating advanced breast cancer in order to achieve some form of local control [5]. Although local excision with adjunctive chemotherapy and/or radiotherapy are used in early stage disease, mastectomy is still necessary for large, multifocal or central tumours. Occasionally it is used for an inflammatory or an advanced, ulcerating and fungating tumour. The wide excision necessary to clear the tumour may involve a radical procedure, removing the breast and affected surrounding tissue. This, together with an axillary procedure, supplemented with adjuvant chemo/radiotherapy, is used despite a poor prognosis. Reconstruction of the resulting defect may then be carried out using a myocutaneous graft. Significant radiation skin damage or rib necrosis are rare nowadays, but in the event, a plastic procedure is required for local symptom control.

As the trend has been towards breast-conserving therapy with wide excision, the role of salvage mastectomy has been considered for local recurrence. With 80% of these recurrences occurring in the first 5 years, the use of salvage mastectomy following a local procedure has been successful. Ninety per cent of these cases are operable, with a 65–80% 5-year survival rate. In conclusion, breast recurrences treated with salvage mastectomy have only a small adverse impact on patient prognosis.

Treatment of locoregional recurrence following mastectomy, which occurs in 5% of cases, is by excisional biopsy. Complete excision of gross disease reduces tumour burden and may improve local control [6]. Radical excision is advised in the absence of distant recurrence. This may require resection of chest wall, including muscle and bone. Appropriate patient selection is important and this surgery is indicated in those with a disease-free interval greater than 5 years, and no distant metastases or medical contraindications. Five-year survival with locoregional recurrence after mastectomy ranges from 10% to 50% [7, 8].

Axillary recurrences are ideally treated with surgery and then radiotherapy. Surgical treatment of distant metastases is seldom indicated, as the nature of the disease leads to multiple deposits. Solitary brain metastases can be resected with good benefit, but these occur in less than 50% of CNS involvement and more than 50% of solitary lesions are surgically inaccessible or associated with uncontrolled systemic disease [9]. A solitary lung lesion deserves investigation to rule out a primary lung carcinoma, but the role of thoracotomy in breast metastases is not recommended.

Gynaecological Pelvic Malignancy

The annual UK incidence of pelvic gynaecological malignancy is 15 000, with approximately 8000 dying from their cancer. In most of these cases surgery has a specific role, either with curative or palliative intent. Once pelvic cancer becomes incurable, various complications will develop, related to the type of primary tumour. Those women with ovarian cancer will gradually develop progressive intestinal obstruction and cachexia, leading to death. Patients with cervical carcinoma will develop obstructive uropathy and renal failure. Occasionally they may develop either rectovaginal or vesicovaginal fistulae. Vulvar cancer is associated with sepsis due to the fungating primary or groin lymphadenopathy. There may be haemorrhage which can be massive in both cervical and vulvar cancer or continuous and troublesome in endometrial cancer.

Ovarian Cancer

Seventy-five per cent of women with ovarian cancer will ultimately die of their disease. The prognosis is related to stage. Although there have been improvements in 5-year survival due to developments in chemotherapy and the use of platinum-related drugs, the overall 5-year survival at present is approximately 35% [10]. Clinically the initial presentation in advanced disease is with abdominal distension and ascites, and occasionally intestinal obstruction. Large bulky solid tumours may be present and resection of these alone may give symptomatic relief. Although the present standard surgical treatment for ovarian cancer is debulking via a radical oophorectomy procedure [11], which consists of total abdominal hysterectomy, bilateral salpingo-oophorectomy, omentectomy and resection of abdominopelvic masses, the place of surgery is being questioned [12]. Therefore, an individualized approach for each patient is required, as radical surgery may not improve outcome. All surgery in advanced ovarian disease may be regarded as non-curative, but at present we feel that there is a survival advantage in removing all or most of the disease. However, even with the most aggressive intent, this ideal cytoreduction to under 1 cm is only achievable in less than half of the cases presenting to gynaecological oncologists. This figure is lower if the woman is managed by general obstetrician/gynaecologists or general surgeons.

A large mass may cause pressure symptoms. More diffuse disease may result in subacute or complete obstruction. Large masses may be removed and intestinal obstruction relieved, either by surgical resection and re-anastomosis of the gastrointestinal tract, or by a bypass procedure. The debulking procedure often reduces the rate of ascites formation. On occasions a terminal colostomy or ileostomy may be all that is practical when there is evidence of widespread disease throughout the gastrointestinal tract. The mesentery is often infiltrated with diffuse retroperitoneal tumour strangulating the mesenteric vessels of the coeliac plexus, making extensive surgical resection impractical. In the situation of primary cytoreduction, the role of bowel surgery in the absence of obstructive symptoms is being questioned. Potter et al. [13] reported that the utilization of bowel resection to reduce tumour burden did not improve survival. In fact, those patients who had a bowel resection to achieve optimal cytoreduction had a survival similar to those with residual disease. Bowel obstruction needs to be managed jointly by the medical oncologist and the gynaecological surgeon. Initially, reports suggested that surgery for relief of bowel obstruction was effective. Rubin et al. [14] reported a series of 54 operations. In nearly 20% no relief was possible. Successful palliation of symptoms was achieved in 63% of cases, with a median survival of 6.8 months compared with 1.8 months for the group where no relief was possible. However, the authors could not define criteria for selection of those patients who would benefit from surgery. In one series, persistent symptoms of intestinal obstruction were present up until the time of death in 58% of the patients who underwent successful bypass surgery and only 32% of those explored survived without symptoms for more than 60 days [15].

The use of a bowel obstruction protocol, with details for the management of symptoms such as pain and nausea, allows a uniform approach to this distressing and frequent problem. Using this conservative approach to bowel obstruction at the Royal Marsden, London, we found that a good outcome could be anticipated if early resolution of the obstruction occurred. In an audit of 36 cases of bowel obstruction in 1993, surgery was associated with a very poor outcome and conferred no survival advantage over those managed medically. However, some of these women who had colostomies or bypass surgery were more independent of hospitals than the women who were managed conservatively. This conservative approach has been validated at other centres where patients who had ascites and/or palpable masses and bowel obstruction lived no longer despite surgical intervention compared to those managed medically (median time to death 36 days versus 33 days) [16].

The use of gastrointestinal drainage via a percutaneous endoscopically placed gastrostomy [17] has been advocated in ovarian cancer despite the usual contraindications for its placement of intra-abdominal malignancy and prior surgery. This allows the woman to continue with a light semi-liquid diet without nasogastric intubation, especially if vomiting is her major symptom. The endoscopic placement avoids the need for open surgery. However, in our experience, we feel that this technique has a limited role due to leakage.

The management of intractable ascites may be improved by inserting a permanent drain [18] or a peritoneovenous shunt of the LeVeen [19] or the Denver type [20]. The Denver shunt features a compressible pump chamber bearing a pressure-sensitive valve. There were no cases of disseminated intravascular coagulopathy and the shunt remained patent in over 60% of cases at death [20]. There is less likelihood of shunt blockage in ascites with a low cell count.

Secondary surgical treatment with palliative intent in advanced ovarian cancer requires careful planning as well as experience and knowledge of the disease. An isolated chemoresistant nodule can be excised at surgery, giving a better quality of life, but probably does not confer a survival advantage. However, there is usually evidence of further recurrence which has not been detected either clinically or radiologically.

There may be a limited place for parenteral feeding, which may be controlled at home in certain individuals who are well motivated and whose disease is slowly growing [21]. A review of home total parenteral nutrition in terminal ovarian cancer [22] advised that there was no useful role for this technique as the patients died very rapidly compared to a group with advanced gastrointestinal malignancy. Due to the psychological and emotional difficulties in cessation of this treatment and also its high cost, we feel that parenteral nutrition in terminal ovarian cancer is only indicated for the short term to allow a successful operative intervention. Consequently, there is a very limited use of parenteral nutrition in our hospitals.

It may be seen, therefore, that the main reasons for carrying out tumour debulking are as follows:

1. To improve a potential response to chemotherapy. At present, chemotherapy for stages III and IV ovarian cancer must be seen as palliative. Maximal cytoreduction provides a survival advantage but is not curative.
2. To reduce the uncomfortable abdominal distension due to tumour and ascites. Psychologically, this active treatment helps the woman in the initial phase of the treatment.
3. To relieve obstruction that may have occurred. It appears that radical debulking surgery involving bowel resection does not reduce the incidence of subsequent bowel obstruction [23].

Cervical Cancer

When recurrence of cervical cancer occurs, this may be situated either centrally within the pelvis, locoregionally on the pelvic side wall, or distally in the para-aortic region, lungs or liver. Rarely, bony or brain metastases may occur. If recurrence occurs following primary surgery, then radiotherapy will be the main form of treatment. If further recurrence occurs centrally, then surgical extirpation by exenteration will need to be considered [24]. Although exenteration is considered for curative intent, the aggressive surgical but histologically incomplete removal of tumour can give a useful palliation. Stanhope and Symmonds [25] report a 46% 2-year survival rate. Despite the poor prognosis associated with exenteration with positive margins, it can be hard both for the surgeon and the woman concerned to forgo the potential cure offered. Forty to 50% of laparotomies will fall into this poor prognosis group despite our best attempts to exclude women with inoperable disease. By combining aggressive surgery with intraoperative radiotherapy, several groups have published promising reports [26, 27].

At the time of exenteration, we feel that consideration should be given to reconstruction as well as the destructive surgery. The dilemma of the cosmetically better but more extensive and complicated surgery to provide a continent urinary stoma, vaginoplasty and continent faecal reservoir must be weighed against the risk of morbidity, failure and recurrence of the tumour. The more complex surgery has a greater morbidity which increases hospitalization, but in the event of recurrence it would be unusual for the gynaecological oncologist to offer reconstruction if the initial operation had been merely a diversion of the urinary and faecal stream.

The place of a salvage central radical hysterectomy following radiotherapy is small. The majority of patients with recurrence will present within 2 years of their initial treatment and diagnosis. Most of these patients will die within a further 12 months from renal failure due to ureteric obstruction. Urinary diversion is not usually offered to women with terminal cervical cancer for treatment of increasing uraemia due to obstructive uropathy. Simple percutaneous nephrostomies allow rapid reversal of the uraemia, but they are difficult to manage in the long term and are not an appropriate solution. A review of our results at the Royal Marsden was similar to those published by Soper et al. [28]. We concluded that the use of nephrostomies was acceptable in advanced cases of pelvic malignancy when there was a useful treatment option remaining, but was unacceptable when there was not. The use of cutaneous ureterostomy has been reported as a reasonably successful technique in the palliative situation [29]. However, our personal experience of this surgery has been a miserable failure. Central progression of disease may lead to fistula formation, either as vesicovaginal or rectovaginal fistula, or a three-way connection giving rise to a cloaca. Palliative exenteration may be ncessary in these cases, but a simpler procedure is usually performed. This is either a colostomy or urinary diversion or both. The site of the fistula needs to be carefully assessed by imaging and the presence of recurrence confirmed with histology. Urinary diversion using a bowel segment such a ileum or sigmoid is only relevant for the management of a urinary fistula. This may be appropriate to relieve the distressing symptom of continuous incontinence. The surgeon has to balance the magnitude of the operation, length of hospital stay and presence of a stoma with a limited life span remaining. Consideration should be given to possible surgical repair at a later date.

A small urinary fistula from the bladder may be repaired vaginally using a Martius labial fat pad as a rotational graft. This is not a very morbid procedure. Alternatively, the omentum may be utilized, providing adequate healthy tissue to separate both the bladder and the vagina after their separate closure. This abdominal procedure requires a longer hospital stay. Ureteric fistulae may be dealt with by reimplantation using a Boari flap or transureterourostomy. The more practical procedure is a urinary diversion by using an ileal conduit with a right iliac fossa urostomy. The Wallace technique is preferred in irradiated cases. An augmentation cystoplasty using terminal ileum will increase the volume of a bladder contracted by radiotherapy. However, in the palliative setting, the problem of frequency and incontinence can be overcome by a long-term indwelling catheter. A rectal fistula may be tackled using the same principles. Extensive recurrence will necessitate diversion via a left iliac fossa terminal colostomy. In cases of radionecrosis, however, closure of the fistula may then be performed vaginally or abdominally. The healing tissues usually have been compromised by the radiotherapy and the repair or anastomosis should be covered with a diverting transverse colostomy. This colostomy may be closed between 6 and 12 weeks later, provided that the healing is sound.

Haemorrhage from the central recurrence via the vagina or bladder should be managed with palliative radiotherapy. If this fails, then fulguration with diathermy or silver nitrate can be considered. However, these local procedures are rarely sufficient. Arterial embolization under radio-imaging control may be usefully considered, provided that the site of bleeding may be identified. The surgical alternative is bilateral internal iliac artery ligation. The vessels may be identified approximately 2 cm below the bifurcation of the common iliac artery on the pelvic side walls. They should be approached in an extraperitoneal manner. The ureter must be reflected away and care taken to avoid tearing the veins below the artery. In a terminal setting, the resuscitation and emergency surgery required as discussed above is not appropriate even though exsanguination is a horrific terminal event.

Vulvar Cancer

Approximately 900 cases of vulvar cancer occur in the UK every year. Surgery with suitable excision, either by wide local excision with groin dissection or radical vulvectomy, forms the mainstay of primary treatment. Recurrence may occur many years later and will be either central at the introitus or perineum, or locoregional involving the groin or pelvic lymph nodes. Rarely more distal metastases will occur in the para-aortic lymph nodes, liver or lungs. The cancer is usually slowly progressive which may result in huge tumours if the primary is neglected. The disturbing symptoms are discharge, gross malodour and pain, especially if the clitoris, perineal body or anus are involved. Surgical excision should always be considered. It may not be possible to obtain primary closure, especially if there has been prior surgical excision and scarring. This defect will need to be closed by a graft. Split thickness skin grafts result in further scarring and do not fill the defect satisfactorily. There is also scarring at the donor site. Musculocutaneous flaps are very useful. The gracilis or gluteus maximus muscles are limited by their relatively short pedicles. Large defects may be closed using a part of the rectus abdominis muscle which provides a large bulk of tissue with a good blood supply via the deep branch of the inferior epigastric artery. Sometimes this pedicle has been compromised by previous surgical procedures [30]. Bilateral flaps can be used to cover a midline defect. The importance of these plastic techniques is that fresh tissue with a good blood supply is brought into the damaged area. Tension, both on suture lines and pedicles, should be avoided to obtain the best results. Huge defects may be closed using the rectus abdominis, with only a small risk of abdominal wall herniation occurring and a very good cosmetic result.

Recent developments with combination chemo/radiotherapy have resulted in 35% complete response rates, even in cases with extensive recurrence of vulvar carcinoma [31]. This has reduced the need for exenteration. If this chemo/radiotherapy fails, then surgical excision and subsequent tissue healing will have been compromised and necessitate extensive grafting. The relief of pain and continence, obtained by exenteration in this setting, is important in the palliative setting and surgery will allow the patient to be mobile, pain free, and to enjoy an active life.

Endometrial Cancer

Exenteration may be the only option for a central pelvic recurrence of this tumour type. However, as there is often distant disease present, surgery is not usually advocated other than local excision of a vaginal metastasis.

Miscellaneous

Occasional enormous tumours may occur on the abdominal wall from other sites such as the cervix [32] and ovary. Rotational flaps, from the latissimus dorsi, gluteus maximus or rectus abdominis, usually will cover the defect. Sister Mary Joseph's nodule is associated with a poor prognosis. If surgery is used for the management of the intra-abdominal malignancy, then excision of the umbilicus is warranted. Consent for this part of the operation should be specifically obtained to avoid later dissatisfaction.

Conclusions

Palliative treatment for advanced or recurrent gynaecological malignancy must be carefully considered on an individual basis to alleviate symptoms. The patient must be involved in the decision-making process relating to her treatment. Surgery should be used to manage symptoms effectively, but at the same time to avoid unnecessary morbidity, allowing the woman to return to her home and family environment with a decent quality of life.

References

1. OPCS Cancer Statistics Registration, England and Wales MBI no. 16. HMSO, London.
2. Marshall E (1990) Experts clash over cancer data: news and comment. Science 250:900–902.
3. Pollock A (1994) The future of cancer registries – purchasers need to recognise how important they are for monitoring services. Br Med J 309:821–822.
4. Baum M, Breach NM, Shepherd JH, Shearer RJ, Meiron Thomas J, Ball A. Surgical palliation. Sympt Manage 129–140.
5. Halstead WJ (1907) The results of radical operations for the cure of cancer of the breast. Ann Surg 46:1–27.
6. Ghossein NA, Alpert S, Barba J, Pressman P, Stacey P, Lorenz E, Schulman M, Sadarangani GJ (1992) Breast cancer: importance of adequate surgical excision prior to radiotherapy in the local control of breast cancer in patients treated conservatively. Arch Surg 127:411–415.
7. Danoff BF, Coia LR, Cantor RI, Parjac T, Kramer S (1983) Locally recurrent breast carcinoma: the effect of adjuvant chemotherapy on prognosis. Radiology 147:849–852.
8. Magno L, Bignardi M, Micheletti E, Bardelli D, Plebani F (1987) Analysis of prognostic factors in patients with isolated chest wall recurrence of breast cancer. Cancer 60:240–244.
9. Patchell RE, Cirrinione C, Thaler HT (1986) Single brain metastases: surgery plus radiation or radiation alone. Neurology 36:447–453.
10. FIGO Annual Report (1991) FIGO, Stockholm.
11. Shepherd JH (1990) Surgical management of ovarian cancer. In Shepherd JH, Monaghan JM (eds) Clinical gynaecological oncology, 2 ed. Blackwell Scientific Publications, Oxford, pp 218–246.
12. Hunter RW, Alexander NDE, Soutter WP (1992) Meta-analysis of surgery in advanced ovarian carcinoma: is maximum cytoreductive surgery an independent germinant of prognosis? Am J Obstet Gynecol 166:504–511.
13. Potter ME, Partridge EE, Hatch KD, Soong SJ, Austin JM, Shingleton HM (1991) Primary surgical therapy of ovarian cancer. How much and when. Gynecol Oncol 40:195–200.
14. Rubin SC, Hoskins WJ, Benjamin I, Lewis JL Jr (1989) Palliative surgery for intestinal obstruction in advanced ovarian cancer. Gynecol Oncol 34:16–19.
15. Lund B, Lundwall F, Hansen HJ (1989) Intestinal obstruction in patients with advanced carcinoma of the ovaries treated with combination chemotherapy. Surg Gynecol Obstet 169:213–218.
16. van Ooijen B, van der Burg ME, Planting AS, Siersema PD, Wiggers T (1993) Surgical

treatment or gastric drainage only for intestinal obstruction in patients with carcinoma of the ovary or peritoneal carcinomatosis of other origin. Surg Gynecol Obstet 176:469–474.
17. Marks WH, Perkal MF, Schwartz PE (1993) Percutaneous endoscopic gastrotomy for decompression in metastatic gynecological malignancies. Surg Gynecol Obstet 177:573–576.
18. Belfort MA, Stevens PJ, DeHaek K, Soeters R, Krige JE (1990) A new approach to the management of malignant ascites: a permanently implanted abdominal drain. Eur J Surg Oncol 16:47–53.
19. Osterlee J (1980) Peritoneovenous shunting for ascites in cancer patients. Br J Surg 67:663–666.
20. Roussel JG, Kroon BB, Hart GA (1986) The Denver type for peritoneovenous shunting of malignant ascites. Surg Gynecol Obstet 162:235–240.
21. Chapman E, Bosscher J, Remmenga S, Park R, Barnhill D (1991) A technique for managing terminally ill ovarian carcinoma patients. Gynecol Oncol 41:88–91.
22. August DA, Thorn D, Fisher RL, Welchek CM (1991) Home parenteral nutrition for patients with inoperable malignant bowel obstruction. J Parent Ent Nutr 15:323–327.
23. Hammond RJ, Houghton CR (1990) The role of bowel surgery in the primary treatment of epithelial ovarian cancer. Aust NZ J Obstet Gynaecol 30:166–169.
24. Shepherd JH, Ngan HYS, Neven P, Fryatt I, Woodhouse CRJ, Hendry WF (1994) Multivarate analysis of factors affecting survival in pelvic exenteration. Int J Gynecol Cancer 4:361–370.
25. Stanhope CR, Symmonds RD (1985) Palliative exenteration – what, when, and why? Am J Obstet Gynecol 152:12–16.
26. Hochel M, Knapstein PG (1992) The combined operative and radiotherapeutic treatment (CORT) of recurrent tumours infiltrating the pelvic wall: first experience with 18 patients. Gynecol Oncol 46:20–28.
27. Garten GR, Gunderson LL, Webb MJ, Wilson TO, Martensen JA, Cha SS, Podratz KC (1993) Intraoperative radiation therapy in gynecologic cancer: the Mayo Clinic experience. Gynecol Oncol 48:328–332.
28. Soper JT, Blaszczyk TM, Oke E, Clark-Pearson D, Creasman WT (1988) Percutaneous nephrostomy in gynecologic oncology patients. Am J Obstet Gynecol 158:1126–1131.
29. Kearney GP, Docimo SG, Doyle CJ, Mahoney EM (1992) Cutaneous ureterostomy in adults. Urology 40:1–6.
30. Shepherd JH, Van Dam P, Jobling T, Breech N (1990) The use of rectus abdominis musculocutaneous flaps following radical excision of vulvar cancer. Br J Obstet Gynaecol 97:1020–1025.
31. Sebag-Montefiore DJ, McLean C, Arnott SJ, Blake P, Van Dam P, Hudson CN, Shepherd JH (1994) Treatment of advanced carcinoma of the vulva with chemo/radiotherapy – can exenterative surgery be avoided? Int J Gynecol Cancer 4:150–155.
32. Neven P, Shepherd JH, Tham KF, Fisher C, Breach N (1993) Reconstruction of the abdominal wall with a latissimus dorsi musculocutaneous flap: a case of a massive abdominal wall metastasis from a cervical cancer requiring palliative resection. Gynecol Oncol 49:403–406.
33. Cavanagh D, Shepherd JH (1982) The place of pelvic exenteration in the primary management of advanced carcinoma of the vulva. Gynecol Oncol 13:318.

4 – Non-Curative Urological Surgery for Cancer

W.F. Hendry

Introduction

The urologist can do a great deal to help the patient with cancer, particularly the maintenance of adequate renal function, to allow the oncologist to give chemotherapy or radiotherapy which may significantly alter the course of the disease. However clearcut the disease state may appear to be, it is always worth checking to make sure that any significant or unexpected deterioration in renal function is really due to the malignant process. Retroperitoneal fibrosis, post-radiation change and non-opaque stones can all mimic ureteric obstruction due to cancer: it is indeed a pity to miss such eminently curable causes of uraemia in a patient who happens to have cancer; full investigation is therefore always worth while before deciding that nothing could or should be done. Perhaps the most difficult decision is whether to treat or not treat a uraemic patient with advanced cancer. For many years, progressive uraemia has been seen as a preferable means of death for the cancer patient, to lingering demise with multiple metastases, and this has delayed or contraindicated relief of uraemia. In fact, modern urological technology allows definition of its cause and drainage of renal obstruction so quickly and painlessly that it is only a minor incident in the overall management of the disease process.

Ureteric Obstruction

Ultrasound or CT scanning will often demonstrate dilatation of one or both pelvicalyceal systems, and can be expected to show up as part of the staging procedure of the malignant process. If measurement indicates impairment of overall renal function, which will significantly reduce the amount of chemotherapy that can be effectively given, or if the degree of obstruction is severe and likely to progress rapidly while the patient is on treatment and before response can reliably be assessed, the urologist should be contacted. In an emergency, percutaneous nephrostomy can be inserted either by the radiologist or the urologist, to allow recovery of renal function. Once the patient is fit for general anaesthetic, which is desirable though not essential, the bladder is examined cystoscopically and dye is injected up each ureter for a retrograde ureterogram. This will demonstrate exactly where the block is situated, and will give a very good indication of its cause [1].

Having identified the problem, the guidewire is inserted up the obstructed ureter or ureters and J stents inserted and positioned under fluoroscopic control; these can be left in for 6 months before being replaced or removed. The patient passes urine normally, without the need for bags or drainage tubes, and is free to go about their everyday activities. Occasionally, pelvic cancers make identification of the ureteric orifices difficult or impossible: under these circumstances, antegrade placement of ureteric stents may be possible in collaboration with radiological colleagues. These stents cause minimal discomfort, apart from some trigonal irritation which can be minimized by using stents manufactured from soft rather than stiff materials.

It is generally desirable to anticipate the need for ureteric drainage prior to starting chemotherapy or radiotherapy, rather than waiting until the patient is leucopenic, and possibly infected and ill, before asking the urologist to intervene.

Occasionally, investigation reveals surprise findings. After radical radiotherapy and Wertheim hysterectomy, for example, it has been estimated that ureteric obstruction is due to fibrosis in over one-third of women [2]. Similarly, in women treated for ovarian cancer, postoperative fibrosis not uncommonly turns out to be the cause of hydroureter and hydronephrosis. It should be remembered that approximately 1 in 400 people have only one functioning kidney; sudden deterioration in renal function, or even anuria, may be due to unexpected impaction of a ureteric stone which may be composed of uric acid and hence invisible on plain radiograph. This is a true surgical emergency which can be successfully treated endoscopically using modern non-invasive techniques; the really important thing is to think of the diagnosis in a patient who already has extensive malignant disease.

Occasionally, the ureter draining a solitary kidney may be so involved in the disease process that it cannot be successfully stented. Under these circumstances, long-term kidney drainage can be provided by nephrostomy. This can be placed percutaneously, although this requires careful aftercare in case it falls out, or inserted by open surgery in the form of a ring nephrostomy which is suitable for long-term drainage and can be replaced as and when required. If both ureters are extensively involved in the disease process, or damaged by post-radiation fibrosis, then interposition of ileum between upper ureters and bladder can provide more permanent drainage [3], although this is seldom required nowadays.

Fistula

Perhaps the most miserable complication of gynaecological cancer is fistula formation. Often accompanying necrosis of the tumour itself, the result is a foul-smelling discharge which is almost impossible to collect or control. Under these circumstances, urinary diversion will provide great symptomatic relief [1]. Ileal conduit is now such a standard procedure that it can be offered to women with even quite advanced disease; if the tumour is mobile, it can be accompanied by palliative exenteration to get rid of the necrotic tumour mass [4]. There has been aversion to double stoma formation for many years; in fact, with modern stoma care facilities this is not a great burden, and is infinitely preferable to a mixture of urine and faeces being lost uncontrollably, either from the perineum or from a single wet colostomy. For the same reason, ureterocolic urinary diversion has fallen into disuse in recent years: when the tumour does recur, terminal nursing care can be a nightmare if the patient becomes incontinent.

Vesicovaginal fistula may follow radiation treatment for gynaecological cancer, and ureteric fistula is not uncommon after a difficult extended hysterectomy. The urologist likes to be involved at the earliest opportunity in these cases, so that the site of the lesion can be defined by cystoscopy and ascending ureterograms; effective urinary drainage by appropriate stenting may sometimes allow the leak to heal spontaneously. In others, modern methods of repair by ureteric reimplantation, transuretero-ureterostomy or closure of bladder fistula with omental interposition give reliable results [5].

Accurate definition of the lesion, use of well-vascularized tissue for the repair, control of primary or superadded infection and a meticulously careful operative technique remain the cornerstones of success.

Urological Tumours

Renal Carcinoma

About 10% of renal tumours have extrarenal metastases at presentation and hence are technically incurable, although it is occasionally possible to remove solitary lesions, with long-term survival. More often, staging investigations show multiple lesions, often in the lungs. The question then arises, should the primary tumour be removed or not? The urologist should be asked to see the patient and review the relevant scans. Some renal tumours can be removed relatively easily, whereas others will obviously present a difficult and dangerous problem, for example if the vena cava is involved [6] or if there are many enlarged para-aortic or para-caval lymph nodes surrounding the renal pedicle. In general, the patient feels better once the primary tumour is out, and occasionally metastases may disappear [7].

Immunological function is altered with renal tumours: the normal helper/suppressor T-cell ratio is often reversed, and one-third of patients show signs of systemic illness with anaemia and raised erythrocyte sedimentation rate. This syndrome is often improved by removal of the primary tumours, and further benefit can be derived from giving interferon and interleukin-2; this is the subject of ongoing trials, and although expensive, early results are showing promise [8]. Spontaneous regression is rare, usually occurring with lung deposits, but is virtually never seen with bone lesions or in the presence of obvious lymph node metastases.

Chemotherapy has little to offer the patient with widespread disease, although hormone therapy with progestational agents such as medroxyprogesterone acetate can produce subjective improvement, and objective regression has been reported in 14% of 80 such patients [9]. Radiotherapy can be very effective in the management of localized bone deposite, particularly in the spine where collapse of a vertebra can have catastrophic consequences. Surgery has little to offer, although the neurosurgeon may be asked to decompress the spinal cord or biopsy a suspicious brain lesion, especially if it is the only evidence of disseminated disease.

Renal carcinoma continues to provide the oncologist with real opportunities to help the patient with incurable disease; the underlying reason for suppressed immunological responsiveness remains obscure, but is receiving much attention at present. Strangely enough, the urologist may still have a role in the management of incurable disease, since removal of the primary lesion has been shown to produce significant improvement in lymphocyte function [10].

Bladder Tumours

One of the most difficult problems to confront the urologist and the oncologist is recurrent and often heavy bleeding from an irradiated bladder. This is always worth cystoscopic assessment, as not uncommonly a single patch of telangiectasia can be identified and diathermized. The opportunity is taken to do a careful bimanual examination, which remains the most sensitive way of determining operability of a recurrent bladder tumour, or indeed of a bladder which is the seat of post-radiation cystitis and contracture. Drug therapy with antifibrinolytic agents such as cyclokapron (1 g t.d.s.) can be tried, but often simply produces rubbery clots that are difficult to pass and impossible to clear with a catheter. Washouts and irrigation may help to keep the bladder clear of clot, but instillations of formalin are now thought to be too dangerous to be used in anything other than life-threatening situations. Emergency cystectomy may be the only answer.

Metastatic disease is often radiosensitive. Local recurrence in the pelvis or distant disease in bone may respond well to irradiation [11]. Chemotherapy promised much but has delivered little as yet; nevertheless, prolonged remission can be achieved with single agents such as methotrexate [12], and multiple drug therapy with combinations such as MVAC have given prolonged and complete remission in up to 15% of patients [13].

Prostatic Cancer

The availability of the prostate-specific antigen (PSA) assay [14] now means that no elderly man with disseminated carcinomatosis need be denied the benefits of accurate diagnosis and effective treatment for this disease. Spinal metastases may present with paraplegia, or extensive local disease may lead to development of chronic retention, incontinence and uraemia. The effects of hormone treatment can be magical: total disappearance of all identifiable disease, relief of urinary symptoms (perhaps after a month or so of catheter drainage), and even recovery from paraplegia are often seen. The best method of obtaining effective androgen ablation remains controversial [15]. Stilboestrol carries a significant risk of cardiovascular side-effects and is best avoided, except in countries where other alternatives are either too expensive or not acceptable. Antiandrogens such as cyproterone, flutamide or casodex are expensive, less effective than other treatment modalities and have significant side-effects. LHRH analogues such as goserilin or leuprolin are effective, but their introduction must be covered by a 3-week course of antiandrogen, starting 1 week before the initial LHRH injection and continuing for 2 weeks thereafter [16]. They are extremely expensive, although there is some evidence that prices are coming down.

For the ill patients with advanced disease, bilateral orchidectomy has the advantage that it is quick and effective, with few side-effects other than the psychological sequelae of castration; in fact, most of these patients readily volunteer that they have finished with their testicles and are glad to be rid of them, once they understand that the procedure is likely to produce significant benefit.

For patients in relapse after primary hormone therapy, medical adrenalectomy with a small dose of cortisone (25 mg mane, 12.5 mg nocte) can produce a second worthwhile remission lasting many months [17].

Some patients with prostate cancer have difficulty passing urine and may develop incontinence. An ultrasound scan of the bladder will indicate whether it is emptying completely or not, and obstruction at the bladder neck can be relieved by transurethral resection or local radiotherapy [18]. A urine culture will demonstrate any urinary infection, which should be treated vigorously, as this will often ameliorate symptoms. Chronic retention in patients weak with advanced disease may be relieved by catheterization, and a modern silastic catheter can be left in for 6 weeks or more without needing to be changed.

Conclusions

Much of the suffering associated with advanced malignant disease is related to urinary complications, and impaired renal function can interfere with the delivery of effective treatment with chemotherapy or radiotherapy. The urologist is always pleased to see these patients, advise on what is possible with a modern technical armamentarium, and get on with relief of upper urinary tract obstruction or ameliorate symptoms of lower tract dysfunction as effectively as possible.

References

1. Hendry WF (1978) Management of urinary complications of recurrent pelvic malignancy in gynaecological practice. J R Soc Med 71:516–519.
2. Jones CR, Woodhouse CR, Hendry WF (1984) Urological problems following treatment of carcinoma of the cervix. Br J Urol 56:609–613.
3. Hendry WF, Christmas TJ, Shepherd JH (1991) Anterior pelvic reconstruction with ileum after cancer treatment. J R Soc Med 84:709–713.
4. Woodhouse CRJ, Plail RO, Schlesinger PE, Shepherd JE, Hendry WF, Breach NM (1995) Exenteration as palliation for patients with advanced pelvic malignancy. Br J Urol 76:315–320.
5. Hendry WF (1985) Urinary tract injuries during gynaecological surgery. In: Studd J (ed) Progress in obstetrics and gynaecology, vol 5. Churchill Livingstone, Edinburgh, pp 362–377.
6. Vale JA, Hendry WF, Kirby RS, Whitfield HN, Lumley JS (1991) Diagnostic and surgical aspects of renal carcinoma with involvement of the inferior vena cava. Br J Urol 68:345–348.
7. Couillard DR, deVere RW (1993) Surgery of renal cell carcinoma. Urol Clin North Am 20:263–275.
8. Taneja SS, Pierce W, Figlin R, Belldegrun A (1994) Management of disseminated kidney cancer. Urol Clin North Am 21:625–637.

9. Bloom HJG, Hendry WF (1982) Special oncology: kidney influence of hormones. In: Chisholm GD, Williams DI (eds) Scientific foundations of urology, 2 ed. Heinemann, London, pp 684–690.
10. Dadian G, Riches PG, Henderson DC, Taylor A, Moore J, Atkinson H et al. (1994) Immunological parameters in peripheral blood of patients with renal cell carcinoma before and after nephrectomy. Br J Urol 74:15–22.
11. Oliver RTD, Hendry WF, Bloom HJG (1981) Bladder cancer: principles of combination therapy. Butterworths, London.
12. Turner AG, Hendry WF, Williams GB, Bloom HJ (1977) The treatment of advanced bladder cancer with methotrexate. Br J Urol 49:673–678.
13. Perry JJ, Muss HB (1994) Management of disseminated disease in the patient with bladder cancer. Urol Clin North Am 21:661–672.
14. Smith DS, Catalona WJ (1994) The nature of prostate cancer detected through prostate specific antigen based screening. J Urol 152:1732–1736.
15. Kaisary AV, Tyrrell CJ, Peeling WB, Griffiths K (1991) Comparison of LHRH analogue (zoladex) with orchiectomy in patients with metastatic prostatic carcinoma. Br J Urol 67:502–508.
16. Waxman J, Man A, Hendry WF, Whitfield HN, Besser GM, Tiptaft RC et al. (1985) Importance of early tumour exacerbation in patients treated with long acting analogues of gonadotrophin releasing hormone for advanced prostatic cancer. Br Med J 291:1387–1388.
17. Bloom HJG, Hendry WF (1973) Treatment of prostatic carcinoma. In: Raven RW (ed) Modern trends in oncology. Butterworths, London, pp 143–180.
18. Fellows GJ, Clark PB, Beynon LL, Boreham J, Keen C, Parkinson MC et al. (1992) Treatment of advanced localised prostatic cancer by orchiectomy, radiotherapy, or combined treatment. A Medical Research Council study. Br J Urol 70:304–309.

5 – Non-Curative Neurosurgery for Malignant Brain Tumours

D.G. Porter and D.G.T. Thomas

Introduction

Malignant intracranial neoplasms are one of the most distressing conditions which present to the neurosurgeon. The management of these tumours is multidisciplinary, with surgery having a central role. Surgical options that are generally available include biopsy, be it freehand or stereotactically guided and open procedures. Conventional external beam radiotherapy is widely available as an adjuvant following surgery and is the only therapy to have consistently improved survival. Brachytherapy and focused radiation are available in specialized centres.

In 1977, the National Institute of Neurological and Communicative Disorders and Stroke received the results of a survey of intracranial neoplasms in the USA. They subsequently reported a national incidence of 25 000 new brain tumour cases per year of which 29% were glioblastoma multiforme and 11% anaplastic astrocytomas [1].

In the UK, gliomas have an average annual incidence of 3.94 per 100 000. Grade 3–4 astrocytomas have a peak incidence of 7.53 per 100 000 in the 50–59 years age group. The peak incidence for oligodendrogliomas was also 50–59 years, but for grade 1–2 gliomas it was 30–39 years [2].

Historical Background

The first reported instance of intracranial surgery for a glioma was reported by Bennett and Godlee in 1884 [3]. The patient concerned was a farmer, with a history of seizures affecting the left side of the body and more recently severe headaches, vomiting with accompanying dehydration and a marked bilateral papilloedema. A trephine was performed over a Rolandic fissure and an abnormal gyrus noted; a subsequent resection of a sub-cortical tumour was performed. The patient awoke with resolution of his symptoms and remained well for 4 weeks, but then succumbed to meningitis. The case provoked considerable discussion: Hughlings Jackson, Ferrier, MacEwen and Horsley all agreed that surgical excision was feasible [4]. In the same decade Horsley reviewed ten cases and suggested that early diagnosis, referral and surgery should be performed. Indeed he concluded by saying, "the operation of exposing and removing considerable portions of the brain is not to be ranked amongst the 'dangerous' procedures of surgery" [5].

Horsley and MacEwen favoured external decompression of a tumour by removing portions of the overlying cranium. This might obviate distressing symptoms of visual failure and headache. However, unfortunately this allowed herniation of the cortex through the defect with subsequent unsightly and unpleasant swellings. These disadvantages led Cushing to develop the subtemporal decompression, whereby the bony defect is hidden beneath the temporal muscles and floor of the middle cranial fossa [6].

One of the main surgical limitations of this era was the ability to localize the tumour. Dandy introduced ventriculography in 1918 and pneumencephalography the following year. Moniz developed the technique of angiography in 1927. These three methods became widely adopted procedures for establishing the location of a lesion.

Improvements in the allied specialities of anaesthesia and blood transfusion, together with improving surgical technique, meant the surgical morbidity and mortality for many brain operations were improving, but the prognosis for cerebral malignancy remained poor.

A pathological classification for brain tumours was introduced by Bailey and Cushing in 1926 [7]. Cushing used the intraoperative diagnosis, obtained by biopsy, to refine the surgical procedure. Dandy relied on the macroscopic appearance to determine the extent of the resection.

McKenzie performed his first internal decompression, for a tumour, in 1936 [8]. He condemned the use of external decompression and this surgical philosophy was agreed with by Sachs [9]. However, Maxwell contested this and suggested that only a subtemporal decompression and radiotherapy be performed because of the frequency of interhemispheric extension of tumour he encountered in his series [10].

Hitchcock and Sato [11] reviewed 225 cases of glioblastomas and noted that partial or complete resection should be restricted to those patients with the symptoms or signs of raised intracranial pressure. However, they acknowledged that a radical procedure may lengthen survival. Jelsma and Bucy [12], in 1967, reviewed 167 patients who had been treated during the last 20 years and concluded that the largest single factor that had reduced operative mortality was dexamethasone. Other factors which improved patient outcome were: age 30–50, extensive resections and an astrocytoma with glioblastomatous change rather than pure glioblastomas. Hitchcock and Bucy agreed that radiotherapy improved both quality and length of patient survival. In 1985, Bucy et al. reported on a single case from the 1967 series who remained alive and well 25 years following resection of a malignant glioma [13].

Independent Factors

There is now overwhelming evidence that age and preoperative performance score have a strong influence on patient survival [14–16]. Histological grade of malignancy which adheres to an accurate classification system and tumour location are also prognostic variables which influence patient outcome in the majority of series [12, 16–18] although their influence is contested by certain authors [15, 19]. These factors have been found to maintain their prognostic significance when subjected to multivariate analysis using the Cox's proportional hazards [14, 20] or Weibull model [21]. Other factors, which appear to have prognostic influence during univariate analysis, failed to demonstrate significance in a multivariate model.

A retrospective review of surgically treated, low-grade astrocytomas demonstrated that the age of the patient at the time of diagnosis had an overwhelming influence on patient outcome which eclipsed all other variables and management forms [22].

In a retrospective series of 560 patients who had a clinical and radiological diagnosis of an intrinsic supratentorial tumour, 164 presented with epilepsy. This latter group appear to have a relatively better clinical course, with a median survival of 37 months as opposed to 6 months in those presenting with other symptoms [23, 24], and this has been supported by other studies [20, 25].

In comparing surgical series, these factors must be controlled for, if the role of alternative surgical approaches is to be elucidated.

Operative Treatment

Principal Aims

The objectives of conventional surgery for primary malignant brain tumours were succinctly summarized by Garfield in 1980 [26]:

1. Establishment of a pathological diagnosis.
2. Relief of distressing symptoms.
3. Improvement of quality of life.
4. Improvement in survival.

Factors which require specific consideration are:

5. The limitations of clinical localization and the importance of accurate radiological localization.
6. The general techniques and hazards of surgery.

To these criteria must be added the controversial issue of cytoreduction of the malignant tissue to aid adjuvant therapy. The first variable to consider is the reduction in tumour load and the second is the effect of surgery on tumour cell behaviour and kinetics. Salcman has analysed a series of patients with a glioblastoma, who were treated with various modalities [27]. He noted that the survival curve followed an exponential shape and suggested that this was in keeping with both clinical observation and the disseminated, slowly growing tumour model of Shackney et al. [28]. This model proposes that responses to therapy of this tumour group are usually not durable and improvements in therapy will increase median survival without producing a cure.

The influence of histopathological classification on patient survival was recognized by Jelsma and Bucy [12]. They noted that all patients who survived beyond 2 years has "astrocytomas with glioblastomatous change" rather than "pure glioblastomas".

The establishment of a tissue diagnosis allows for planning of further treatment and a prognosis to be provided. Neither CT nor MRI scanning features provide a reliable definitive diagnosis and the responsibility rests with the neurosurgeon to obtain a suitable tissue sample for analysis. The available options are either biopsy or an open procedure. Prior to CT scanning, freehand biopsy via a burr hole was a common procedure. However, Hitchcock and Sato reported a morbidity and mortality of 27% for a burr hole biopsy in comparison to 5% for a craniotomy [11].

Once a histological diagnosis has been obtained, further intervention to alter the course of the disease rests with the neurosurgeon. In the presence of a severe neurological deficit, for example dysphasia in an otherwise alert patient or a hemiplegia, then further operative intervention is seldom justified because of the poor quality of life experienced by the patient.

Symptoms of raised intracranial pressure, headache, nausea and vomiting, deterioration in conscious level and failing visual acuity, may temporarily be relieved by corticosteroids supplemented by osmotic diuretics like mannitol. This has, to a great extent, removed the need for an emergency craniotomy. Whether further intervention is warranted will be dictated by the patient's clinical condition. A craniotomy and debulking of the lesion can provide good symptomatic relief as a palliative procedure.

The factors alluded to above – age at the time of diagnosis, neurological disability, preoperative performance rating and whether symptoms of raised intracranial pressure are present – will all be influential in deciding on the operative procedure in an individual case. However, no conclusive evidence exists to demonstrate that survival in high-grade gliomas is improved by a craniotomy as opposed to a biopsy [29, 30]. It is recognized that elderly patients with a high-grade glioma have a poor outcome, despite aggressive therapy [31, 32]. Kelly and Hunt [33] retrospectively reviewed 128 elderly patients, aged over 65 years, who had a high-grade glioma treated by either stereotactic biopsy or volumetric resection and postoperative radiotherapy. They found that the overall median survival was 15.4 weeks in the biopsy group and 27 weeks in the resection group. They concluded that although a prolongation in survival was evident, it was also modest. Therefore the question of resection in this group, regardless of preoperative status, must be questioned.

Perioperative Care

A brain tumour gives rise to altered cerebral physiology. The presence of the mass and the surrounding vasogenic oedema leads to an alteration in cerebral autoregulation in both the tumour and adjacent brain. The zone of ischaemia is increased by the brain shift and distortion of local blood vessels. Continuing expansion of the mass leads to a further reduction in cerebral compliance and another small increase in size can cause acute decompensation and precipitate a crisis for the patient.

The altered cerebral physiology must be rectified and optimized prior to any surgical intervention. The use of mannitol, steroids, a smooth induction, use of anaesthetic agents that do not interfere with cerebral flow, prevention of hypoxia or hypercapnia, close attendance to position on the table, minimal brain retraction and meticulous attention to haemostasis with careful postoperative monitoring will ensure the optimum outcome for the patient.

Tumour Biopsy

Freehand biopsy has largely fallen into disuse. Image-directed techniques have demonstrated improved accuracy of biopsy with subsequent improved levels of histopathological diagnosis and reduced morbidity and mortality [34, 35]. A variety of stereotactic frames are available, including the BRW (Brown, Roberts and Wells), Hitchcock and Lexsell. In this institution, the CRW (Cosman, Roberts and Wells) arc system, a "target-centred" stereotactic apparatus, is favoured. In this system the stereotactic target is located at the centre of the circular arc. These procedures can be performed under a local or general anaesthetic.

The head ring is attached to the patient's head by means of four metal screws attached to carbon head ring posts. To this is attached the CT localizer which comprises three N-shaped structures. A CT scan taken through the head will include nine fiducials; each of their two-dimensional X and Y co-ordinates can be calculated from the CT scanner console. These co-ordinates define the slice plane and allow calculation of the target co-ordinates in relation to the base ring by a lap-top computer. The localizer is removed, the CRW frame attached to the base ring and the target co-ordinates transcribed to the apparatus.

The trajectory to the chosen target can be at any point along the radius of the arc and is calculated to avoid passing the needle across an area of eloquent cortex. The biopsy can be obtained via a twist drill or burr hole approach. The advantage of the latter is that it allows direct inspection of the cortical surface and thereby avoidance of surface vessels. A side-cutting needle is introduced within a protective sheath and passed to the target. Multiple biopsies can be taken, from different regions of interest on the scan, and forwarded for histology. In reported series, histological analysis of the tissue has yielded a result in up to 94% of cases [36].

The commonest complications are haemorrhage at the site of biopsy and postoperative swelling of the lesion, which is most commonly encountered in high-grade gliomas. A recent survey by Cook and Gutherie demonstrated that the morbidity and mortality of the procedure varies with the eloquence of the brain in which the lesion lies. They report an overall complication rate of 6.5%, 2.7% of which were permanent. However, in their series, patients with lesions in eloquent brain who had a pre-existing deficit could expect to be immediately worse up to 31% of the time. One-half of the patients retained some increased neurological deficit [37].

If the biopsy is an uncomplicated procedure, then the patient should be closely observed for a period of 12–24 h for complications due to haemorrhage, brain swelling or epilepsy. They are then safe to be discharged.

Lesions that are not demonstrated on a CT scan but are evident on MRI can be biopsied under MRI guidance [38]. The basic principles remain the same, except that for MRI compatibility the head ring is replaced by one constructed to be compatible with the strong magnetic field in the scanner.

A direct surgical attack on a brainstem lesion, via the retromastoid, subtemporal or suboccipital route, is a major operation. While using image-directed surgery it is possible to biopsy lesions in such surgically inaccessible areas and provide a high yield of histological material with a low morbidity and mortality [39, 40]. In a similar way lesions of the basal ganglia or of the dominant hemisphere may be biopsied with relative safety.

Open Procedures

The available options are an intratumoral debulking procedure which may be partial or more extensive. Sometimes extensive procedures may involve lobectomy.

Lobectomy

Tumours wich appear to be macroscopically confined to the frontal, temporal or occipital lobe can be resected beyond the apparent tumour margin. In theory this should provide excision of tumour, infiltrative edge and a margin of uninvolved brain, but this is seldom achieved. In practice, this operation often only provides a generous decompression. The general principles remain the same, but there are important landmarks which must be borne in mind. It is possible to perform a frontal, temporal or occipital lobectomy. The extent of safe resection varies between the non-dominant and dominant hemisphere. Methods of surgical resection and detailed surgical considerations can be found in a number of dedicated surgical texts [41, 42].

The influence of lobectomy on survival is controversial; a number of studies have failed to show an advantage over intratumoral resection [29]. The issue has not been addressed in a randomized trial. What is apparent is that some cases of partial tumour removal may result in dangerous brain swelling postoperatively and that if resection, rather than biopsy, is performed, adequate debulking is indicated.

Gliomas in Specific Sites

Gliomas of the basal ganglia or brainstem present a difficult management problem. The vital nature of this tissue has led to advocates of treatment without obtaining a pathological diagnosis [43–45]. It is now obvious that evaluation of pathological tissue is mandatory to direct future therapy and prevent the possibility of inappropriate management [39, 46]. Computed tomographic and MRI-directed biopsies via a transfrontal approach have demonstrated a high yield of positive pathological diagnoses with a relatively low morbidity and mortality [39, 47].

Intra-axial brainstem lesions have been resected via an open operation [11, 48]. A major series of open operations for brainstem tumours classified tumours as diffuse, focal or cervicomedullary [49]. All tumours that appeared diffuse on a MRI scan were grade 3 or 4 tumours and tumours rostral to the medulla were almost all grade 3 or 4. No patient with a grade 3 or 4 tumour benefited from the operation. In contrast, a grade 1 or 2 tumour would usually be rostrally confined to the lower two-thirds of the medulla, although caudally the tumour may extend into the cervical cord. Patients with cervicomedullary junction tumours may show improved neurological recovery and extended longevity following radical excision of the tumour [50].

Technical Advances

Improvements in surgical techniques are directed towards improving the accuracy of resection and therefore reducing the associated morbidity and mortality, especially if the lesion lies within an eloquent area.

Microscope

The operative microscope with its coaxial illumination and magnification allows visualization in the depth of the operative field. This means that cortical incisions can be considerably smaller than the tumour to be resected. The microscope is frequently used in conjunction with self-retaining retractors and bipolar coagulation. The improved visualization provides the surgeon with a better appreciation of tumour extent, but even this apparent advantage is usually not confirmed by postoperative scanning.

Laser

Operative lasers allow for the precise vaporization of malignant tissue. Due to the limited penetration of energy beyond the resection margin, adjacent normal brain is spared. Therefore, accurate resection can be performed while the function of adjacent brain is preserved. The two lasers which have found favour in neurosurgical practice are the carbon dioxide and Nd:YAG lasers. Despite the advantages outlined above, there are a number of disadvantages to using the laser. The carbon dioxide laser is a time-consuming procedure with inadequate haemostasis and the Nd:YAG laser allows for more rapid tumour removal but with less precision. A recent report suggests other hazards [51].

Continuous Ultrasonic Aspirator

High-frequency ultrasonic sound waves combined with a system of irrigation and suction means glioma tissue can be sequentially fragmented and aspirated. It is possible to adjust the intensity of vibration, flow rate or irrigation and magnitude of suction, thus allowing for a high degree of precision. The aspirator does not provide for haemostasis and hence bipolar coagulation is required. However, this method does not divide vessels with an elastic wall, which are skeletonized and exposed for subsequent diathermy.

Ultrasound

Real-time B-mode ultrasonography allows intraoperative localization and characterization of a pathological lesion. This method relies on the fact that high-frequency sound waves are reflected from substances of differing density, which can then be displayed as an image. Interpretation of the received image is fairly simple and allows a precise estimation of the location of the lesion and its surrounding anatomy.

Compass (Volumetric Stereotactic Surgery)

The compass stereotactic system has evolved during the last 10 years under the guidance of P. Kelly, currently at the Mayo Clinic. It is an interactive, multi-modality hardware and software system which enables volumetric resection of deep-seated central or peripherally located tumours. The patient's head is fixed to a rigid headframe compatible with the imaging method chosen - CT, MRI, PET or DSA can be utilized [52].

Image-Directed Interactive Surgery

Recent advances in diagnostic imaging allow demonstration of a pathological lesion at an earlier stage and improved discrimination between the lesion and surrounding brain.

The combination of advanced neuroimaging and the principles of stereotaxy have led to the development of image-directed neurosurgery, which can incorporate an interactive free arm, ISG viewing wand (ISG Technologies, Ontario, Canada) or a powered robotic system [53].

In the management of malignant lesions, these systems allow for excision of small or centrally located lesions or those found within eloquent areas with improved accuracy.

Results of Surgery

The average survival following the diagnosis of a malignant glioma is 2 months [11]. The influence of surgery alone on these survival statistics is now difficult to judge because of the influence of adjuvant therapy and independent prognostic factors on survival, which are not always accounted for in published series. Differing therapeutic regimens have been shown to prolong survival without ever producing a cure.

The Brain Tumour Study Group [16] studied the effects of postoperative radiotherapy and chemotherapy on 467 patients with histologically proven malignant glioma, within 3 weeks of surgical intervention, which varied from a biopsy to a total resection and lobectomy. The survival curves for patients receiving radiotherapy alone and those receiving radiotherapy plus carmustine were practically superimposed for the first 12 months, although in the latter group there was a greater survival rate at 18 months, with 15–20% still alive at that time.

Lieberman et al. [54] found a 2-year survival of eight out of 57 (14%) patients with a malignant astrocytoma. All the patients were treated with surgery, radiotherapy and chemotherapy. Four patients succumbed to tumour regrowth. In the three patients who survived for the longest period, he reported the development of diffuse cortical dysfunction. This development was not related to tumour regrowth, hydrocephalus, endocrine or metabolic abnormalities, but was thought to be due to the delayed effects of radiotherapy on normal brain tissue.

Role of Surgical Intervention Following Recurrence

It provides a grim reminder for the patient and their family when a malignant glioma recurs. The first signs of recurrence usually appear between 6 and 12 months. Frequently there is therapeutic nihilism on the part of the responsible physician. The operative options of further craniotomy and debulking of tumour, intratumoral brachytherapy or stereotactic radiosurgery should all be considered. The use of chemotherapy or radiotherapy, if not already prescribed, must be utilized.

Reoperation

There is little information regarding the definitive role of reoperation. A series reported by Salcman et al. [55] of 74 patients, who were all initially treated with surgery, radiotherapy and chemotherapy and 40 of whom received second operations following tumour recurrence, demonstrated a median survival, from the time of reoperation, of 37 weeks. Length of survival after the second operation was independent of patient age, performance status, tumour grade and interoperative interval. There was minimal morbidity and no mortality. They concluded that reoperation for malignant astrocytoma is safe, feasible and of potential benefit in combination with other therapies.

Stromblad et al. [40], Ammirati et al. [56] and Harsh et al. [57] agree that patients with a performance score which exceeds 70 will have survival prolonged by a second operation. The time elapsed between operations has been found to be influential on patient survival by Harsh et al. [57] but not by other authors. In Stromblad et al.'s series [40], univariate analysis demonstrated that reoperation was associated with a significant improval in median survival. However, when incorporated into a multivariate analysis, which simultaneously corrected for other potential prognostic factors, no significant effect could then be demonstrated.

Rehabilitation

The diagnosis of a cerebral glioma has physical, psychological and social implications for both the patient and their family. A review of the literature will reveal that glioma research is directed towards the diagnosis, therapeutic manipulation and survival of this patient group. In the majority of papers, patient function is assessed against the Karnofsky Index and although this provides a rapid and relatively simple assessment, it suffers from interobserver variability.

Support and counselling are required by both patient and family to understand the wider implications of the diagnosis. The general practitioner will be faced with the day-to-day anxieties and it is essential that they are informed of the diagnosis and plan of management at an early stage.

The terminal stages of the disease are often accompanied by a rapid deterioration in the clinical status of the patient, with an attendant increase in their dependency, frequently requiring hospitalization or transfer to a hospice.

When further medical intervention is felt inappropriate and the patient has died, then bereavement counselling for the family should be provided.

Conclusions

Current surgical aims are the relief of distressing symptoms, improvement in the quality of survival, provision of a tissue diagnosis and a possible aid to adjunctive therapy. The infiltrative nature of this neoplasm means that surgery is unlikely to provide a curative role. However, the technological advances in image-directed surgery may allow resection of all the malignant tissue visible on a scan, with minimum compromise of the surrounding intact tissue.

In the foreseeable future any substantial impact on the prognosis of a patient harbouring a malignant glioma is more likely to be provided by a greater understanding of tumour biology than a surgical advance.

References

1. Mahaley MS, Mettlin C, Natarajan N et al. (1989) National survey of patterns of care for brain tumour patients. J Neurosurg 71:826–836.
2. Barker DJP, Weller RO, Garfield JS (1976) Epidemiology of primary brain tumours of the brain and spinal cord: a regional survey in Southern England. J Neurol Neurosurg Psychiat 39:290–296.
3. Bennett AH, Godlee RJ (1884) Excision of a tumour from the brain. Lancet 2:1090–1091.
4. Ferrier D, Horsley V, Hughlings-Jackson J, MacEwen W (1885) Discussion of paper by AH Bennett and RJ Godlee. Case of cerebral tumour – the surgical treatment. Br Med J 1:988–989.
5. Horsley V (1887) Remarks on ten consecutive cases of operations upon the brain and cranial cavity to illustrate the details and safety of the method employed. Br Med J 1:863–865.
6. Cushing H (1905) The establishment of cerebral hernia as a decompressive measure for inacessible brain tumours. Surg Gynecol Obstet 1:297–314.
7. Bailey P, Cushing H (1926) A classification of the tumours of the glioma group on a histogenic basis with a correlated study of prognosis. Lippincott, Philadelphia.
8. McKenzie KG (1936) Glioblastoma. Arch Neurol Psychiat 36:542–546.
9. Sachs E (1950) The problem of glioblastoma. J Neurosurg 7:185–189.
10. Maxwell HP (1946) The incidence of interhemispheric extension of glioblastoma multiforme through the corpus callosum. J Neurosurg 3:54–57.
11. Hitchcock E, Sato FJ (1964) Treatment of malignant gliomata. J Neurosurg 21:497–506.
12. Jelsma RK, Bucy PC (1967) The treatment of glioblastome multiforme of the brain. J Neurosurg 27:388–400.
13. Bucy PC, Oberhill MR, Sigueira EB et al. (1985) Cerebral glioblastoma can be cured! Neurosurgery 16:714–717.
14. Burger PC, Green SB (1987) Patient age, histologic features and length of survival in patients with glioblastoma multiforme. Cancer 59:1617–1625.
15. Chang CH, Horton J, Schoenfield D et al. (1983) Comparison of postoperative radiotherapy and combined postoperative radiotherapy and chemotherapy in the multidisciplinary management of malignant gliomas. A joint Radiation Therapy

Oncology Group and Eastern Cooperative Oncology Group study. Cancer 52:997–1007.
16. Walker MD, Green SB, Byar DP et al. (1980) Randomized comparisons of radiotherapy and nitrosoureas for the treatment of malignant glioma after surgery. N Engl J Med 303:1323–1329.
17. Burger PC, Vogel FS, Green SB et al. (1985) Glioblastoma multiforme and anaplastic astrocytoma: pathological criteria and prognostic implications. Cancer 56:1106–1111.
18. Coffey PC, Lundsford LD, Taylor FH (1988) Survival after stereotactic biopsy of malignant gliomas. Neurosurgery 22:465–473.
19. Nelson JS, Tsukada Y, Schonfield D et al. Necrosis as a prognostic criterion in malignant supratentorial astrocytic gliomas. Cancer 52:550–554.
20. Adams GE, Ayoub Bey AMA, Barnard RO et al. (1990) Prognostic factors for high-grade malignant glioma: development of a prognostic index. Report of the MRC Brain Tumour Working Party. J Neuro-Oncol 9:47–55.
21. Byar DP, Green SB, Strike TA (1983) Prognostic factors for malignant glioma. In: Walker MD (ed) Oncology of the nervous system. Martinus Nijhoff, Boston.
22. Laws ER, Taylor WF, Clifton MB et al. (1984) Neurosurgical management of low-grade astrocytoma of the cerebral hemispheres. J Neurosurg 61:665–673.
23. Hutton JL, Smith DF, Sandemann D et al. (1992) Development of prognostic index for primary supratentorial intracerebral tumours. J Neurol Neurosurg Psychiat 55:271–274.
24. Smith DF, Hutton JL, Sandemann D et al. (1991) The prognosis of primary intracerebral tumours presenting with epilepsy: the outcome of medical and surgical management. J Neurol Neurosurg Psychiat 54:915–920.
25. Scott GM, Gibberd FB (1980) Epilepsy and other factors in the prognosis of gliomas. Acta Neurol Scand 61:227–239.
26. Garfield JS (1980) Surgery of cerebral gliomas. In: Thomas DGT, Graham DI (eds) Brain tumours: scientific basis, clinical investigation and current therapy. Butterworth, London, pp 301–321.
27. Salcman M (1980) Survival in glioblastoma: historical perspective. Neurosurgery 7:435–439.
28. Shackney SE, McCormack GW, Cuchural GH (1978) Growth rate patterns of solid tumours and their relation to responsiveness to therapy: an analytical review. Ann Intern Med 89:107–121.
29. Nazzaro JM, Neuwelt EA (1990) The role of surgery in the management of supratentorial intermediate and high-grade astrocytomas in adults. J Neurosurg 73:331–344.
30. Quigley JR, Maroon JC (1991) The relationship between survival and the extent of the resection in patients with supratentorial malignant gliomas. Neurosurgery 29:385–389.
31. Ampil F, Fowler M, Kim K (1992) Intracranial astrocytomas in elderly patients. J Neuro-Oncol 12:125–130.
32. Winger MJ, Macdonald DR, Cairncross JG (1989) Supratentorial anaplastic gliomas in adults. The prognostic importance of extent of resection and prior low-grade glioma. J Neurosurg 71:487–493.
33. Kelly PJ, Hunt C (1994) The limited value of cytoreductive surgery in elderly patients with malignant gliomas. Neurosurgery 34:62–67.
34. Apuzzo MLJ, Chandrosoma TT, Cohen D et al. (1987) Computer imaging stereotaxy; experience and perspective related to 500 procedures related to brain masses. Neurosurgery 28:792–800.
35. Thomas DGT, Nouby RM (1989) Experience with 300 cases of CT-directed stereotactic surgery for lesion biopsy and aspiration of haematoma. Br J Neurosurg 3:321–326.
36. Revesz T, Scaravilli F et al. (1993) The reliability of histological diagnosis including grading in gliomas biopsied by image guided stereotatic techniques. Brain 116:781–793.

37. Cook RJ, Gutherie BL (1994) Complications of stereotactic biopsy. In: Pell MF, Thomas DGT (eds) Handbook of stereotaxy using the CRW apparatus. Williams & Wilkins, Baltimore.
38. Bradford R, Thomas DGT, Bydder GM (1987) MRI-directed stereotactic biopsy of cerebral lesions. Acta Neurochir suppl 39:25–27.
39. Hood TW, Gebarski SS, McKeever PE, Venes JF (1986) Stereotaxic biopsy of intrinsic lesions of the brain stem. J Neurosurg 65:172–176.
40. Stromblad LG, Anderson H, Malmstrom P, Salford LG (1993) Reoperation for malignant astrocytomas. Br J Neurosurg 7:623–633.
41. McCabe JJ (1979) Treatment of gliomas by surgery. In: Symon L (ed) Operative neurosurgery, 3 ed. Butterworths, London, pp 111–120.
42. Schmidek HH, Sweet WH (1996) Operative neurosurgical techniques. Indications, methods and results. Grune & Stratton, Orlando.
43. Bray PF, Carter S, Taveras JM (1985) Brainstem tumours in children. Neurology 8:1–7.
44. Lassman LP (1974) Tumours of the pons and medulla oblongata. In: Vinken PH, Brunken GW (eds) Tumours of the brain and skull, part 2. Handbook of clinical neurology, vol 17. North Holland, Amsterdam, pp 693–706.
45. Villani R, Gaini SM, Tomei G (1975) Follow-up study of brainstem tumours in children. Child Brain 1:126–135.
46. Hoffman MG, Becker L, Craven MA (1980) A clinically and pathologically distinct group of benign brain stem gliomas. J Neurosurg 7:243–248.
47. Thomas DGT, Bradford R, Gill S, Davis CH (1988) Computer-directed stereotactic biopsy of intrinsic brainstem lesions. Br J Neurosurg 2:235–240.
48. Heffez DS, Zinreich SJ, Long DM (1990) Surgical resection of intrinsic brain stem lesions: an overview. Neurosurgery 27:789–798.
49. Epstein F, McCleary EL (1986) Intrinsic brain-stem tumours of childhood: surgical indications. J Neurosurg 64:11–15.
50. Epstein F, Wisoff J (1987) Intra-axial tumours of the cervicomedullary junction. J Neurosurg 67:483–487.
51. Jain KK (1985) Complications of use of the neodymium: yttrium-aluminium-garnet laser in neurosurgery. Neurosurgery 16:759–762.
52. Kelly PJ, Kall BA (1994) Contemporary issues in neurological surgery. Computers in stereotactic neurosurgery. Blackwell Scientific Publications, Cambridge, USA.
53. Drake JM, Prudencio J, Holowka S (1996) A comparison of the PUMA robotic system and the ISG viewing wand for neurosurgery. In: Maciunas RJ (ed) Neurosurgical topics. Interactive image-guided neurosurgery. AANS Publications Committee,
54. Lieberman AN, Foo SH, Ranshoff J et al. (1982) Long term survival among patients with malignant brain tumours. Neurosurgery 10:450–453.
55. Salcman M, Kaplan RS, Ducker TB et al. (1982) Effect of age and reoperation on survival in the combined modality treatment of malignant astrocytoma. Neurosurgery 10:454–463.
56. Ammirati M, Vick N, Llao Y et al. (1987) Effect of the extent of surgical resection on survival and quality of life in patients with supratentorial glioblastomas and anaplastic astrocytomas. Neurosurgery 21:201–206.
57. Harsh GR, Levin VA, Gutin PH et al. (1987) Reoperation for recurrent glioblastoma and anaplastic astrocytoma. Neurosurgery 21:615–621.

6 – Non-Curative Surgery for Thoracic Malignancies

Ugo Pastorino and Peter Goldstraw

Introduction

The poor surgical curability of most thoracic malignancies and the lack of effective systemic therapies has led to greater emphasis being placed upon palliative management, to control symptoms and thereby improve the quality of life, and treatments aimed at prolonging the survival of those patients who have no chance of cure.

This chapter reviews the role of non-curative surgery in the management of chest tumours: from the results of surgical resection for locally advanced or metastatic disease, to the efficacy of symptom palliation compared to other less invasive procedures.

Lung

Primary Lung Cancer

The overall proportion of patients amenable to curative surgery, i.e. complete resection, has not significantly changed over the last 20 years. Potentially 20–30% of all primary lung cancers in the USA are treated surgically, but only 10% of cases in the UK. In the vast majority of cases surgery is not possible because of local extension, or is not advised because of distant metastases, or the poor general condition or inadequate respiratory reserve of the patient.

In historical series, the 5-year survival of resected T_4 or bulky N_{2-3} disease is 0% [1, 2]. Induction chemotherapy or chemo/radiotherapy have been reported to improve the proportion of patients with advanced non-small cell lung cancer (stage IIIa–b) who can undergo resection. Long-term survival may also be improved by such an approach, and in phase II studies was reported to be 18% at 5 years, compared to 9% in historical series [3, 4]. However, in the group with bulky N_2 disease the 5-year survival after induction chemotherapy was only 4%.

Although the presence of a pleural effusion does not represent *per se* a contraindiction for surgery, lung resection in the presence of cytological positive pleural effusion has been associated with a mean survival of 3–6 months [5, 6]. Analogously, long-term survival is almost unknown after resection for T_4 tumours invading mediastinal structures such as the superior vena cava, aorta, myocardium or oesophagus [7, 8].

Lung cancer patients presenting with an isolated distant metastasis may benefit from combined resection of both tumour foci (a more common problem now that CT scans of brain and abdomen are routinely performed for preoperative evaluation).

A solitary brain metastasis in a patient with otherwise operable non-small cell lung cancer is the most typical indication for such a combined surgical approach. The probability of long-term survival after resection of the brain metastasis and the lung primary is between 10% and 20% at 5 years. A large retrospective series of 185 cases so treated at Memorial Sloan Kettering showed a 13% 5-year survival, with no significant difference in survival between patients with synchronous and metachronous presentation of brain lesions [9]. On the other hand, a prospective randomized trial comparing surgery plus brain irradiation versus radiotherapy alone has demonstrated a significant improvement of median survival (19 vs. 9 months) with better quality of life in the surgical arm [10]. These results emphasize two distinct aspects of brain metastasectomy: a better control of CNS symptoms, and a small but definite possibility of cure for metastatic lung cancer. The palliative aspect is prominent, however, and in patients with synchronous disease the priority of treatment should be given to brain resection.

Occasional long-term survivors have been reported after resection of isolated adrenal metastases [11]. In the presence of a solitary adrenal mass associated with resectable non-small cell lung cancer, tissue diagnosis is mandatory, as a high proportion of these lesions are benign. The pathological confirmation can be usually achieved by fine-needle aspiration biopsy under CT or ultrasound guidance. Concurrent resection of primary lung tumour and adrenal metastasis with curative intent may be justified in very selected cases [12].

More difficult is the assessment of prognosis after resection of synchronous intrapulmonary metastases. A Japanese paper has reported a 25% 5-year survival in 42 patients with resected synchronous intrapulmonary lesions [13]. In fact, there is no way to differentiate on the basis of the appearance at surgery or on conventional histopathology a second primary cancer from an intrapulmonary metastasis. The distinction is further complicated by satellite nodules around the lung primary. Recent data on the molecular biology of synchronous pulmonary lesions support the concept of field cancerization and the diagnosis of multiple primary lung cancers even when the tumours are of similar histology and located within the same lobe [14]. From the clinical point of view, concurrent lung lesions should be considered as independent primary tumours; each lesion should be assessed separately, and surgical treatment with curative intent is appropriate if all can be resected.

For those lung cancer patients in which complete resection cannot be achieved, incomplete or debulking surgery does not appear to influence life expectancy or improve quality of life. The few long-term survivors after incomplete resection are those treated by postoperative radiotherapy, and the outcome is not different from that expected with radiotherapy alone [15, 16].

The role of palliative resection has generally been overemphasized, and the concept of symptomatic surgery is often misleading. In fact, symptoms such as cough, dyspnoea or chest pain may be worse after surgery than they were before.

Bronchial obstruction and haemoptysis are better palliated by radiotherapy or endoscopic treatment. Lung abscess or acute sepsis are rare indications for incomplete resection, and even experienced thoracic surgeons have only anecdotal cases. In paraneoplastic syndromes, the permanent control of hormone-related symptoms can only be achieved by complete excision of the disease. In the vast majority of such cases, radiotherapy with or without chemotherapy is better than incomplete surgery. A particular problem is represented by patients undergoing primary medical treatment for locally advanced lung cancer in whom salvage lung resection may occasionally be indicated to manage acute life-threatening complications, such as the massive necrosis of heavily irradiated lung parenchyma.

In conclusion, major surgery in the management of primary lung cancer is rarely justified on palliative grounds alone.

Lung Metastases

The resection of pulmonary metastases is considered today a potentially curative procedure, and many studies have proved that pulmonary metastasectomy can achieve a 20–30% long-term survival, even in cases presenting with multiple bilateral lung metastases [17–19], although permanent control of disease may often require multiple thoracotomies. In some specific tumours such as sarcomas, the concept of metastasectomy is based on the natural history of organ-restricted metastatic spread. In fact, lung metastases are often the only site of distant relapse, occurring in 60–80% of osteosarcomas, and 30–50% of soft-tissue sarcomas. Systemic therapy appears ineffective in advanced or relapsing disease, and median survival of patients with lung metastases from sarcomas treated with chemotherapy only ranges between 6 and 10 months, with no survivors beyond 36 months.

The general criteria of curative resection also apply to metastasectomy: thorough preoperative staging, careful intraoperative reassessment and complete resection with adequate margins. Debulking surgery, i.e. partial resection of lung metastases leaving obvious residual disease, is not justified. The minimum eligibility criteria for the resection of lung metastases include: assured locoregional control of the primary site, exclusion of extrathoracic metastatic disease, and surgeon's assessment that all lesions detectable on CT scan can be resected by one or more operations. The number of metastases and the length of disease-free interval do not represent useful criteria for patient selection for surgery.

In patients with metastatic sarcomas and unilateral disease on CT scan, the role of median sternotomy, allowing the exploration of both lungs and the resection of unsuspected contralateral lesions, is still debated [20, 21]. Although the occurrence of radiologically occult disease is generally accepted, some surgeons are not convinced that early resection of small pulmonary nodules, undetectable on CT scan, may improve the long-term results.

For some metastatic tumours where the chances of cure are minimal, such as breast cancer, melanoma, or even sarcomas with a large number of metastatic deposits, complete resection may be beneficial in terms of improvement of survival. Non-randomized studies suggest that even in the subset of patients who ultimately die due to recurrence of metastatic disease, median survival is longer than that of unresected cases with similar histology and clinical extent of disease.

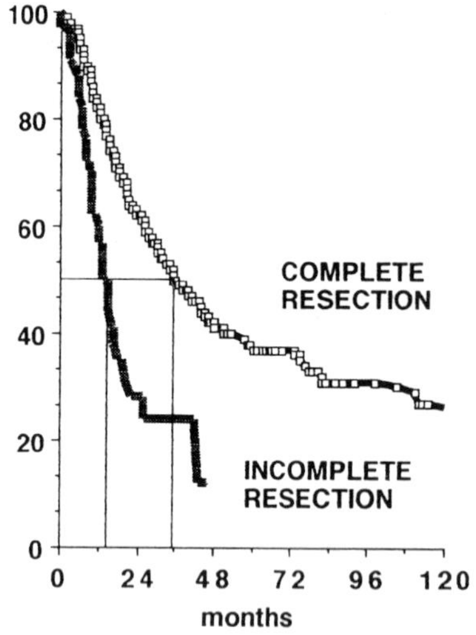

Figure 6.1 Overall survival after resection of lung metastases: results of complete resection (445 cases) vs. incomplete resection (64 cases). (After National Cancer Institute, Milan)

The experience of metastasectomy at the Royal Brompton Hospital, London, and National Cancer Institute of Milan is summarized in Figures 6.1–6.3. A total of 509 patients underwent pulmonary resection for lung metastases between 1974 and 1993 in Milan. The overall survival for the 445 cases where complete resection proved feasible was 32% at 10 years (Figure 6.1). Of the other 64 cases where only incomplete resection was possible, the survival was 25% at 3 years. Median survival was respectively 32 months and 13 months. Among the 445 patients undergoing complete resection, 276 (62%) developed further metastases isolated to the lungs. The overall median survival of this group was 28 months, but was 47 months for the 69 patients who underwent further surgery and 20 months for those in whom this was not possible (Figure 6.2).

Similar results have been observed in 280 patients operated upon at the Royal

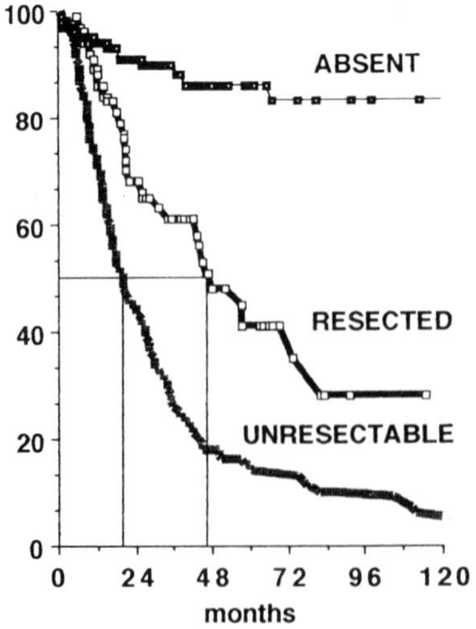

Figure 6.2 Overall survival after metastasectomy (all sites) according to the presence and resectability of relapse: absent (169 cases), resected (69 cases), unresectable (207 cases). (After National Cancer Institute, Milan)

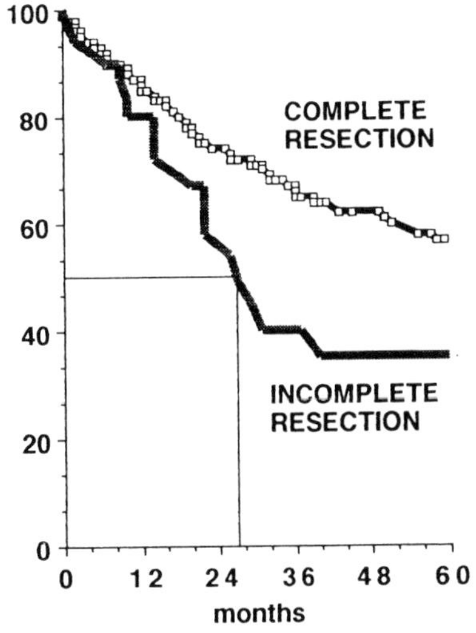

Figure 6.3 Overall survival after metastasectomy: results of complete resection (243 cases) vs. incomplete resection (37 cases). (After Royal Brompton Hospital, London)

Brompton Hospital between 1980 and 1992. Both median survival (27 months) and 5-year survival (35%) after incomplete resection were higher in the Brompton experience owing to the large number of testicular tumours in this particular series (Figure 6.3).

These results indicate that metastasectomy may prolong median survival, and second-phase surgery is of value in those cases relapsing with further lung metastases after the first lung resection. In our experience, the median survival appears to be two to three times that expected after medical treatment or supportive care only. The relative influence of biological selection on such results is obviously unknown.

Pleura

Mesothelioma

Diffuse malignant mesothelioma remains incurable, despite combination therapy using surgery, radiotherapy and chemotherapy in very aggressive regimens [22].

Pleurectomy/decortication and extrapleural pneumonectomy represent two extremes of surgical management with curative intent [23]. Pleurectomy and decortication is the most common type of surgical treatment, generally applied with cytoreductive intent.

Extrapleural pneumonectomy has been associated with significant morbidity and mortality but no comparable advantage in the local control of disease. Although theoretically attractive in cases with limited extent of disease (stages I and II), extrapleural pneumonectomy has resulted in very high local recurrence rates and poor survival. There are no randomized trials comparing surgery with other treatment modalities, or studies evaluating the quality of life of tumour-reductive therapies compared to best supportive care. A large retrospective survey conducted in Ontario on 332 patients showed no survival advantage for surgical treatment [24]. The median survival of 23 patients treated by extrapleural pneumonectomy was 9.3 months, compared to 9.8 months for 63 patients treated by decortication/pleurectomy, and 8 months for those not receiving any surgery. Pneumonectomy, however, was associated with a 30% morbidity and 13% mortality. There was a significant difference in survival for patients who received chemotherapy compared with no chemotherapy (12.3 vs. 7.3 months). Another non-randomized study conducted in the UK in the early 1980s provided very similar results, comparing 52 treated with 64 untreated patients [15]. In particular, the median survival of 28 patients treated by decortication alone was 20 months, compared to an overall median survival of 18 months for the 64 untreated patients.

A single report from the Brigham and Women's Hospital of Boston, based on 52 cases of extrapleural pneumonectomy, has shown a more favourable outcome, with an overall mortality of 5.8% and a 5-year survival of patients with epithelial histological variant and negative mediastinal lymph nodes as high as 45% [25]. These results appear encouraging, but must be interpreted cautiously as they are derived from a very selected series of patients.

Recently, decortication/pleurectomy has been tested in a phase II study in combination with intrapleural and systemic chemotherapy with cisplatin and mitomycin [26]. Of 36 patients entered in the study, only 28 have completed the planned treatment. Median survival was 17 months and disease-free survival at 3 years approximately 10%.

Taking into account the obvious selection of patients who are candidates for thoracotomy, there is no evidence that marginal or incomplete resection of diffuse malignant mesothelioma is significantly better than other non-surgical modalities.

Metastatic Effusion

In pathologically proven metastatic pleural effusion, surgical treatment aims to prevent troublesome recurrence by achieving complete expansion of the lung and pleurodesis.

A few studies have demonstrated that surgical pleurodesis, achieved by talc poudrage at thoracoscopy or thoracotomy, yields the best results, with permanent control of pleural effusion in excess of 90% of cases [27]. Medical pleurodesis with intercostal chest drainage and the intrapleural instillation of tetracycline or other chemicals may be accepted as a valid alternative in compromised patients, although the success rate is lower (50–60%).

Failure of pleurodesis may be due to several factors: inadequate drainage of the effusion, the choice of an ineffective agent, adhesion or fibrin from previous pleural interventions preventing contact between the agent and the pleural surface, and restriction of lung re-expansion due to a cortex which may be malignant or benign, or indeed a mixed variant. Such a cortex does not allow apposition of the two surfaces, which must adhere for pleurodesis to be obtained. In patients in whom the lung will not expand sufficiently to allow apposition, all the attempts of pleurodesis will fail, but the insertion of a pleuroperitoneal shunt may provide effective palliation (Figure 6.4).

The experience of the Royal Brompton Hospital has been summarized in a recent paper reporting on 180 patients treated with talc pleurodesis (117 cases) or

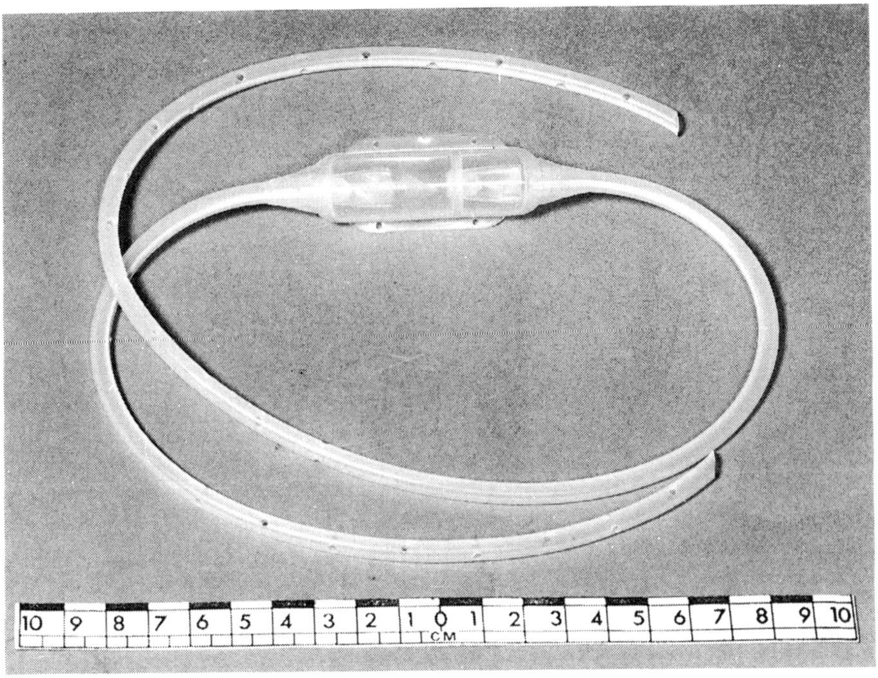

Figure 6.4 The pleuroperitoneal Denver shunt

pleuroperitoneal Denver shunt (63 cases). In both groups effective palliation was achieved in over 95% of patients [28]. There was no intraoperative mortality, and the median survival was 5 months (range 1–53 months). There were nine (5%) early deaths occurring 2–30 days after surgery, as a consequence of respiratory or multisystem organ failure associated with advanced malignant disease. These results are of particular interest, considering that three-quarters of the patients had previously been treated with various modalities before referral to our department.

From our experience we would advocate the early referral for surgical treatment of any patient with good performance status and recurrent malignant effusion. At thoracoscopy, using video assistance, the situation can be assessed fully and talc pleurodesis performed or a pleuroperitoneal shunt inserted as appropriate. Both procedures provide reliable long-term control of effusion, without the need for repeated readmission and pleural aspiration, with its consequent danger of infection.

Chest Wall

Primary Tumours

Primary sarcomas of the chest wall are a rare but challenging disease for the thoracic surgeon. Complete resection can be accomplished in previously untreated patients, with limited mortality. Long-term survival is good, particularly in low-grade sarcomas.

A more complex therapeutic problem is represented by patients with extensive recurrence after prior treatment, secondary sarcoma arising in an area of chest wall previously irradiated for prior malignancy, or those with lung metastases at presentation. Although the chances of cure are less under such circumstances, surgical resection may be of value in relieving pain or preventing ulceration and bleeding.

In one large series of soft-tissue sarcomas of the chest wall treated surgically, neither positive surgical margins (in high-grade tumours) nor subsequent local recurrence had a significant impact on long-term survival [29]. However, in the experience of NCI-Bethesda, patients with positive resection margins had a median survival of only 6 months and none survived 5 years [30].

The presence of lung metastases, synchronous or metachronous, is a negative prognostic factor. However, when both primary and metastatic deposits can be completely resected, a median survival of nearly 3 years has been reported, and the 5-year survival was greater than 20% [29].

Locally Advanced Lung Cancer

Chest wall resection for locally advanced lung cancer yields excellent results, provided that tumour excision is macroscopically and microscopically complete. In fact, the 5-year survival for T_3N_0 is approximately 50%.

Palliative surgery is often advocated in superior sulcus or Pancoast tumours. However, there is little evidence that incomplete resection in these circumstances affords better control of chest pain after radiotherapy. Median survival after incomplete resection of Pancoast tumours is only 7 months, with 10–15% of patients surviving 3 years and none alive at 5 years [31]. Survival is poorer in patients whose pain did not respond to preoperative radiotherapy [32]. However, at Memorial Sloan Kettering, where postoperative brachytherapy has been systematically used as an adjuvant for patients undergoing resection of superior sulcus tumours, 9% of patients survived 5 years after incomplete resection [33], but there was no difference in survival between these patients and those who did not undergo resection. Median survival was dismal (11 months).

For patients with chest wall invasion due to lung cancer there is no benefit in terms of symptomatic relief and survival from incomplete resection compared to radiotherapy alone [34, 35].

Recurrent Breast Cancer

Local recurrence after surgical treatment of breast cancer occurs in 2–10% of cases, depending upon the extent of disease, the volume of resection and the type of adjuvant treatment applied [36, 37]. Local relapse is more frequent after limited resection with lumpectomy or simple quadrantectomy, but in these cases surgical rescue by mastectomy can usually achieve local control. Local relapse is more difficult to treat after radical mastectomy, and may prove refractory to further surgery and radiotherapy. Chest wall invasion can be a problem in such unsuccessful cases, and this may represent the only site of persistent disease.

The management of these patients may be further complicated by the distressing late sequelae of thoracic irradiation with extensive radionecrosis which may involve soft tissues and bone. Skin is invariably ulcerated with various degrees of inflammation and oedema, and direct exposure of the ribs or the sternum is not uncommon. Chronic pain and infection may be so disabling as to justify chest wall resection, which usually achieves a long-term relief of symptoms with occasional cure.

In a large series, overall 5-year survival after full-thickness chest wall resection ws 35–40%, with a median survival of 36–48 months [38, 39]. A disease-free interval from primary treatment of less than 24 months, the presence of positive mediastinal nodes or concurrent extrathoracic metastases were found to be unfavourable prognostic factors [39, 40]. Disease-free survival was less, in the order of 25–30% at 5 years, with a median disease-free survival of 12–18 months. However, relapse was usually at distant sites, local control was satisfactory, and the large majority of patients were free from local symptoms for their remaining life [41].

Bone Metastases

Radiotherapy remains the primary treatment for symptomatic bone secondaries. However, rib or sternal resection is occasionally advised if relapse occurs after radiotherapy and the prognosis is otherwise reasonable, or if there are no other sites of disease and the primary tumour is controlled.

One may occasionally resect a rib lesion in a patient with no known extrathoracic malignancy, only to find it is a metastasis. Usually, however, if an extensive resection is contemplated, open biopsies will be performed as a preliminary, to avoid surgery in this situation.

Survival after resection of bone metastases depends on the tumour type and the extent of primary disease. Where effective chemotherapy is available, as in osteosarcoma or Ewing's sarcoma, complete resection may result in prolonged survival or even cure.

Surgical Technique

The development of safe techniques for chest wall reconstruction, including prosthetic materials and soft-tissue reconstruction using myocutaneous flaps, has expanded the role of surgery in this field [42]. Extensive chest wall resection, including total sternectomy, can now be performed with virtually no operative mortality.

Polypropylene mesh (Marlex) has proved to be a good prosthetic material for bone reconstruction. This can be used alone if the defect is limited to one or two ribs, but for larger defects, particularly those involving the lateral aspect or the apex of the chest, a methyl methacrylate composite prosthesis within two layers of mesh offers superior mechanical strength and external profile. The mesh-methacrylate composite is manufactured at the time of surgery when the size and shape of prosthesis can be determined, and provides excellent functional and cosmetic results. Paradoxical movement of the chest can be prevented with such prostheses, even with very large defects.

When there is limited skin involvement, the soft-tissue defect can be repaired by primary closure or sliding flaps. However, for larger soft-tissue defects, and where the viability of the residual skin has been reduced by prior radiotherapy, myocutaneous rotation flaps are necessary. The latissimus dorsi offers an excellent flap even for extensive anterior defects, such as after total sternectomy. Our experience confirms the efficacy and safety of this technique, with no perioperative mortality on over 200 cases of chest wall resection.

Mediastinum

Advanced Thymoma

Locally advanced thymoma or thymoma with pleural and pericardial dissemination (stages IIIb and IV according to Masaoka [43] is probably the best example of thoracic malignancy in which incomplete resection or debulking surgery may improve long-term survival and provide prolonged local control [44–46].

Median sternotomy is the preferred approach, and surgical treatment should be aimed at complete or near complete removal of the tumour. This may necessitate resection of a large portion of pericardium, of superior vena cava or left innominate vein, as well as lung resection. All efforts should be made to preserve the phrenic nerves, particularly in patients with myasthenic syndrome.

Survival following resection for stage IV thymoma ranged from 17% to 59% at 5 years from 11% to 50% at 10 years, with a median survival exceeding 5 years in most series (Table 6.1). Even when resection is macroscopically incomplete, the 5-year survival may be as high as 70% [47]. There is a high risk of local relapse, but reoperation for recurrent disease yields good results, with limited morbidity and long-term survival greater than 50% [47, 48].

The role of postoperative radiotherapy and induction or adjuvant chemotherapy has not been clearly established. However, postoperative radiotherapy is recommended after incomplete resection, and to this purpose it is useful to mark the residual tumour with metal clips.

Although some authors suggest that radiotherapy alone can achieve similar or better results than surgery in such advanced stage disease [49, 50], the overwhelming opinion supports complete resection or cytoreductive surgery in these circumstances.

Table 6.1 Results of surgical resection of advanced thymoma: stage III vs. IV

Reference	Stage III survival				Stage IV survival			
	No. pts.	5-year	10-yr	Median*	No. pts.	5-yr	10-yr	Median*
Maggi et al. [47]	52	71	64	n.r.	21	59	39	78
Fuentes et al. [45]	19	35	35	18	4	50	50	120
Etienne et al. [44]	9	33	33	10	18	17	11	12
Park et al. [46]	35	71	47	130	44	46	21	60

* Median survival in months.

SVC Syndrome

The role of surgery in the palliation of malignant superior vena cava (SVC) syndrome is marginal. Resection and reconstruction of the SVC or innominate vein is indicated for primary germ cell tumours of the mediastinim or invasive thymoma, where surgery is aimed at cure or long-term survival. Under these circumstances, replacement or bypass of the SVC with expanded polytetrafluoroethylene grafts has proved to be safe and effective with prolonged patency [8, 51]. For other malignancies chemo- and/or radiotherapy offer good palliation without the risk of surgery.

The recent development of intravascular stenting techniques has provided new possibilities for the management of persisting or recurrent SVC obstruction after medical treatment [52, 53]. The percutaneous transvenous insertion of expandable wire stents, with or without prior balloon dilatation, can be a safe and effective alternative to conventional therapy.

Late salvage surgery may be indicated for SVC syndromes caused by recurrent thymomas if long-term control has been achieved with radiotherapy.

Pericardial Involvement

Surgical management is often required in patients with malignant pericardial involvement where constriction or effusion leads to cardiac tamponade. Conventional technique consists in pericardiectomy for constriction and pericardial fenestration for effusion [54]. Both operations can be performed through thoracotomy or video-assisted thoracoscopy.

The sub-xiphoid approach has been advocated for pericardial fenestration as a safer alternative to the thoracic approach [55], bearing less complication (10% vs. 67%) and relatively longer survival (2.7 vs 1.2 months). However, given the retrospective type of analysis, such a difference is likely to be related to other factors than the technique.

Alternative management techniques include percutaneous balloon pericardiotomy [56] and pericardioperitoneal shunt [57].

Airway Obstruction

Obstruction of the trachea and main bronchi causes severe dyspnoea and stridor which can prove life threatening. Intraluminal growth is usually due to a primary airway malignancy or lung cancers, and if localized may be susceptible for resection with curative intent. Rarely, such intraluminal tumours are metastatic [58]. More commonly, obstruction results from compression of the airway due to metastatic involvement of mediastinal nodes at the carina or in the paratracheal chains. This is most usually due to lung cancer, where there may also be an intraluminal component, but can occur secondary to other extrathoracic malignancies such as lymphoma or carcinoma of the breast. Cure for the majority of cases is not possible and palliative therapy is usually given by external irradiation. In an emergency, however, or if relapse occurs after external irradiation, the surgeon may be involved in palliation.

Where the major component is endoluminal, endoscopic disobliteration can be achieved by various techniques including simple "core out" [59], Nd:YAD laser photocoagulation [60, 61], cryotherapy [62] or diathermy resection [63]. Although laser photocoagulation can be applied through the fibreoptic bronchoscope, all these modalities of endoscopic treatment are usually performed under general anaesthesia, with the use of rigid bronchoscope and Sanders Venturi ventilation. In fact, through the rigid bronchoscope it is possible to maintain an adequate ventilation during the whole procedure even in case of significant bleeding, to secure the haemostasis at the end of resection, and to consider other modalities, such as the insertion of an endobronchial stent if required. Once relief has been obtained, consolidation treatment may be achieved by a high dose of intraluminal radiotherapy [64].

In most cases the major component of obstruction is due to extrinsic compression. If relapses occur after external irradiation, then the insertion of an endoluminal support can relieve symptoms. This was formerly undertaken using a T tube or T–Y tube inserted at the tracheostomy operation (Figure 6.5). More recently, adequate support has been provided by endobronchial silicone stents, manufactured from T tubes at the time of surgery [16] or commercially available [65]. Such stents may subsequently be removed if obstruction is relieved by further irradiation, external or endobronchial, and reinserted at subsequent relapse [66]. Wire stents have been used in these circumstances, but tumour regrowth remains a problem and covered expanding stents have been developed. Currently, at one endoscopic procedure a combination of therapies is used to treat separately the intraluminal and extraluminal components of the obstruction (Table 6.2).

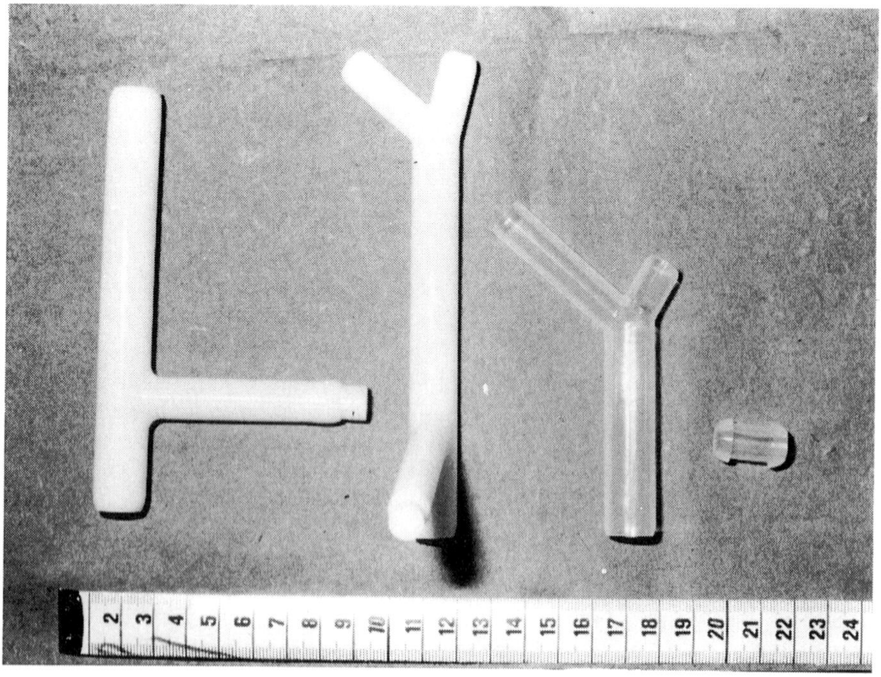

Figure 6.5 Examples of T tube and T–Y tube to be inserted by tracheostomy

Table 6.2 Endoscopic techniques in the palliation of malignant airways obstruction

		Advantages	Disadvantages	Comment
Disobliteration	Nd:YAG laser Diathermy Cryotherapy	Effective Effective Effective	Costly Not widely available Repeated application	Choice depends mainly on availability
Brachytherapy	Iridium afterload	Day-case treatment	Not widely available	Can be used when external RXT is contraindicated by normal tissue tolerance
Silicone stents	T or T–Y tubes Endobronchial stents	Cheap, stable Cheap	Tracheostomy needed Can displace	
Metal stents	Gianturco Wallstent Covered	Expandable Thin wall High internal/external ratio	Tumour ingrowth can displace	Covered wire stents to be developed

The experience of the Royal Brompton Hospital on endoscopic palliation of tracheobronchial malignancies has been summarized in a paper analysing 29 patients treated with bronchoscopic diathermy and stent insertion [67]. It appears that diathermy resection is an effective and safe method for relieving the intraluminal component of the obstruction at appreciably less cost than laser resection, and can be combined with silicone stent insertion if there is an extraluminal component or obstruction.

Advanced Oesophageal Cancer (Stage III–IV)

Surgical resection for locally advanced (stage IIb–III) oesophageal cancer provides poor long-term survival, in the order of 20% at 2 years and 5–10% at 5 years [68, 69]. These figures are not substantially different from those obtained by radiotherapy alone. Therefore, in most cases of advanced oesophageal cancer, oesophagectomy should be considered a palliative procedure, whose risks and benefits have to be carefully evaluated for each individual patient. Oesophagectomy may indeed provide a good quality of swallowing, which is usually sustained until death from advanced metastatic disease. Preoperative chemo/radiotherapy has obtained a remarkable frequency of complete pathological responses (15–30%) and a higher 2-year survival (35–40%) in phase II studies, but these results need to be confirmed by properly controlled prospective studies.

Bypass procedures for unresectable cancer can achieve effective and long-lasting relief of dysphagia. However, the results of oesophageal bypass are poor even in experienced hands, with perioperative mortality of 11–36% and median survival of about 6 months in most series (range 5–10, Table 6.3 [70–74]). Although the majority of patients are reported as having a significant improvement of dysphagia, the overall impact on quality of life is difficult to evaluate in such retrospective experiences. Oesophageal bypass may be advisable for occasional good-performance status patients, especially in the presence of tracheo-oesophageal fistula.

Radiation therapy can achieve a significant palliation of dysphagia in 60–80% of patients with oesophageal carcinoma, which usually lasts 5–10 months [75, 76]. Local relapse is, however, frequent after radiotherapy, and recurrent dysphagia represents a common clinical problem.

The insertion of an endoprosthesis or endoscopic laser resection are the main alternatives in this situation. Even in experienced hands, oesophageal intubation is associated with average 10% mortality and 20% morbidity, and a median survival of 4–6 months [77, 78]. A recent paper [79] has illustrated the results

Table 6.3 Results of surgical bypass for oesophageal cancer

Reference	No. pts.	Mortality (%)	Morbidity (%)	Symptoms relief (%)	Survival (median, months)
Orringer [70]	37	24	59	25	6
Mannell et al. [71]	124	11	50	82	5
Hirai et al. [72]	93	36	33	60	6
Segalin et al. [73]	49	20	46	71	6
Sawant and Moghissi [74]	70	22	NS	NS	10

NS = not specified.

achieved on 409 patients who underwent push-through intubation for cancer of the thoracic oesophagus and cardia, using different types of prosthesis (Celestin, Wilson-Cook, Atkinson). The hospital mortality was 3.4% (14/409). Perforation occurred in 20 cases (4.9%), resulting in the patients' death in six cases and requiring emergency bypass in four because of large perforation and effusion. Tube dislocation occurred in 52 patients (13%), requiring repositioning in 24, and removal of the tube in 19. Resumption of semi-solid oral feeding was possible in 80% of the discharged patients. The survival was 8% at 1 year, with a median of 4 months. Laser ablation has provided similar levels of symptomatic palliation (60–80%) with minimal or no mortality [73, 80–82]. The applicability and success of laser resection depends, however, on the location and extent of oesophageal stricture [83]. Recently, a randomized study [84] has shown that new expandable metal stents may be more effective than conventional plastic prostheses in terms of complication rate (0 vs. 43%), average hospital stay after the procedure (4 vs. 9 days) and 30-day mortality (14% vs. 29%). This observation is based on a total of 42 patients and needs to be confirmed by other studies, but the results appear encouraging.

Conclusions

Major thoracic surgery is rarely justified if the prospects for permanent cure are poor, as long-term survival is not improved. Advanced thymoma represents an exception to this rule. There are, however, several clinical conditions where the thoracic surgeon can be of help, relieving symptoms and improving the quality of life, with minor palliative procedures.

References

1. Naruke T, Goya T, Tsuchiya R, Suhemasu K (1988) Prognosis and survival in resected lung carcinoma based on the new international staging system. J Thorac Cardiovasc Surg 96:440–447.
2. Van Raemdonck DE, Schneider A, Ginsberg RJ (1992) Surgical treatment for higher-stage non-small-cell lung cancer. Ann Thorac Surg 54:999–1013.
3. Burkes RL, Ginsberg RJ, Shepherd FA, Blackstein ME, Goldberg ME, Waters PF, Patterson GA, Todd T, Pearson FG, Cooper JD, Jones D, Lockwood G (1993) Induction chemotherapy with MVP (mitomycin C + vindesine + cisplatin) for stage iii (t13, n2, m0) unresectable nonsmall cell lung cancer: the Toronto experience. Lung Cancer, 9:377–382.
4. Martini N, Kris MG, Flehinger BJ, Gralla RJ, Bains MS, Burt ME, Heelan R, McCormack PM, Pisters KM, Rigas JR et al. (1993) Preoperative chemotherapy for stage IIIa (N2) lung cancer: the Sloan-Kettering experience with 136 patients. Ann Thorac Surg 55:1365–1373.
5. Decker DA, Dines DE, Payne WS, Bernatz DE, Pairolero PC (1978) The significance of cytologically negative pleural effusion in bronchogenic carcinoma. Chest 6:640–642.
6. Martini N, McCormack PM (1983) Therapy of stage III non-metastatic disease. Semin Surg Oncol 10:95–110.
7. Burt M, Pomerantz AH, Bains MS, McCormack PM, Kaisr LR, Hilaris BS, Martini N

(1987) Results of surgical treatment of stage III lung cancer invading the mediastinum. Surg Clin North Am 67:987–1000.
8. Dartevelle PG, Chapelier AR, Pastorino U, Corbi P, Lenot B, Cerrina J, Bavoux EA, Verley JM, Neveux JY (1991) Long-term follow-up after prosthetic replacement of the superior vena cava combined with resection of mediastinal pulmonary malignant tumors. J Thorac Cardiovasc Surg 102:259–265.
9. Burt M, Wronski M, Arbit E, Galichich GH (1992) Resection of brain metastasis from non-small cell lung carcinoma. J Thorac Cardiovasc Surg 103:399–410.
10. Patchell RA, Tibbs PA, Walsh JW, Dempsey RJ, Maruyama Y, Kryschio RJ, Markesbery WR, MacDonald JS, Young B (1990) A randomized trial of surgery in the treatment of single metastases to the brain. N Engl J Med 322:494–500.
11. Reyes L, Parves Z, Nemoto T, Regal AM, Takita H (1990) Adrenalectomy for adrenal metastasis from lung carcinoma. J Surg Oncol 44:32–34.
12. Burt M (1994) Treatment of the solitary brain or adrenal metastasis in patients with non-small cell lung cancer. In: Motta G (ed) Lung cancer frontiers in science and treatment. Grafica LP, Genova, pp 513–521.
13. Shimizu N, Ando A, Date H, Teramoto S (1993) prognosis of undetected intrapulmonary metastases in resected lung cancer. Cancer 71:3868–3872.
14. Sozzi G, Miozzo M, Pastorino U et al. (1995) Genetic evidence for an independent origin of multiple preneoplastic and neoplastic lung lesions. Cancer Res 55:135–140.
15. Law MR, Gregor A, Hodson ME, Bloom HJG, Turner-Warwick M (1984) Malignant mesothelioma of the pleura: a study of 52 treated and 64 untreated patients. Thorax 39:255–259.
16. Tsang V, Goldstraw P (1989) Endobronchial stenting for anastomotic stenosis after sleeve resection. Ann Thorac Surg 48:568–571.
17. Goldstraw P (1987) Surgical management of pulmonary metastases. Baillière's clinical oncology. Ballières, London, 1:601–615.
18. McCormack PM (1990) Surgical resection of pulmonary metastases. Semin Surg Oncol 6(5):297–302.
19. Pastorino U, Gasparini M, Tavecchio L, Azzarelli A, Mapelli S, Zucchi V, Morandi F, Fossati-Bellani F, Valente M, Ravasi G (1991) The contribution of salvage surgery to the management of childhood osteosarcoma. J Clin Oncol 9:1357–1362.
20. Pastorino U, Valente M, Santoro A, Gasparini M, Azzarelli A, Casali P, Tavecchio L, Ravasi G (1990) Results of salvage surgery for metastatic sarcoma. Ann Oncol 1:269–273.
21. Roth JA, Pass HI, Wesley MN, White D, Putnam JB, Seipp C (1986) Comparison of median sternotomy and thoracotomy for resection of pulmonary metastases in patients with adult soft-tissue sarcomas. Ann Thorac Surg 42:134–138.
22. Rusch VW (1990) Diagnosis and treatment of pleural mesothelioma. Semin Surg Oncol 6:279–285.
23. Sugarbaker DJ, Mentzer SJ, Strauss G (1992) Extrapleural pneumonectomy in the treatment of malignant pleural mesothelioma. Ann Thorac Surg 54:941–946.
24. Ruffie P, Feld R, Minkin S, Cormier Y, Boutan-Laroze A, Ginsberg R, Ayoub J, Shepherd FA, Evans WK, Figueredo A (1989) Diffuse malignant mesothelioma of the pleura in Ontario and Quebec: a retrospective study of 332 patients. J Clin Oncol 7:1157–1168.
25. Sugarbaker DJ, Strauss GM, Lynch TJ, Richards W, Mentzer SJ, Lee TH, Corson JM, Antman KH (1993) Node status has prognostic significance in the multimodality therapy of diffuse, malignant mesothelioma. J Clin Oncol 11:1172–1178.
26. Rusch V, Saltz L, Venkatraman E, Ginsberg R, McCormack P, Burt M, Markman M, Kelsen D (1994) A phase II trial of pleurectomy/decortication followed by intrapleural and systemic chemotherapy for malignant pleural mesothelioma. J Clin Oncol 12:1156–1163.
27. Webb WR, Ozmen V, Moulder PV, Shabahang B, Breaux J (1993) Iodized talc

pleurodesis for the treatment of pleural effusions. J Thorac Cardiovasc Surg 103:881–886.
28. Petrou M, Kaplan D, Goldstraw P (1995) The management of recurrent malignant pleural effusion: the complementary role of talc pleurodesis and pleuroperitoneal shunting. Cancer 75:801–805.
29. Gordon MS, Hajdu SI, Bains MS, Burt ME (1991) Soft tissue sarcomas of the chest wall. Results of surgical resection. J Thorac Cardiovasc Surg 101:843–854.
30. Perry RR, Venzon D, Roth JA, Pass HI (1990) Survival after surgical resection for high-grade chest wall sarcomas. Ann Thorac Surg 49:363–368.
31. Maggi G, Casadio C, Pischedda F, Giobbe R, Cianci R, Ruffini E, Molinatti M, Mancuso M (1994) Combined radiosurgical treatment of Pancoast tumor. Ann Thorac Surg 57:198–202.
32. Sartori F, Rea F, Calabro F, Mazzucco C, Bortolotti L, Tomio L (1992) Carcinoma of the superior pulmonary sulcus. Results of irradiation and radical resection. J Thorac Cardiovasc Surg 104:679–683.
33. Ginsberg RJ, Martini N, Zaman M, Armstrong JG, Bains MS, Burt ME, McCormack PM, Rusch VW, Harrison LB (1994) Influence of surgical resection and brachytherapy in the management of superior sulcus tumor. Ann Thorac Surg 57:1440–1445.
34. Komaki R, Roh J, Cox J (1981) Superior sulcus tumors: results of irradiation of 36 patients. Cancer 48:1563–1568.
35. Van Houtte P, MacLennan I, Poulter C (1984) External radiation in the management of superior sulcus tumor. Cancer 54:223–227.
36. Fisher B, Redmond C, Fisher E et al. (1985) Ten-year results of a randomised clinical trial comparing radical mastectomy and total mastectomy with or without radiation. N Engl J Med 312:674–681.
37. Veronesi U, Saccozzi R, Del Vecchio M et al. (1981) Comparing radical mastectomy with quadrantectomy, axillary dissection, and radiotherapy in patients with small cancers of the breast. N Engl J Med 305–6–11.
38. McCormack PM, Bains MS, Burt ME, Martini N, Chaglassian T, Hidalgo DA (1989) Local recurrent mammary carcinoma failing multimodality therapy. A solution. Arch Surg 124:158–161.
39. Miyauchi K, Koyama H, Noguchi S, Inaji H, Yamamoto H, Kodama K, Iwanaga T (1992) Surgical treatment for chest wall recurrence of breast cancer. Eur J Cancer 28A:1059–1062.
40. Muscolino G, Valente M, Lequaglie C, Ravasi G (1992) Correlation between first disease-free interval from mastectomy to second disease-free interval from chest wall resection. Eur J Surg Oncol 18:49–52.
41. Dahlstrom KK, Andersson AP, Andersen M, Krag C (1993) Wide local excision of recurrent breast cancer in the thoracic wall. Cancer 72:774–777.
42. McCormack PM, Bains MS, Beattie ED Jr et al. (1981) New trends in skeletal reconstruction after resection of chest wall tumours. Ann Thorac Surg 31:45–56.
43. Masaoka A, Monden Y, Nakahara K, Tanioka T (1981) Follow-up study of thymoma with special reference to their clinical stages. Cancer 48:2485–2492.
44. Etienne T, Deleaval PJ, Spiliopoulos A, Megevand R (1993) Thymoma: prognostic factors. Eur J Cardiothorac Surg 7:449–452.
45. Fuentes P, Leude E, Ruiz C, Bordigoni L, Thomas P, Giudicelli R, Gastaud JA, Morati N (1992) Treatment of thymomas. A report of 67 cases. Eur J Cardiothorac Surg 6:180–188.
46. Park HS, Shin DM, Lee JS, Komaki R, Pollack A, Putnam JB, Cox JD, Hong WK (1994) Thymoma. A retrospective study of 87 cases. Cancer 73:2491–2498.
47. Maggi G, Casadio C, Cavallo A, Cianci R, Molinatti M, Ruffini E (1991) Thymoma: results of 241 operated cases. Ann Thorac Surg 51:152–156.
48. Kirschner PA (1990) Reoperation for thymoma: report of 23 cases. Ann Thorac Surg 49:550–555.

49. Cohen DJ, Ronningen LD, Graeber JM et al. (1984) Management of patients with malignant thymoma. J Thorac Cardiovasc Surg 87:301–307.
50. Ichinose Y, Ohta M, Yano T, Yokoyama H, Asoh H, Hata K (1993) Treatment of invasive thymoma with pleural dissemination. J Surg Oncol 54:180–183.
51. Shimizu N, Moriyama S, Aoe M, Nakata M, Ando A,Teramoto S (1992) The surgical treatment of invasive thymoma. Resection with vascular reconstruction. J Thorac Cardiovasc Surg 103:414–420.
52. Oudkerk M, Heystraten FM, Stoter G (1993) Stenting in malignant vena caval obstruction. Cancer 71:142–146.
53. Watkinson AF, Hansell DM (1993) Expandable wallstent for the treatment of obstruction of the superior vena cava. Thorax 48:915–920.
54. Piehler JM, Pluth JR, Schaff HV, Danielson GK, Orszulak TA, Puga FJ (1985) Surgical management of pericardial disease: influence of extent of pericardial resection on clinical course. J Thorac Cardiovasc Surg 90:506–516.
55. Park JS, Rentschler R, Wilbur D (1991) Surgical management of pericardial effusion in patients with malignancies. Comparison of subxiphoid window versus pericardiectomy. Cancer 67:76–80.
56. Keane D, Jackson G (1992) Managing recurrent malignant pericardial effusions. Br Med J 305:729–730.
57. Wang N, Feikes JR, Mogensen T, Vyhmeister EE, Bailey LL (1994) Pericardioperitoneal shunt: an alternative treatment for malignant pericardial effusion. Ann Thorac Surg 57:289–292.
58. Shepherd MP (1982) Endobronchial metastatic disease. Thorax 37:362–365.
59. Mathisen DJ, Grillo HC (1989) Endoscopic relief of malignant airway obstruction. Ann Thorac Surg 48:469–475.
60. Cavaliere S, Foccoli P, Farina PL (1988) Nd-YAG laser bronchoscopy. A five-year experience with 1396 applications in 1000 patients. Chest 94:15–21.
61. Dumon JF, Shapshay S, Bourcereau J, Cavaliere S, Meric B, Garbi N, Beamis J (1984) Principles for safety in application of neodymium-YAG laser in bronchology. Chest 86:163–168.
62. Walsh DA, Maiwand MO, Naith AR, Lockwood P, Lloyd MH, Saab M (1990) Bronchoscopic cryotherapy for advanced bronchial carcinoma. Thorax 45:509–513.
63. Ledingham SJM, Goldstraw P (1989) Diathermy resection and gold grains for palliation of obstruction due to recurrence of bronchial carcinoma after external irradiation. Thorax 44:48–51.
64. Burt PA, O'Driscoll BR, Notley HM, Barber PV, Stout R (1990) Intraluminal irradiation for the palliation of lung cancer with the high dose rate micro-Selectron. Thorax 45:765–768.
65. Dumon JF (1990) A dedicated tracheobronchial stent. Chest 97:328–332.
66. Goldstraw P (1995) Endobronchial stents. In: Etzel M (ed) Minimally invasive therapies in thoracic medicine and surgery. Chapman and Hall, London.
67. Petrou M, Kaplan D, Goldstraw P (1993) Bronchoscopic diathermy resection and stent insertion: a cost effective treatment for tracheobronchial obstruction. Thorax 48:1156–1159.
68. Siewert JR, Fink U, Beckurts KT, Roder JD (1994) Surgery of squamous cell carcinoma of the esophagus. Ann Oncol 5 (supp 3): 1–7.
69. Wilke H, Siewert JR, Fink U, Stahl M (1994) Current status and future directions in the treatment of localized esophageal cancer. Ann Oncol 5 (suppl 3): 27–32.
70. Orringer MB (1984) Substernal gastric bypass of the excluded esophagus: results of an ill-advised operation. Surgery 96:467–470.
71. Mannell A, Becker PJ, Nissenbaum M (1988) Bypass surgery for unresectable esophageal cancer: early and late results in 124 cases. Br J Surg 75:283–286.
72. Hirai T, Yamashita T, Mukaida H et al. (1988) Bypass operation for unresectable oseophageal cancer: early and late results in 124 cases. Br J Surg 75:283–286.
73. Segalin A, Little AG, Ruol A, Ferguson MK, Bardini R, Norberto L, Skinner DB,

Peracchia A (1989) Surgical and endoscopic palliation of esophageal carcinoma. Ann Thorac Surg 48:267–271.
74. Sawant D, Moghissi K (1994) Management of unresectable oesophageal cancer: a review of 537 patients. Eur J Cardiothorac Surg 8:113–116.
75. Kelsen D, Minsky B, Smith M, Beitler J, Niedzwieki D et al. (1990) Preoperative therapy for esophageal cancer: a randomized comparison of chemotherapy versus radiation therapy. J Clin Oncol 8:1352–1361.
76. Morita K, Takagi I, Watanabe M, Niwa K, Kazanawa H (1985) Relationship between radiologic features of esophageal cancer and the local control by radiation therapy. Cancer 55:2668–2676.
77. Buset M, De Marez B, Baize M et al. (1987) Palliative endoscopic management of obstructive esophageal cancer: laser or prosthesis. Gastrointest Endosc 33:357–361.
78. Pattison CW, Griffin SC, Cocker C, Townsend ER, Fountain SW (1990) Palliative intubation of malignant oesophageal strictures. Scand J Thorac Cardiovasc Surg 24:153–155.
79. Cusumano A, Ruol A, Segalin A (1992) Push-through intubation: effective palliation in 409 patients with cancer of the esophagus and cardia. Ann Thorac Surg 53:1010–1014.
80. Carter R, Smith JS, Anderson JR (1993) Palliation of malignant dysphagia using the Nd:YAG laser. World J Surg 17:608–613.
81. Hahl J, Salo J, Ovaska J, Haapiainen R, Kalima T, Schroder T (1991) Comparison of endoscopic Nd:YAG laser therapy and oesophageal tube in palliation of oesophagogastric malignancy. Scand J Gastroenterol 26:103–108.
82. Reed CE, Marsh WH, Carlson LS, Seymore CH, Kratz JM (1991) Prospective, randomized trial of palliative treatment for unresectable cancer of the esophagus. Ann Thorac Surg 51:552–555.
83. Shmueli E, Myszor MF, Burke D, Record CO, Matthewson K (1992) Limitations of laser treatment of malignant dysphagia. Br J Surg 79:778–780.
84. Knyrim K, Wagner HJ, Bethge N, Keymling M, Vakil N (1993) A controlled trial of an expansile metal stent for palliation of esophageal obstruction due to inoperable cancer. N Engl J Med 329:1302–1307.

Section 2

Non-Curative Radiotherapy

7 – Non-Curative Radiotherapy for Lung Cancer

D.J. Boote and N.M. Bleehen

Introduction

Lung cancer is the commonest malignancy in the Western world. In the UK it is the commonest malignancy in men and the second commonest in women after breast cancer. In the UK, lung cancer accounted for 40 000 deaths in 1990. In Scotland and parts of northern England, lung cancer has recently overtaken breast cancer as the main cause of female cancer death.

There are four main histological types: squamous (40%), small cell (25%), adenocarcinoma (20%) and large cell (15%). Small cell carcinoma is the most malignant and many patients have extrathoracic disease at presentation. For treatment purposes, it is useful to divide patients into two groups: those who have non-small cell lung cancer (NSCLC) and those with small cell lung cancer (SCLC).

The treatment of choice for NSCLC is surgery. However, only a small proportion of patients have operable tumours and are fit for surgery. Radical radiotherapy is an alternative for those with small tumours who are unfit or refuse surgery. Unfortunately, the majority of patients with NSCLC are unsuitable for either of these treatments and are considered for palliative radiotherapy.

The treatment of choice for SCLC is chemotherapy, except for the rare patients with $T_1M_0M_0$ disease. Some of these patients may benefit from adjuvant radiotherapy to the chest and this will be discussed later.

Non-Small Cell Lung Cancer

Most patients (80%) with NSCLC are unsuitable for radical treatment and are considered for palliative radiotherapy. The most common symptoms are cough (70%), dyspnoea (45%), haemoptysis (40%), chest pain (40%) and weight loss (30%).

The aim of palliative radiotherapy is to relieve distressing symptoms without treatment-related morbidity and this can usually be achieved very rapidly. In this context, the questions that need to be addressed are:

1. Does radiotherapy improve quality of life and/or duration of survival?
2. When should the radiotherapy be given?
3. What is the optimal dose and fractionation?

There is a paucity of randomized trials addressing the relevant questions and only the most recent studies have included quality-of-life assessments. There is little doubt that radiotherapy can control many of the symptoms associated with lung cancer, either at presentation or during its course. Thus, in a recent MRC study [1], palliation of major symptoms was achieved for a useful time for cough (52%), haemoptysis (40%), chest pain (66%) and dysphagia (63%). In addition, most patients (70%) with superior vena caval obstruction due to NSCLC get good symptomatic relief from palliative radiotherapy. However, palliative radiotherapy is less useful for hoarseness due to recurrent laryngeal nerve involvement and non-metastatic symptoms such as weight loss.

The earliest study looking at survival in patients with inoperable lung cancer was organized by the US Veterans Administration [2] and used survival as the end-point. A total of 308 patients received 40–50 Gy in 4–6 weeks, while 246 received placebo capsules. Symptomatic relief was not assessed, but the median survival time (MST) was 112 days and 1-year survival 13.9% in the control group, and 142 days and 18.2% in the radiotherapy group ($p = 0.01$). A major problem with this study was that the level of supportive care for the radiotherapy group (in-patients) was better than for the control group who were treated as out-patients.

In contrast, another trial [3] found no advanced in survival or quality of life, as assessed by an arbitrary index, for immediate radiotherapy over supportive care. The high MST (240 days) suggested considerable selection of better prognosis patients.

Berry et al. [4] compared radiotherapy versus control arms which were treated with chemotherapy. They found no difference in survival between the three regimens. A more recent study [5] found that thoracic radiotherapy did not prolong survival in patients with locally advanced NSCLC. However, the radiotherapy technique used in this study has been criticized, as simulation was not routinely used in treatment planning. Kubata et al. [6] gave a group of patients with locally advanced NSCLC chemotherapy and then randomized them to receive or not receive radiotherapy (50–60 Gy). Radiotherapy significantly prolonged the time to progression and increased the 2-year survival from 6% to 29% ($p < 0.05$).

There is controversy as to whether patients with inoperable tumours, with no or minimal symptoms, should have thoracic radiotherapy immediately or whether this should be reserved for symptom control. Some radiotherapists advocate a policy of immediate radiotherapy in the belief that local control will improve quality of life and may prolong survival. In contrast, others recommend waiting until symptoms develop, since there is no convincing evidence that immediate radiotherapy prolongs survival or improves quality of life. Randomized trials are needed to determine the role and timing of radiotherapy in these patients. An MRC study is currently under way in patients with inoperable NSCLC where patients receive supportive care and are randomized either to immediate thoracic radiotherapy or to radiotherapy delayed until the onset of symptoms. The end-points are both quality of life and survival.

Several studies have shown that equal palliation and survival may be achieved with different radiotherapy doses and fractionation [7, 8]. A sequence of three MRC studies since 1985 have investigated the dose/fraction requirements for palliation. In the first MRC study [9], 369 patients with inoperable NSCLC, too advanced for radical radiotherapy, were randomized to receive either a conventional regimen of 30 Gy in 10 fractions over 2 weeks, or 17 Gy given as two 8.5 Gy fractions 1 week apart.

Prior to treatment, 93% of patients complained of cough, 58% anorexia, 57% chest pain, 47% haemoptysis and 11% dysphagia. Symptom palliation was achieved in a high proportion of patients, e.g. 65% for cough and 81% for haemoptysis in the two-fraction group, and 56% for cough and 86% for haemoptysis in the ten-fraction group. For the major symptoms, the median duration of palliation was $\geqslant$50% of survival. For poor performance status patients there was an improvement in performance status in about 50% of patients. Quality of life, as assessed by diary cards, deteriorated slightly during treatment but improved over the following month. The number of patients complaining of severe dysphagia increased from about 5% to about 40% during treatment. The results were similar in the two treatment groups. The median survival time was 179 days in the two-fraction group and 177 days in the ten-fraction group. There was one case of possible radiation myelopathy in a patient who had received the two-fraction regimen. In this study, a local radiographic response to radiotherapy was recorded in 30% of patients.

The ensuing study [1] in 233 patients investigated whether a single fraction of 10 Gy could provide equal palliation to 17 Gy in two fractions (as used in [9]), in patients with inoperable NSCLC. This study was limited to patients with a rather worse performance status (WHO 2–4) than in the first study. At entry to the study, 95% of patients had cough, 64% anorexia, 59% chest pain, 47% haemoptysis and 16% dysphagia. The rate of symptom palliation varied from 48% to 75%. The median duration of palliation was $\geqslant$ 50% of survival. All these results were similar in the two treatment groups. The median survival time was 100 days in the two-fraction group and 122 days in the single fraction group. The only significant difference was in radiation-induced dysphagia which occurred in 56% of the two-fraction regimen and in 23% of the single fraction regimen.

A further study [10] was completed in 1992 on 509 patients with good performance status (WHO 0–2) with localized, inoperable NSCLC too advanced for radical radiotherapy. These patients were randomized to receive 17 Gy in two fractions 1 week apart or 39 Gy in 13 fractions over 2.5 weeks. A preliminary analysis showed that palliation was similar in both groups, but there was a significant increase ($p = 0.06$) in the MST of 275 days in the 13-fraction group over the 222 days for patients receiving two fractions. The 1-year survival was 31% in the two-fraction group and 37% in the 13-fraction group. The 2-year survival was 10% in the two-fraction group and 11% in the 13-fraction group. Dysphagia was more severe in the 13-fraction group. It was reported by 43% of patients in the two-fraction group and lasted for a median of 5 days. In the 13-fraction group, dysphagia was reported in 59% of patients and lasted for a median of 10 days. Two patients in the 13-fraction group developed radiation myelopathy. It is uncertain at this time whether the small increase in MST at 1 and 2 years justifies the use of the longer treatment regimen. Detailed analysis of quality-of-life assessments will help, but these results are not yet available.

Adverse Effects of Palliative Radiotherapy

The only common adverse effect is dysphagia. This occurs in approximately 40% of patients and lasts for up to 2 weeks. This is usually controlled with a local anaesthetic preparation such as mucaine liquid 10 ml t.d.s. The incidence of radiation myelopathy in the first two MRC studies was approximately 0.5% for patients receiving either 17 Gy in two fractions a week apart or a single fraction of 10 Gy.

Specific Problems

Superior Vena Cava Obstruction (SVCO)

This syndrome develops in about 5% of patients with lung cancer, and lung cancer (especially small cell carcinoma) accounts for 85% of cases of SVCO, with approximately 10% of cases of SVCO being due to malignant lymphoma. The commonest symptoms are dyspnoea and swelling of the upper half of the body. On examination, these patients usually have distension of the veins in the neck and chest, facial oedema and cyanosis. The usual finding on chest X-ray is of a mass in the right superior mediastinum. Histological diagnosis is important and can usually be obtained by bronchoscopy, lymph node biopsy or mediastinoscopy. Treatment depends on tumour type. Chemotherapy is given for chemosensitive tumours such as lymphoma and SCLC. Radiotherapy is given when the cause is NSCLC.

All patients should be commenced on dexamethasone. Oxygen is administered if the patient is hypoxic. Radiotherapy should be given promptly, to include the mediastinal mass and superior vena cava. A dose of 20 Gy in five fractions over 5 days or 17 Gy in two fractions over 8 days is adequate. Radiotherapy relieves symptoms in about 70% of patients. The median survival is 4 months for NSCLC and 10 months for SCLC.

Respiratory obstruction caused by extensive tumour compression or by intrinsic tumour growth is an acute emergency and is treated with high-dose dexamethasone and palliative radiotherapy. Alternatively, the obstruction can be relieved using a laser or endobronchial brachytherapy (see later).

Pancoast Tumours

Tumours at the lung apex are sometimes known as superior sulcus tumours. When this occurs with Horner's syndrome and pain in the arm they are called Pancoast tumours. They are caused by invasion by tumour of the brachial plexus and the cervical sympathetic plexus. Most patients present with pain in the upper chest and shoulder region.

Pancoast tumours require a higher dose of radiotherapy than for other palliative treatments [11]. In addition, it is important that for these tumours the whole of the adjacent vertebrae are included in the radiotherapy treatment field. A typical dose would be 40 Gy in 20 fractions over 4 weeks followed by treatment to the tumour only (not including spinal cord) with a further 20 Gy in ten fractions over 2 weeks.

Re-treatment

There are very few studies that have looked at retreatment with radiotherapy. Jackson and Ball [12] re-treated patients with a dose of 20–30 Gy over 2–3 weeks. Symptoms improved in 52% of patients. Montebello et al. [13] re-treated 30 patients who had previously received radiotherapy (median dose 60 Gy in 6 weeks). The median time from initial radiation to recurrence was 12 months. The median retreatment dose was 3030 cGy over 3 weeks. Symptoms improved in 70% of patients. Re-treatment toxicity included oesophagitis (20% patients), dry desquamation (13%) and pneumonitis (3%).

Trials suggest that haemoptysis and pain are palliated more effectively than other symptoms such as dyspnoea. In our experience, a single fraction of 8 Gy is effective for re-treatment in lung cancer, provided that the volume of spinal cord in the field is kept to a minimum.

Small Cell Lung Cancer

Chemotherapy is the standard treatment for patients with SCLC. For patients with limited disease (defined as disease confined to one side of the thorax), giving thoracic radiotherapy reduces the risk of local recurrence from approximately 75% to 30%. The effect of radiotherapy on survival is controversial, as the results of several randomized studies addressing this question have been inconsistent. A meta-analysis [14] showed that thoracic radiotherapy moderately improves survival by about 5% at 3 years.

It is recommended that thoracic radiotherapy is given following chemotherapy only to patients with limited disease who have had either a complete or good partial response to chemotherapy. A dose of 40–50 Gy (conventional fractionation) is usually given.

For patients with symptomatic relapse or progressive SCLC, radiotherapy is often useful, and response rates of 60% or more have been seen [15]. For these patients, a dose of 17 Gy in two fractions over 8 days or a single fraction of 10 Gy is recommended.

The brain is a common site for metastases in patients with SCLC. Prophylactic cranial irradiation (PCI) reduces the incidence of cerebral metastases from 22% to 8% [16]. However, it is not known whether PCI confers a survival benefit, and in addition PCI may cause neurological abnormalities such as memory loss and ataxia. In view of this uncertainty, PCI should only be given to patients with limited disease who achieve a complete response to chemotherapy and ideally these patients should be included in the current UKCCR trial which is looking at the value of PCI.

Endobronchial Techniques

Several methods of endobronchial treatment have been tried, including stents, laser therapy and endobronchial radiotherapy. Laser therapy is effective and rapidly relieves symptoms. However, it is associated with more morbidity than endobronchial brachytherapy and may produce a shorter duration of response

[17]. Endobronchial radiotherapy delivers a high dose of radiotherapy to the tumour using a catheter placed next to the tumour. It produces a very localized treatment and spares the surrounding normal tissues from the effects of radiation. Treatment is given using a miniature high-activity iridium source via a remote afterloading system (e.g. the micro Selectron-HDR). The treatment catheter (2 mm diameter) is inserted under local anaesthetic using a fibreoptic bronchoscope, and usually this can be performed as a day-case procedure. A typical dose is 15 Gy prescribed at 1 cm from the course. Treatment takes approximately 15 min, and can relieve the symptoms of bronchial obstruction by tumour or extraluminal pressure by lymph nodes.

A study in the USA [18] reported on 80 high-dose-rate endobronchial treatments in 32 patients. Half of the patients (group 1) received endoscopic brachytherapy as a boost to primary external-beam radiotherapy. The other half (group 2) were treated for endobronchial recurrence after prior external beam radical radiotherapy. The usual dose was 15 Gy in three fractions at weekly intervals. The median follow-up was 9 months. Symptomatic improvement was observed in haemoptysis (100%), cough (86%) and dyspnoea (100%). In ten patients, follow-up endoscopy was performed and revealed a pathological complete response. At 6 months after treatment local control was obtained in 88% of the patients in group 1 and in 70% of the patients in group 2. The treatment was well tolerated and without complications.

In a recent study from the Christie Hospital in Manchester [19], 406 patients with inoperable symptomatic bronchial carcinoma were given intraluminal radiotherapy (ILT). Most patients (80%) were previously unirradiated and received a single fraction of ILT as their primary treatment. A dose of 15–20 Gy was delivered at 1 cm from the centre of the treatment source. At 6 weeks following treatment there was an improvement in stridor (92%), haemoptysis (88%), cough (62%), dyspnoea (60%), pain (50%) and pulmonary collapse (46%). A large proportion (67%) of these patients required no further treatment during their lifetime. A second group of 65 patients (16%) consisted of patients whose disease had recurred following prior external beam radiotherapy. Symptom palliation at 6 weeks was similar to that seen in the first group, although the duration of palliation was shorter. A third group of 17 patients (4%) received concurrent ILT with external beam radiotherapy and achieved similar levels of symptom palliation as in the first group of patients. Overall the treatment was well tolerated apart from a temporary exacerbation of cough lasting about 2 weeks.

Randomized trials are under way to investigate the usefulness of endobronchial radiotherapy in combination with external beam treatment to try to improve local control, and also its use as second-line treatment in previously irradiated patients.

Conclusions

Palliative radiotherapy is worth while in patients with advanced lung cancer. It leads to an improvement in symptoms in most patients and does not cause significant morbidity. In addition to helping the primary tumour, radiotherapy is also effective in the treatment of symptoms due to metastases. Palliative radiotherapy is being made more acceptable to patients by a considerable reduction in its overall duration.

References

1. Bleehen NM, Girling DJ, Machin D et al. (1992) A Medical Research Council randomised trial of palliative radiotherapy with two fractions or a single fraction in patients with inoperable non-small cell lung cancer (NSCLC) and poor performance status. Br J Cancer 65:934–941.
2. Roswit B, Paton ME, Rapp R et al. (1968) The survival of patients with inoperable lung cancer: a large scale randomized study of radiation therapy versus placebo. Radiology 90:688–697.
3. Durrant KR, Berry RJ, Ellis F et al. (1971) Comparison of treatment policies in inoperable bronchial carcinoma. Lancet 1:715–719.
4. Berry RJ, Laing AH, Newman CR et al. (1977) The role of radiotherapy in treatment of inoperable lung cancer. Int J Radiat Oncol Biol Phys 2:422–439.
5. Johnson DH, Einhorn LH, Bartolucci et al. (1990) Thoracic radiotherapy does not prolong survival in patients with locally advanced, unresectable, non-small cell lung cancer. Ann Intern Med 113:33–38.
6. Kubata K, Furuse K, Kawahara M et al. (1990) Randomized trial of chemotherapy with or without thoracic radiation therapy for treatment of locally advanced non-small cell lung cancer. Proc Am Soc Clin Oncol 9:226.
7. Simpson JR, Francis ME, Pérez-Tamayo R et al. (1985) Palliative radiotherapy for inoperable carcinoma of the lung. Final report of a RTOG multi-institutional trial. Int J Radiat Oncol Biol Phys 11:751–758.
8. Teo P, Tai TH, Choy D et al. (1988) A randomized study on palliative radiation therapy for inoperable non-small cell carcinoma of the lung. Int J Radiat Oncol Biol Phys 14:867–871.
9. Medical Research Council (1991) Inoperable non-small cell lung cancer (NSCLC): a Medical Research Council randomised trial of palliative radiotherapy with two fractions or ten fractions. Br J Cancer 63:265–270.
10. Medical Research Council (1994) Randomised trial of two radiotherapy policies for patients with inoperable non-small cell lung cancer and good performance status. Lung Cancer 11:131.
11. Van Houtte P, Maclennan I, Poulter C et al. (1984) External radiation in the management of superior sulcus tumour. Cancer 54:223–227.
12. Jackson M, Ball D (1987) Palliative retreatment of locally recurrent lung cancer after radical radiotherapy. Med J Aust 147:391–394.
13. Montebello JF, Aron BS, Manatunga AK et al. (1993) The reirradiation of recurrent bronchogenic carcinoma with external beam irradiation. Am J Clin Oncol 16(6):482–488.
14. Pignon J, Arriagada R, Ihde D et al. (1992) A meta-analysis of thoracic radiotherapy for small cell lung cancer. N Engl J Med 327:1618–1624.
15. Ochs JJ, Tester WJ, Cohen MH et al. (1983) Salvage radiation therapy for intrathoracic small cell carcinoma of the lung progressing on combination chemotherapy. Cancer Treat Rep 67(12):1123–1126.
16. Bleehen NM (1986) Radiotherapy for small cell lung cancer. Chest 89 (suppl): 268s–276s.
17. Hetzel MR, Nixon C, Edmonstone WM et al. (1985) Laser therapy in 100 tracheobronchial tumours. Thorax 40:341–345.
18. Nori D, Allison R, Kaplan B et al. (1993) High dose-rate intraluminal irradiation in bronchogenic carcinoma: technique and results. Chest 104(4):1006–1011.
19. Gollins SW, Burt PA, Barber PV et al. (1994) High dose rate intraluminal radiotherapy for carcinoma of the bronchus: outcome of treatment of 406 patients. Radiother Oncol 33:31–40.

8 – Non-Curative Radiotherapy for Bone Metastases

M.E.B. Powell and P.J. Hoskin

Introduction: Prognosis and Clinical Course

Bone metastases account for more than 95% of malignant bone tumours. Although virtually all cancers can give rise to bone metastases it is carcinoma of the breast, prostate, bronchus and kidney that show a particular propensity for dissemination to bone and may be present in up to 50% of patients with these malignancies.

In general, once bone metastases have developed the overall prognosis is poor and the patient is considered to have incurable disease. There are exceptions to this and these include germ-cell tumours, well-differentiated thyroid cancer and high-grade non-Hodgkin's lymphoma. In these malignancies curative systemic treatment is available. However, for the majority of patients who have incurable bone metastases, survival is greatly influenced by primary histology, patients with melanoma and lung cancer having a median survival of less than 6 months compared with 2 years for breast and prostatic cancer. For this latter group of patients, where the disease may run a long clinical course and in whom bone may be the only clinically detectable site of metastases, effective palliation is of particular importance in maintaining function and improving quality of life.

Pathophysiology

Tumour cells reach bone primarily through blood-borne spread, although direct invasion can also take place, mainly from pharyngeal, lung and pelvic cancers. The process of haematogenous dissemination into the medullary cavity of bone is not simply random. It is characterized by a complex sequence of interactions between host and tumour cells controlled at the molecular level [1].

The distribution of metastases is influenced by many tumour- and host-related factors that will include anatomical considerations, chemotactic factors and organ susceptibility. Although any bone may be involved, it is the axial skeleton that is predominantly affected and this is probably a reflection of the distribution of red marrow in the adult. The majority of patients will have radiological evidence of widespread disease at the time of clinical presentation, but in a few patients solitary metastases can be found. These are classically associated with renal cell carcinoma and neuroblastoma, but may occur in any tumour type.

Once tumour cells reach bone they are able to disrupt the normal bone remodelling process and much work has been performed to elucidate the cellular mechanisms by which this occurs. Normal bone is in a dynamic state of formation and resorption, and the balance between these two processes is finely regulated by changing mechanical stresses and mineral homeostasis. It is thought that many of the mediators important in regulating normal bone remodelling are produced in abnormal amounts in the presence of malignant cells [2].

Most tumour-induced skeletal destruction is mediated by osteoclasts and the initial step in the malignant process is osteoclast proliferation [3], which leads to increased bone resorption. This is stimulated by numerous factors secreted by or in response to the tumour. Examples of such factors include prostaglandins, epidermal growth factor, osteoclast activating factor (OAF), tumour growth factor α and β, interleukin-1 and parathormone. Prostaglandins, in particular PGE_2, are considered to be among the most potent inducers of bone resorption in epithelial cancer, whereas OAF, a cytokine produced by lymphocytes, is important in the development of lytic lesions in haematological malignancies.

Osteoblastic activity is also enhanced in the presence of tumour cells, although the regulation of this is far less clearly defined. Osteoblasts are attracted to sites of bone resorption where they produce focal osteoid that fills in defects caused by the osteolytic process. Various factors have been identified that stimulate this activity, and these include transforming growth factor-β, platelet derived growth factor, macrophage colony stimulating factor and prostaglandins [2].

Both osteoclastic and osteoblastic activity is evident in all bone metastases, and it is the relative proportion of bone resorption and formation that determines the radiographic appearances of bone lesions. If bone resorption predominates, the radiographic appearance will be lytic as in myeloma, whereas increased osteoblastic activity, as in carcinoma of the prostate, will give rise to dense sclerotic lesions. This spectrum is illustrated in Figure 8.1.

Symptoms

Although pain is the cardinal feature of bone metastases, most, in fact, do not cause symptoms [4]. The pain is characteristically dull, unremitting and exacerbated by movement. Although usually localized, it may be referred or induce symptoms of nerve compression. It is well recognized that the extent of disease does not always correlate with the severity of symptoms. Patients may have widespread osseous metastases with minimal symptoms or conversely may have severe pain in the presence of only a solitary bone lesion.

The actual mechanism by which bony involvement causes pain is poorly understood. It is postulated that two components contribute to the development of symptoms [5]. First, the presence of tumour may cause local oedema, distortion of the periosteum and growth into surrounding tissues. Secondly, chemical mediators such as bradykinins, histamine and substance P, released by the damaged bone in response to the neoplastic process, may result in stimulation of nociceptors in the endosteum. However, no data are yet available to substantiate these hypotheses.

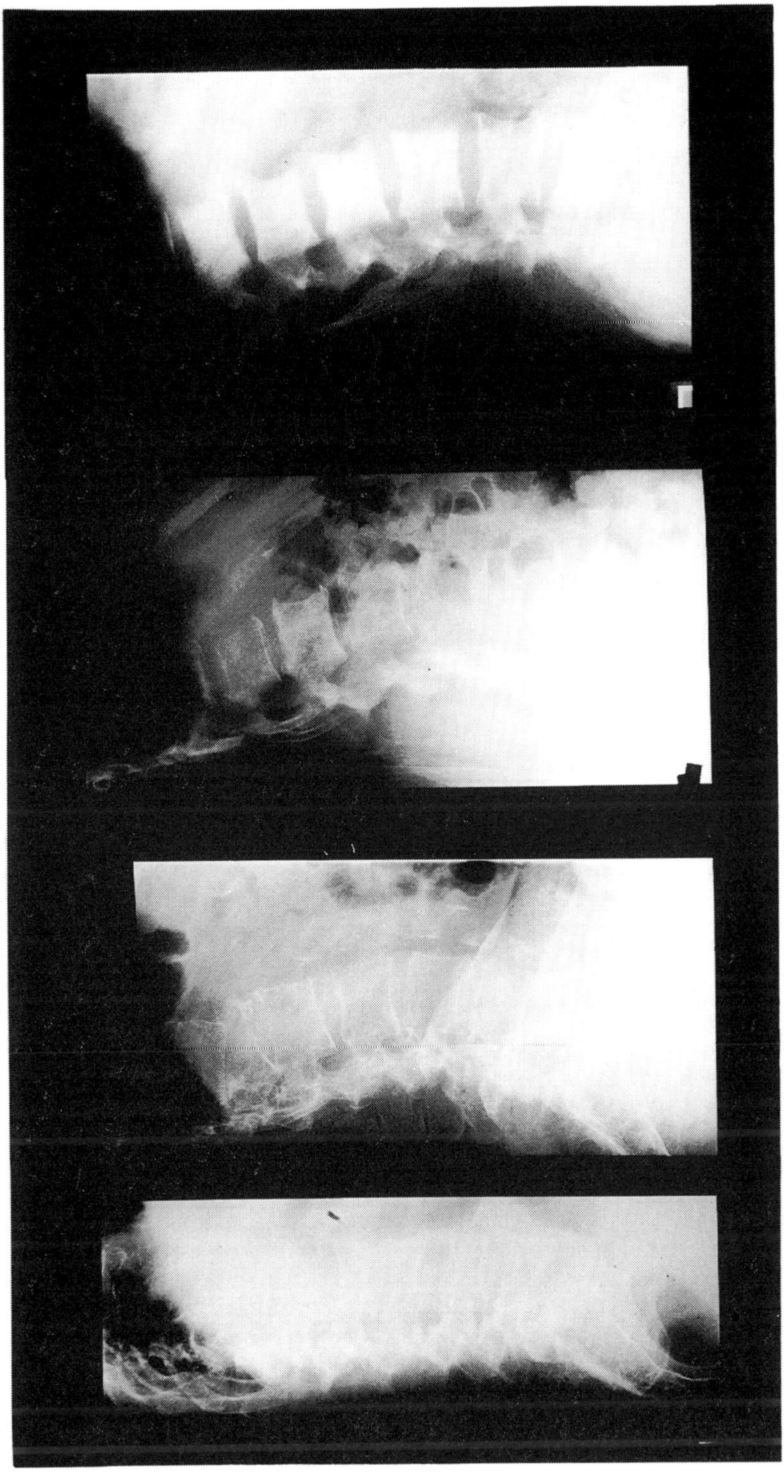

Figure 8.1 X-rays demonstrating the spectrum of change following the development of bone metastasis from diffuse lytic disease to extensive sclerotic disease, both appearances reflecting a different balance of osteoclastic and osteoblastic activity in response to the tumour cells

Radiotherapy in the Treatment of Bone Metastases

The primary objectives of treatment of bone metastases are relief of painful symptoms, prevention of pathological fractures and treatment of spinal cord or nerve compression. Effective treatment will result in pain control with improved function, mobility and quality of life.

Ionizing radiation has long been recognized as a useful means of treating bone pain, and by the mid-1920s it became established as a highly effective method of relieving pain, with reported response rates of 80% [6]. Despite this, the biological basis of its action in promoting analgesia remains a matter of conjecture.

Following irradiation, radiographic features of bone healing, with recalcification and reossification, can be observed in up to 75% of patients and occur within 2 months of treatment [7]. These changes, while stabilizing the bone, are probably only partly responsible for the control of symptoms. Very low doses can confer significant pain relief, often occurring within hours of treatment [8]. It has been suggested that this rapid analgesic effect is mediated by a cytotoxic response, with inhibition of the release of substances such as prostaglandins and kinins which are known to modulate the pain response [9, 10].

Local External Beam Radiotherapy

A wide range of dose fractionation schedules have been evaluated in a number of retrospective studies [11]. These have shown that local radiotherapy can achieve pain relief in up to 80% of patients, with single doses of 4–15 Gy being as effective as fractionated courses of 40 Gy or more. Many of these surveys conclude that response does not seem to be influenced by either dose of radiotherapy or histology of the tumour and that analgesic effect is not simply based upon tumour radiosensitivity. These studies are of limited value since, in the main, they involve retrospective review of case notes, no pretreatment assessment of pain and unreliable or unvalidated measures of treatment response.

There have been six prospective, randomized trials of local radiotherapy in a palliative setting (Table 8.1). These have set out to determine the optimum dose fractionation schedule and to assess the efficacy of a single fraction of radiotherapy in palliating symptoms.

The largest is the RTOG multicentre study involving over 1000 patients and using physicians' assessment of pain relief. The initial publication of the trial's findings suggested that a protracted high-dose regimen was equivalent to a low-dose 5-day schedule in providing symptom control in patients with both solitary or multiple metastases [12]. The data was reanalysed, with all patients grouped together, and the pain score adapted to include both analgesic requirements and the need for retreatment. It concluded, conversely, that protracted courses offer significantly improved pain relief [13]. These contrary results serve to emphasize that, to create an objective end-point, clearly defined, validated methods of pain assessment are necessary.

The findings of the second analysis are not borne out in a trial carried out in 288 patients at the Royal Marsden Hospital, comparing a single treatment with a fractionated course of radiotherapy [14]. Patients used an independently

Table 8.1 Prospective randomized studies of localized radiotherapy in bone pain

Reference	No. of patients	Dose (Gy)/ fractions/days	Overall response (%)	Complete response (%)
Tong et al. [12]	72	20/5f/5d	90	53
	74	40.5/15f/19d	92	61
	613	15–30/5–10f/ 5–12d	89	53
Madsen [36]	27	20/2f/8d	48	
	30	24/6f/18d	47	
Price et al. [14]	140	8/1f/1d	85	27
	148	30/10f/12d	85	27
Okawa et al. [37]	27	20/10f/5d	78	37
	36	22.5/5f/14	75	42
	29	30/15f/20d	76	41
Cole [15]	16	8/1f/1d	100	
	13	24/6f/14–21d	100	
Hoskin [16]	137	4/1f/1d	53	26
		8/1f/1d	76	23

validated questionnaire to assess pain both before and after radiotherapy. Results from this study suggest that a single 8 Gy fraction is as effective as 30 Gy in ten fractions in providing pain relief, with an overall response rate of 85%. In addition, the speed of onset of pain relief was similar in both treatment arms, with 65% responding at 4 weeks and, in responders, 39–48% remained pain free at 24 weeks.

Concern about increased toxicity from large fractions has been expressed, especially where large field sizes are used. The above study, however, found that neither field size nor fractionation influenced acute toxicity, and a second smaller trial [15], comparing single and multiple fractions, also found that the toxicity associated with treatment was similar in both treatment arms.

Evidence for a dose response in pain relief is sparse. A second trial from the Royal Marsden Hospital attempted to address this question for single fractions of radiotherapy [16]. A total of 270 patients were randomized to receive single treatments of either 4 or 8 Gy. There was a significant difference in the incidence of pain relief between those patients receiving 8 Gy (69% response) and those in the 4 Gy arm (44% response). However, the duration of relief in those responding and the incidence of complete response was comparable in both groups, demonstrating that 4 Gy can be a useful treatment, particularly where tissue tolerance is limited.

Although these randomized, prospective trials appear to confirm the findings of the non-randomized studies, they are open to criticism in two main areas. First, the small number of patients entered into trials, which limits the statistical power of the studies, and secondly, the unreliable methods of measuring response to treatment. The evaluation of pain relief is complex and, by definition, can only be experienced by the patient. The perception of pain is recognized as being altered by subjective influences such as anxiety or depression [17], and by objective factors, such as systemic treatment and analgesic requirement. Patient self-assessment, using validated instruments, accounting for all of these variables, may help to ensure a more accurate evaluation of response.

The questions regarding the relationship between duration of response beyond 3 months and dose of radiotherapy, and the significance of tumour histology on probability of response, remain unanswered. This is of some importance, since patients with carcinoma of the breast or prostate may have a life expectancy of many months. The first question should be answered by an ongoing, randomized study in the UK, where, following randomization to either a single dose or a fractionated course of radiotherapy, patient self-assessment continues for 1 year.

Pathological Fracture

It is estimated that 10–30% of bone metastases will progress to fracture. This can have disastrous consequences for patients and initial management is therefore aimed at prophylactic stabilization of the affected bone. Certain factors which predispose patients to pathological fracture have been identified. These include metastases in weight-bearing bones and lytic lesions, either greater than 2.5 cm in diameter or where more than 50% of the cortex is destroyed. Such situations should be treated by surgical fixation followed by postoperative radiotherapy [18].

When a pathological fracture occurs in a weight-bearing long bone, surgical fixation is usually the best mode of treatment since it allows speedier pain relief and earlier mobilization. Postoperative radiotherapy is usually given as a fractionated course, with the aim of achieving some reduction in tumour burden and a degree of growth delay. Irradiation following surgery, either as part of an elective procedure or following fracture, is given on an empirical basis. In order to evaluate the place of radiotherapy in this situation, prospective, randomized studies are needed to assess its role in stabilizing the bone, ameliorating symptoms and delaying disease progression.

Radiotherapy can be used as the sole method of treatment of a pathological fracture. Indications for this include fracture of bones such as rib, scapula and pelvis which are unsuitable for internal fixation, and those patients who are unfit for surgery. In the first Royal Marsden Hospital bone pain study [14], 43 patients with pathological fractures of a vertebral body were irradiated with either single or multiple fractions. It appeared that analgesic effect was not affected by the presence of a fracture, since 71% of patients with a pathological fracture responded to treatment compared with 82% with no fracture. This was not a statistically significant difference.

Fracture healing will follow a palliative dose of radiotherapy, as shown in Figure 8.2. The dose of radiation required to enable a fracture to heal remains a matter of conjecture, but the usual practice is to deliver a short fractionated course of 20–30 Gy in 1–2 weeks.

Spinal Cord Compression

Direct extension of vertebral bone metastasis into the spinal canal, as shown in Figure 8.3 (*overleaf*), accounts for only 24% of cases of spinal cord compression [19]. The prognosis from this condition is directly related to the speed of diagnosis and performance status at presentation, with only 15% of paraplegic

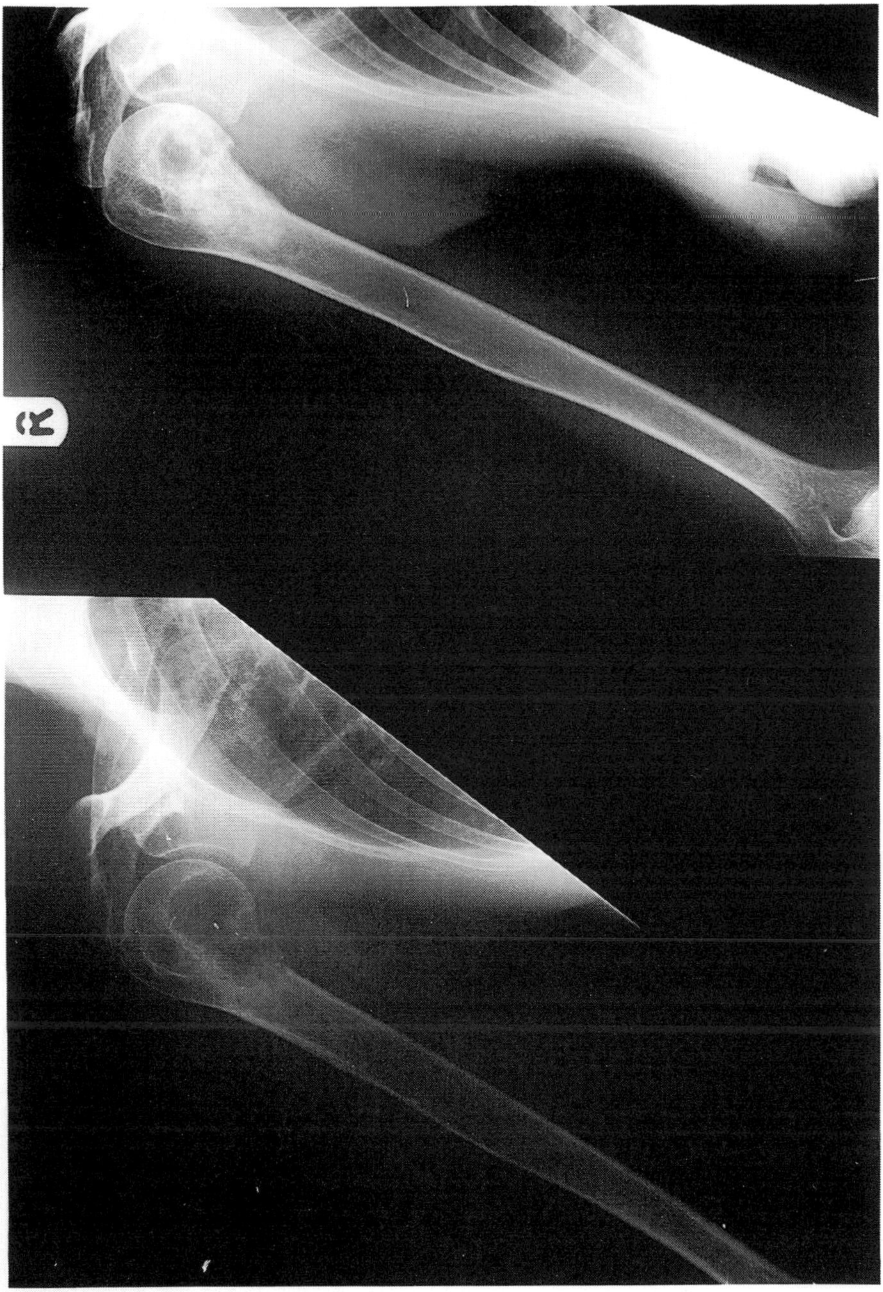

Figure 8.2 Bone healing following local radiotherapy to the upper humerus

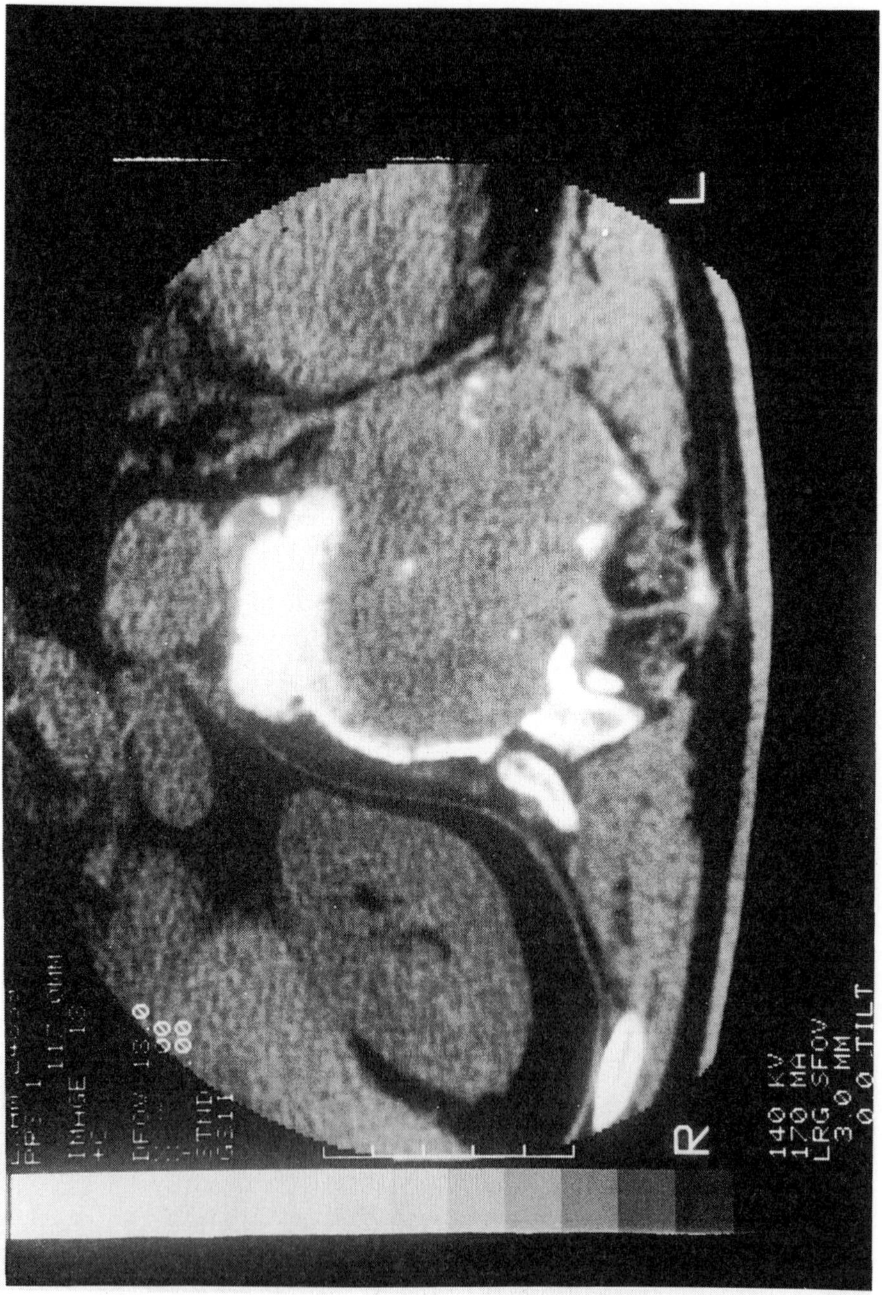

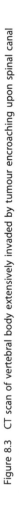

Figure 8.3 CT scan of vertebral body extensively invaded by tumour encroaching upon spinal canal

patients regaining useful function compared to 85% of those who are mobile at presentation. In the absence of vertebral instability, radiotherapy is the treatment of choice [20], preceded if necessary by needle biopsy to confirm the diagnosis of malignancy [21].

As with pathological fracture, there is no clear consensus on the optimal dose for spinal cord compression. The usual clinical practice is for a short course of treatment delivering 20–30 Gy in 2–3 weeks, although there is some evidence supporting the use of single fractions, particularly in patients with poor performance status [22].

Extended Field Radiotherapy

Metastatic bone disease is usually widespread and patients may well have disparate sites of pain. This is particularly true of multiple myeloma, prostatic and breast carcinoma, and in these patients wide-field radiotherapy has been used with some success. In this treatment either one-half or one-third of the patient is encompassed by the radiotherapy field. As with localized irradiation, treatment is carried out on a cobalt unit or linear accelerator. However, in order to ensure the large area is covered by the treatment field, the distance from the origin of the beam to the patient must be extended from the standard 80–100 cm to 300–350 cm, thereby enlarging the area encompassed in the beam, as shown in Figure 8.4.

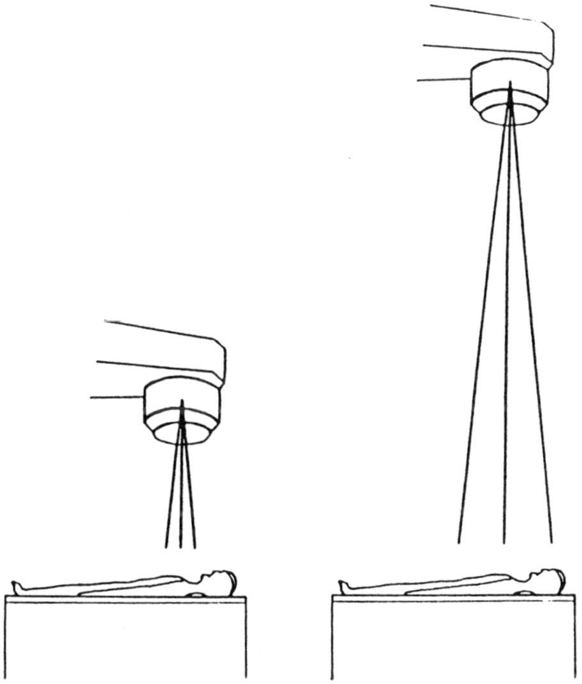

Figure 8.4 Extending the distance from the source of radiation to the patient increases the field size, enabling large areas to be included in the treatment volume.

Table 8.2 Hemibody radiotherapy and pain relief

Reference	No. of patients	Dose (Gy)	Time to response	Response (%)
Reddy et al. [38]	52	7.5 (upper 10 (lower)	24–48 h	80
Rowland et al. [39]	96	7.5 (upper) 10 (lower)	24.48 h	80
Quasim [25]	129	7–8	12–48 h	76
Salazar et al. [23]	168	6–8 (upper) 8–10 (lower)	1–14 days	73
Nag and Shah [40]	19	16/2 f	24–48 h	100
Hoskin et al. [8]	39	6–7 (upper) 8 (lower)		82
Zelefsky et al. [27]	14	6 (upper) 8 (lower)	24–48 h	100
	15	25–30/9–10 f	7–14 days	95

Response rates of 75% have been achieved and the onset of pain relief is surprisingly rapid, with 50% of responding patients having some effect within 48 h of irradiation and 80% within 7 days [23]. A review of published data is shown in Table 8.2. Neither primary tumour type nor previous radiotherapy seem to influence the likelihood of response which, in two-thirds of patients, will last until death [8, 23].

In any patient with limited life expectancy, the fundamental aim of palliation is to ensure that benefit from the treatment outweighs toxicity. Most patients will experience some degree of acute gastrointestinal upset. This is more pronounced in upper hemi-body irradiation (HBI), due to the inclusion of liver and stomach. It may be limited by giving a premedication of intravenous hydration, antiemetics and steroids.

Bone marrow suppression may occur particularly in patients who have either received prior chemotherapy or had low baseline blood counts at the time of radiotherapy. It is transient, with counts returning to pretreatment levels within 4–6 weeks [9]. However, if sequential hemibody radiotherapy is given, prolonged marrow suppression may result, with patients requiring intensive haematological support [24].

The other major complication following upper HBI is pneumonitis. In HBI the lungs are the dose-limiting normal tissue with a tolerance dose, depending upon fractionation and dose rate, of 8–11 Gy [10]. Doses in excess of this will markedly increase the probability of developing pneumonitis. In some early studies, lung toxicity was unacceptably high. In one series a dose of 8 Gy resulted in a 21% incidence of severe, often fatal pneumonitis; a dose of 7 Gy reduced this to 8% [25]. In these patients no correction was made for the fact that, since lung has a reduced density relative to other tissue, the absorbed lung dose will be increased by about 30%. On the basis of these findings, in order to minimize the incidence of pulmonary toxicity, an uncorrected dose of 6 Gy is generally prescribed. With this dose, clinically relevant pneumonitis is rare.

The benefit of HBI in an adjuvant setting has been examined in a RTOG study involving 500 patients with metastatic bone involvement [26]. Patients were randomized to receive local field radiotherapy with, or without, additional HBI.

The results suggest that HBI can offer small but statistically significant improvement in both time to disease progression and time to the development of new disease. In the HBI plus local radiotherapy arm, the median time to new disease was 12.6 months compared with 6.3 months in the local only arm ($p = 0.0014$). Similarly, at 1 year 25% of patients treated with HBI showed signs of disease progression against 46% of patients treated locally ($p = 0.032$).

Data from total body irradiation suggest that fractionated treatment can enhance the therapeutic ratio. This has been looked at with HBI in a small study of 29 patients [27]. The results suggest a small benefit for fractionated HBI, with an improved duration of response, fewer retreatments and equivalent toxicity. Further work using fractionated schedules in HBI may lead to improvement of the therapeutic ratio.

In summary, hemibody radiotherapy is effective in achieving prompt, durable pain relief in patients with extensive, painful bony disease. The side-effects can be significant, but accurate dosimetry, the prescribing of appropriate medication and careful follow-up can enable them to be limited.

Radioisotopes

Systemically administered radionuclides have been used in the treatment of malignant disease for more than 40 years. They allow treatment to be given systemically but targeted to specific sites, thereby delivering a high dose of radiation to the tumour within bone, sparing nearby normal tissue. The isotopes used may be classified into those which are specifically directed against tumour, such as iodine-131 and ^{131}I-meta-iodobenzyl-guanidine, and those that are bone seeking, such as phosphorus-32 and strontium-89.

Iodine-131 (^{131}I) has long been recognized as being an effective, targeted treatment of well-differentiated thyroid cancer. A review of 235 patients treated with ^{131}I showed that while it could be curative in the treatment of pulmonary and lymph node metastases, few patients with painful bone lesions gained improvement in either symptoms or survival [28]. However, patients with bone lesions who were treated with localized external beam radiotherapy obtained good pain relief, and it was concluded that this should be used preferentially in the palliation of bone metastases. Recent work has shown that response to ^{131}I is dose related [29]. Patients with painful bone metastases showing no response to ^{131}I treatment received a mean dose of 20 Gy to the affected site, whereas those that responded absorbed doses in excess of 100 Gy. This suggests that if uptake of ^{131}I into affected bone could be enhanced, palliation might be improved.

Radiophosphorus (^{32}P) was the first radionuclide to be used for the treatment of bone secondaries. It has been most widely used in the treatment of metastatic prostate and breast cancers and, until relatively recently, was the only isotope readily available for systemic treatment of bone metastases. Unfortunately the clinical usefulness of ^{32}P is limited, because it is non-specifically concentrated in both normal and abnormal bone alike. As a result, normal bone marrow receives a significant dose of radiation and this can lead to prolonged marrow suppression. A degree of selective uptake may be achieved by giving testosterone or parathyroid hormone to the patient. This "priming" enhances uptake into neoplastic tissue with the aim of optimizing symptom control and minimizing marrow toxicity. Reported response rates with this technique are 87% [30], with

Table 8.3 Prospective studies of strontium-89 in bone pain

Reference	No. of patients	Dose (MBq)	Overall response (%)	Complete response (%)
Tenvall et al. [41]	11	2.9–4.3/kg	45	9
Robinson et al. [31]	137	1.11–4.3/kg	80	10
Laing et al. [42]	98	0.7–3.0/kg	71	20
Lewington et al. [43]	32	150	70	
Quilty et al. [32]	153	200	66	

no significant marrow toxicity. The effectiveness of ^{32}P in providing pain relief has led to new work evaluating other bone-seeking radioisotopes which, by being more specific, are less marrow suppressive.

One such isotope is the pure β-emitter strontium-89 (^{89}Sr). Although first used in 1940 it is only over the past decade that it has become established as an effective agent in the treatment of bone metastases. It is of similar chemical composition to calcium and is preferentially localized in areas of osteoblastic activity. In addition, at sites of bone metastases the biological half-life may be prolonged by more than three times that of normal bone, with retention at these sites for up to 100 days [31], enabling concentration of radiation at the sites of bone invasion. It has been found that a dose of $1.5\,MBq\,kg^{-1}$ is optimal for achieving pain control and minimizing toxicity and this may be given as a single intravenous injection as an outpatient procedure.

In the clinical setting, ^{89}Sr has primarily been evaluated in the treatment of metastatic prostate cancer. Several retrospective studies have shown it to be effective in the treatment of disseminated bone metastases, with response rates in the region of 75%. Recent randomized trials have confirmed these findings, with an overall response rate of around 70%, and onset of pain relief occurring 2–4 weeks following administration of the ^{89}Sr and lasting for about 30–40 weeks. Published data on strontium use is shown in Table 8.3. Toxicity from strontium is mainly haematological, with reduction in platelet and leucocyte counts of about 30% [32], which are rarely associated with clinical problems.

The role of ^{89}Sr as an adjuvant treatment in the prevention of bone pain has been evaluated in a recent multicentre, randomized, prospective Canadian trial in prostate cancer [33]. Patients were treated with local radiotherapy plus either ^{89}Sr or placebo. The results show that although survival and rates of response were similar in both groups, fewer patients treated with ^{89}Sr developed new sites of bone metastases and the median time to further radiotherapy to a bony site was delayed by about 4 months compared to the control group. This has been corroborated by a multicentred British study of 284 patients with prostate cancer, which compared ^{89}Sr with either local radiotherapy or hemibody irradiation, depending on the number of sites involved [32]. Response rates were similar in all groups at about 65%, but ^{89}Sr was superior to both local and wide-field radiotherapy in delaying the progression of new sites of pain, and in reducing the need for additional local radiotherapy.

Other isotopes can be targeted to bone by conjugation with bone-seeking compounds such as bisphosphonates. Examples of such radioisotopes are samarium-153 (^{153}Sm) and rhenium-186 (^{186}Re). ^{153}Sm is combined with EDTMP and has been demonstrated to be effective in palliating pain, with a reported response rate of 79% [34]. It is currently being evaluated in a multicentre placebo-controlled study.

Clinical experience with ^{186}Re-hydroxyethane-diphosphoric acid is limited; early work has shown that it is significantly more effective than placebo in providing pain relief, with a response rate of 77% [35]. Presently there is an ongoing phase II study evaluating further the efficacy and toxicity of ^{186}Re.

Conclusions

Radiotherapy is established as one of the most effective methods of alleviating bone pain from metastatic disease, although the biological basis of its action in providing symptom relief remains uncertain. The results of recent prospective, randomized trials not only confirm its efficacy but suggest that a single dose of local irradiation will provide some degree of pain relief in the majority of patients. For those with multiple sites of pain, hemibody irradiation can achieve similar rates of response and perhaps delay the inevitable progression of bone disease, although greater toxicity from the gastrointestinal tract and bone marrow may be expected.

There remains considerable therapeutic potential for the use of radioisotopes in malignant disease. It is hoped that, by further evaluation of new isotopes and the identification of methods of enhancing the therapeutic ratio, treatment options available to patients with disseminated bone secondaries can be increased and improved.

Other important indications for radiotherapy in bone metastases include pathological fracture, both after surgical fixation and primary treatment where surgery is not possible, and neurological complications, in particular spinal cord compression.

In the future, further prospective, randomized studies using validated patient assessments of pain are needed to enable individualization of treatment and comparison of the newer radioisotopes with established treatments. In addition, the role and timing of radiotherapy in the management of pathological fracture requires evaluation to determine the optimal treatment.

References

1. Mundy GR, Boyce BF, Yoneda T (1994) Mechanisms of osteolytic bone destruction. In: Diel JS, Kaufmann M, Bastert G (eds) Metastatic bone disease: fundamental and clinical aspects. Springer-Verlag, Heidelberg, pp 86–94.
2. Boyce P, Chen H (1994) Normal bone remodelling and metastatic bone disease. In: Diel JS, Kaufmann M, Bastert G (eds) Metastatic bone disease: fundamental and clinical aspects. Springer-Verlag, Heidelberg, pp 46–58.
3. Carter RL (1985) Patterns and mechanisms of localised bone invasion by tumours: studies with squamous carcinomas of the head and neck. Crit Rev Clin Lab Sci 22:275–315.
4. Twycross R (1983) Analgesics and relief of bone pain. In: Stoll BA, Parbhoo S (eds) Bone metastases: monitoring and treatment. Raven, New York, pp 289–310.
5. Stoll BA (1983) Natural history, prognosis and staging of bone metastasis. In: Stoll BA, Parbhoo S (eds) Bone metastases: monitoring and treatment. Raven, New York, pp 1–20.
6. Burch HA (1944) Osseous metastases from graded cancers of the breast with particular reference to Roentgen treatment. Am J Roentgenol Radium Ther 52:1–23.

7. Garmatis CJ, Chu F, Dwyer AJ (1978) The effectiveness of radiation therapy in the treatment of bone metastases from breast cancer. Radiology 16:235–237.
8. Hoskin PJ, Ford HT, Harmer CL (1989) Hemibody irradiation for metastatic bone pain in two histologically distinct groups of patients. Clin Oncol 1:67–69.
9. Poulsen HS, Nielsen OS, Klee M et al. (1989) Palliative irradiation of bone metastases. Cancer Treat Rev 16:41–48.
10. Hoskin PJ (1989) Scientific and clinical aspects of radiotherapy in the relief of bone pain. Cancer Surv 7:69–86.
11. Nielsen OS, Munro AJ, Tannock IF (1991) Bone metastases: pathophysiology and management policy. J Clin Oncol 9:509–524.
12. Tong D, Gillick L, Hendrickson FR (1982) The palliation of symptomatic osseous metastases. Final results of the study by the radiation therapy oncology group. Cancer 50:893–899.
13. Blitzer PH (1985) Reanalysis of the RTOG study of the palliation of symptomatic osseous metastasis. Cancer 55:1468–1472.
14. Price P, Hoskin PJ, Easton D et al. (1986) Prospective randomised trial of single and multi fraction radiotherapy in the treatment of painful bony metastases. Radiother Oncol 6:247–255.
15. Cole DJ (1989) A randomized trial of a single treatment versus conventional fractionation in the palliative radiotherapy of bone metastases. Clin Oncol 1:59–62.
16. Hoskin PJ, Price P, Easton D et al. (1992) Prospective randomised trial of 4 Gy or 8 Gy single doses in the treatment of metastatic bone pain. Radiother Oncol 23:74–78.
17. Hanks GW, Hoskin PJ (1986) Pain control in advanced cancer: Pharmacological methods. J R Coll Phys Lond 20:276–281.
18. Bates T (1992) A review of local radiotherapy in the treatment of bone metastases and cord compression. Int J Radiat Oncol Biol Phys 23:217–221.
19. Pigott KH, Baddeley H, Maher EJ (1994) Pattern of disease in spinal cord compression on MRI scan and implications for treatment. Clin Oncol 6:7–10.
20. Findlay GFG (1984) Adverse effects of the management of malignant spinal cord compression. J Neurol Neurosurg Psychiat 47:761–768.
21. Findlay GFG, Sandeman DR, Buxton P (1988) The role of needle biopsy in the management of malignant spinal cord compression. Br J Neurosurg 2:479–484.
22. Hoskin PJ (1994) Changing trends in palliative radiotherapy. In: Tobias J, Thomas PRM (eds) Current radiation oncology, vol 1. Edward Arnold, London, pp 342–364.
23. Salazar OM, Rubin P, Hendrickson FR et al. (1986) Single dose half body irradiation for palliation of multiple bone metastases from solid tumours. Cancer 58:29–36.
24. Maclennan I, Hosni MS, Rubin P (1989) Sequential hemibody radiotherapy in poor prognosis localised adenocarcinoma of the prostate gland: a preliminary study of the RTOG. Int J Radiat Oncol Biol Phys 16:215–218.
25. Quasim MM (1989) Half body irradiation in metastatic carcinomas. Clin Radiol 35:215–219.
26. Poulter CA, Cosmatos D, Rubin P et al. (1992) A report of the RTOG 8206: a phase III study of whether the addition of a single dose hemibody irradiation to standard fractionated local field irradiation is more effective than local field irradiation alone in the treatment of symptomatic osseous metastases. Int J Radiat Oncol Biol Phys 23:207–214.
27. Zelefsky MJ, Scher HI, Forman JD et al. (1989) Palliative hemiskeletal irradiation for widespread metastatic prostate cancer: a comparison of single dose and fractionated regimens. Int J Radiat Oncol Biol Phys 17:1281–1285.
28. Brown AP, Greening WP, McReady VR et al. (1984) Radioiodine treatment of metastatic thyroid carcinoma: the Royal Marsden Hospital experience. Br J Radiol 57:323–327.
29. O'Connell MEA, Flower M, Hinton PJ et al. (1993) Radiation dose assessment in radioiodine therapy. Dose-response relationships in differentiated thyroid carcinoma using quantitative scanning and PET. Radiother Oncol 28:16–26.

30. Burnet NG, Williams G, Howard N (1990) Phosphorus-32 for intractable bony pain from carcinoma of the prostate. Clin Oncol 2:220–223.
31. Robinson RG, Blake GM, Preston DF et al. (1989) Treatment results and kinetics in patients with painful metastatic prostate and breast cancer in bone. Radiographics 9:271–281.
32. Quilty PM, Kirk D, Bolger JJ et al. (1994) A comparison of the palliative effects of strontium-89 and external beam radiotherapy in metastatic prostate cancer. Radiother Oncol 31:33–40.
33. Porter AT, McEwan AJB, Powe JE et al. (1993) Results of a randomized phase III trial to evaluate the efficacy of strontium-89 adjuvant to local field external beam irradiation in the management of endocrine resistant metastatic prostate cancer. Int J Radiat Oncol Biol Phys 25:805–813.
34. Turner JH, Claringbold PG (1991) A phase II study of treatment of painful multifocal skeletal metastases with single and repeated dose samarium-153 ethylenediaminetetramethylene phosphate. Eur J Cancer 27:1084–1086.
35. Holmes R (1993) Radiopharmaceuticals in clinical trials. Semin Oncol 20(suppl 2):22–26.
36. Madsen EJ (1983) Painful bone metastasis: efficacy of radiotherapy assessed by the patients: a randomised trial comparing 4 Gy × 6 versis 1- Gy × 2. Int J Radiat Oncol Biol Phys 9:1775–1779.
37. Okawa T, Kita M, Goto M et al. (1988) Randomized prospective clinical study of small, large and twice-a-day fraction radiotherapy for painful bone metastases. Radiother Oncol 13:99–104.
38. Reddy S, Hendrickson FR, Hocksema J (1983) The role of radiation therapy in the palliation of metastatic genitourinary tract carcinomas. A study of the Radiation Therapy Oncology Group. Cancer 52:25–29.
39. Rowland CG, Bullimore JA, Smith PJB, Roberts JBM (1981) Half body irradiation in the treatment of metastatic prostatic carcinoma. Br J Urol 53:628–629.
40. Nag S, Shah V (1986) Once-a-week lower hemibody irradiation for metastatic cancers. Int J Radiat Oncol Biol Phys 12:1003–1005.
41. Tennvall J, Darte L, Lundgren R, el Hassan AM (1988) Palliation of multiple bone metastases from prostate cancer with strontium-89. Acta Oncol 27:365–369.
42. Laing AH, Ackery DM, Bayly RJ et al. (1991) Strontium-89 chloride for pain palliation in prostatic skeletal malignancy. Br J Radiol 64:816–822.
43. Lewington VJ, McEwan AJB, Ackery DM et al. (1991) A prospective randomised double-blind study to examine the efficacy of strontium-89 in pain palliation in patients with advanced prostate cancer metastatic to bone. Eur J Cancer 27:954–958.

9 – *Part 1:* Non-Curative Radiotherapy for Upper Gastrointestinal Tract Cancer

D.J. Sebag-Montefiore and S.J. Arnott

Introduction

Gastrointestinal tract malignancies account for nearly a quarter of deaths in the UK. For most patients surgery remains the treatment of choice as primary management. However, the disappointing results of surgery as a single modality of treatment has led to an evaluation of the use of both chemotherapy and radiotherapy in the adjuvant setting. In spite of this the majority of patients are unsuitable for a curative approach and require effective palliation of their symptoms. Similiarly, many patients who are initially treated by surgery alone relapse and likewise require palliative measures to alleviate their problems.

Unfortunately, in trying to assess the value of palliative radiotherapy for these patients there is a lack of published documentary evidence to support its benefit. This is partly because many of the studies have attempted to evaluate radiotherapy as an alternative to surgery in curative treatment and have not accurately assessed symptom relief. In upper gastrointestinal malignancy this is the case for oesophageal cancer. A further fact which is often discounted is the potential toxicity of radiotherapy and when for many patients survival time is short, this is a factor which must be taken into account when assessing whether treatment is worth while. The concerns of the toxicity of radiotherapy and short survival time are perhaps the major reasons that account for the lack of radiotherapy studies in pancreatic and stomach cancer.

In order to try to make a valid assessment of symptomatic benefit of radiotherapy, information from studies that have mainly reported on improvements in survival have not been included. Such studies have frequently failed to provide adequate information on symptomatic benefit and treatment-related toxicity. In those circumstances where there is a lack of published information, personal experience is described.

Oesophageal Cancer

A particular difficulty in assessing published results in the treatment of oesophageal cancer is the heterogeneity of the extent of disease and fitness of the patients studied. For example, the results of radiotherapy are frequently reported in patients with "inoperable" disease. This will include a spectrum of patients ranging from those with small tumours but who are medically unfit for radical surgery to those patients with extensive primary tumour in the presence of metastatic disease.

Most studies that have attempted to measure symptomatic benefit have focused on dysphagia as one of the most distressing symptoms for patients with oesophageal cancer, commonly resulting in significant weight loss and malnutrition prior to diagnosis. Other symptoms such as chest pain due to mediastinal spread and dyspnoea or haemoptysis due to spread into the tracheobronchial tree may also cause considerable distress but are seldom assessed.

The available non-surgical treatment options include laser, intubation and radiotherapy either as a single modality or used in combination, and the choice of treatment modality has been well reviewed by Bown [1]. The optimal therapeutic choice remains uncertain, with differences in the latent interval prior to symptomatic improvement, the magnitude of improvement, its duration and the treatment-related morbidity. Laser therapy can produce very rapid improvements in dysphagia, but has the disadvantages of the need for frequent repeat treatments, and is most suitable for patients with exophytic tumours rather than malignant strictures and carries a risk of treatment-related morbidity. Intubation can also produce rapid improvement in dysphagia, but there can be problems with tube slippage. Plastic prostheses have a relatively narrow lumen, necessitating a sloppy diet for the patient's remaining life as well as a procedure-related morbidity. Radiotherapy can produce significant improvements in symptoms but suffers from the disadvantage of treatment-induced temporary oesophagitis. Unfortunately, there have been very few randomized trials to compare the different treatment modalities.

Radiotherapy

The main choice is between external beam irradiation, endoluminal brachytherapy or the two in combination. The advantages of external beam radiotherapy include the treatment of extramural disease due to direct primary tumour extension or mediastinal lymphadenopathy, but at the expense of greater treatment-related side-effects. Endoluminal brachytherapy offers the attractions of a short treatment time and minimal treatment-related toxicity, but will undertreat extramural disease.

External Beam Irradiation Alone

Fractionated external beam radiotherapy has the advantage of delivering a homogeneous dose to the primary tumour as well as to extra-oesophageal disease. The disadvantages of this approach include the treatment-related toxicity which predominantly consists of oesophagitis and the risk that severe dysphagia may worsen to absolute dysphagia secondary to radiation-induced oedema. The fractionation schedules used have commonly consisted of a radical course of treatment (55–60 Gy in 20–30 fractions) in the belief that this is necessary to produce prolonged symptomatic benefit.

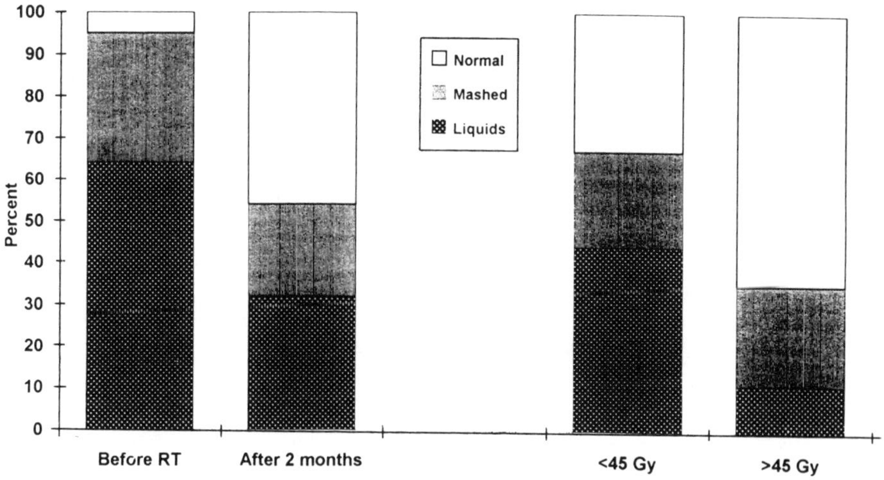

Figure 9.1.1 Improvement in dysphagia following external beam radiotherapy

Most studies using external beam radiotherapy as a single treatment modality have reported on a heterogeneous group of patients with advanced disease. Albertsson et al. [2] evaluated dysphagia in some detail before and 2 months after external beam radiotherapy alone. From a series of 149 patients with inoperable carcinoma of the oesophagus, 110 patients completed radiotherapy using a wide range of total dose (24–65 Gy). Of these, 36% could swallow normal or mashed food prior to radiotherapy compared with 66% 8 weeks after completion of radiotherapy (Figure 9.1.1). An analysis of the effect of total dose on improvement in dysphagia was also performed for patients receiving up to 45 Gy (67 patients) and those receiving 46–64 Gy (43 patients). When compared in this way, 55% of patients receiving up to 45 Gy could swallow normal or mashed food after radiotherapy compared with 86% of those receiving >45 Gy. The greater benefit seen in the patients receiving greater than 45 Gy may be explained as either evidence of a true dose-response relationship or that the patients in the low- and high-dose groups were not comparable with respect to the extent of disease. There is indirect evidence for the latter conclusion, as the median survival of the patients receiving less than 45 Gy was 7 months compared with 15 months for the patients receiving more than 45 Gy. The duration of improvement in dysphagia was not studied in detail, although six out of 67 (10%) patients in the low-dose radiotherapy group required a gastrostomy for progressive dysphagia after a median interval of 27 weeks compared with 9/43 (21%) in the high-dose group after a median of 52 weeks.

Wara et al. [3] studied the improvement in dysphagia and its duration in a group of 103 patients receiving 50–60 Gy of external beam radiotherapy. Although the extent of disease within this patient group is not stated, the median survival was 7 months. Palliation was defined as an improvement in dysphagia which ended with the onset of symptomatic progression. No response was seen in 11%, 66% of patients were palliated for less than 6 months, 11% for 6–12 months and 14% for greater than 1 year.

There is unfortunately a lack of information on symptomatic benefit in patients treated with short palliative courses of radiotherapy. Regimens in common use include 20 Gy in five fractions and 30 Gy in ten fractions. The authors' experience suggests that good symptomatic benefit from dysphagia and chest pain may be obtained using short fractionation courses. Treatment-related toxicity includes mild nausea and radiation-induced oesophagitis, lasting usually 7–10 days. Patients who present with critical dysphagia for liquids may not be suitable for external beam irradiation alone, owing to a high risk of the development of absolute dysphagia due to radiation-induced oedema. Initial treatment should consist of an endoluminal treatment with consideration of the need for subsequent external beam irradiation. Indications would include a high risk of recurrent dysphagia following endoluminal therapy such as dilatation or alcohol injection, to avoid the need for further endoluminal treatment such as laser or the need to palliate symptoms such as chest pain.

Brachytherapy

The technique of delivering a high local dose of irradiation to the oesophagus involves the endoscopic placement of a hollow guide tube through which a radioactive source can be afterloaded. The presence of a high-activity radioactive source in the oesophageal lumen allows the delivery of a high dose to the endoluminal tumour with a rapid fall off in dose to the surrounding heart, mediastinum and spinal cord. This technique is designed to produce the maximal relief of dysphagia with significantly less treatment-related toxicity than that associated with fractionated external beam irradiation. Depending on the type of source used, treatment may be of high dose rate (HDR) with treatment times of 10–30 min or low dose rate with treatment times of 12–48 h. Treatment is either given as a single session or a number of sessions 2–7 days apart.

Rowland and Pagliero [4] reported in 1985 their experience of brachytherapy in 40 patients of a median age of 76 years with advanced oesophageal carcinoma of whom 60% had advanced metastatic disease. Using a single treatment of 15 Gy prescribed 1 cm from the central axis, the treatment time was approximately 75 min. Thirty-five (87%) patients were discharged from hospital within 2 days of treatment and only five (12%) patients experienced oesophagitis for 5–10 days. Unfortunately, the improvement of dysphagia was not reported in detail, but good relief of dysphagia was found in 20 (70%) patients with squamous cell carcinoma and 12 (60%) patients with adenocarcinoma. The median duration of relief was 15 and 12 weeks for the two groups, respectively. Using the same dose and dose rate, Jager et al. [5] treated 36 patients with advanced inoperable disease. The median survival of 4 months and 14 (39%) patients with stage IV disease indicates the very poor prognosis of this patient group. Of the 32 evaluable patients, one (3%) could eat any food prior to brachytherapy compared with 14 (44%) after treatment. When patients who could eat mashed food were evaluated, 15 (47%) could do so prior to brachytherapy compared with 22 (69%) after treatment. The median duration of response was 4.5 months and 16 patients were well palliated for their remaining survival time. Eight patients relapsed with dysphagia and six were treated with brachytherapy, with improvement in five. Only six (17%) of the whole patient group required intubation. Similar studies [6, 7] have reported up to 90% of patients showing improvement of at least one grade of dysphagia, with the median duration of response of

4–5 months. Perhaps 60–80% of patients' survival time has been usefully palliated in these studies.

The Christie Hospital group have recently reported their results using HDR brachytherapy for patients unsuitable for radical treatment [8]. A total of 197 patients were treated over a 4-year period. The brachytherapy dose ranged from 7.5 to 20 Gy at 1 cm, with 83% receiving a single treatment of 15 Gy. Assessment was performed at 6 weeks, and of 161 evaluable patients, 67 (54%) had improved. The median duration of improvement was 17.5 weeks and the median survival for the whole patient group was 19.5 weeks. However, it appears that the improvement observed was unlikely to be more than one grade of dysphagia, as 54% of the whole group could only manage fluids prior to treatment compared with 50% of the assessable patients after treatment. The poor symptomatic benefit in this series may be due to the presence of very advanced disease, although the only evidence to support this is a high median age of 73.

External Beam + Brachytherapy

This combination is designed to maximize the advantages of each treatment modality, but can result in increased treatment-related toxicity. Pakisch et al. [9] treated 48 patients with inoperable disease, using between one and four fractions of brachytherapy from a HDR source followed by external beam irradiation to a total dose of 50–60 Gy for 35 patients of good performance status and 30 Gy for 13 patients of poor performance status. Dysphagia scores were assessed prior to therapy, after brachytherapy and after external beam radiotherapy. Sixty-one per cent of patients had complete dysphagia or could only manage liquids prior to therapy compared with 21% after brachytherapy and 3% after external beam radiotherapy. Only 12% of patients had slight or absence of dysphagia prior to therapy compared with 36% of patients following brachytherapy and 70% of patients following external beam radiotherapy. Unfortunately, the duration of improvement is not stated. Treatment-related toxicity from brachytherapy was reported as slight soreness only, whereas external beam radiotherapy was associated with weariness in four patients, loss of appetite in 12 patients and oesophagitis of mild to moderate severity in 35 patients (73%). Late complications were also noted and included oesophageal ulceration in four patients healing with conservative therapy and oesophagitis in 5 patients occurring 5–10 months after therapy which healed with supportive measures but resulted in benign strictures.

In an interesting study, Sur et al. [10] reported on a total of 50 patients with good performance status and tumours of 6–8 cm length without extra-oesophageal spread. All patients received 35 Gy in 15 fractions of external beam radiotherapy and were alternately allocated to receive a further 20 Gy in 10 fractions or HDR intracavitary irradiation, receiving 12 Gy at 1 cm in two fractions, 1 week apart. Although this was not a randomized study and consisted of a relatively small number of patients, the results were interesting as the two groups were designed to receive similar biological doses of irradiation. Relief of dysphagia was found in 90% and 76% of patients at 6 and 12 months, respectively, for patients treated with external beam plus brachytherapy compared to 53% and 37.5% of patients treated with external beam radiotherapy alone. Eight patients treated with external beam plus brachytherapy developed treatment-related

Table 9.1.1 Measures of symptomatic benefit following external beam radiotherapy plus brachytherapy

	Prior to treatment (%)	After treatment (%)
Performance status:		
0	0	29
1	24	46
2	76	25
Swallowing:		
any food	3	57
soft food	23	29
blended or worse	73	14
Weight:		
loss	91	35
stable	9	37
gain	0	28
Pain:		
no pain	60	83
sometimes	20	14
always	20	3

ulceration which was managed conservatively. Although this study was confined to a selected group of patients, it demonstrates that a 3-week course of external beam irradiation, followed by two intracavitary treatments, merits further study in patients with an expectation of survival of over 6 months.

Flores et al. [11] analysed their results when 171 evaluable patients were treated by a combination of 40 Gy in 15 fractions of external beam irradiation, followed by a single HDR intracavitary treatment of 15 Gy at 1 cm. Of these patients, 153 had either extra-oesophageal disease or distant metastases. The assessment of quality of life was based on performance status, swallowing ability, weight loss and pain on swallowing at 6 months. The improvement in these parameters is summarized in Table 9.1.1 Improvements in swallowing any food were marked, with only 3% of patients in this category prior to treatment compared to 57% after radiotherapy. The duration of improvement is not documented in detail, although 90% had improved swallowing lasting for at least 3 months, with 35% of the total patient group requiring subsequent dilatations. This was also one of the few studies to evaluate pain related to swallowing. The morbidity of radiation oesophagitis is mentioned as being of moderate severity in the majority, although it was severe in 14% of patients and persisted until death. However, the contribution of irradiation to these symptoms is difficult to assess due to the presence of persistent and progressive malignancy.

Chemo/radiotherapy

Combination chemotherapy using cisplatin and 5-fluorouracil have been reported to produce rapid improvement in dysphagia. However, the time spent in hospital and chemotherapy-related toxicity can be considerable. The use of synchronous chemotherapy and external beam irradiation has shown promise when given to patients with disease limited to the mediastinum. For example, the randomized trial of Herskovic et al. [12] has shown an improvement in survival, a reduction in local recurrence and distant metastases when patients were treated with synchronous chemo/radiotherapy. There was, however, significantly greater toxicity from synchronous chemo/radiotherapy compared with radiotherapy alone when patients with good performance status were treated, and there was no significant difference in the improvement in the ability to swallow between the two treatments. At present, the symptomatic benefits of synchronous chemo/radiotherapy compared with irradiation alone remain uncertain, but deserve further study in patients with a survival expectation of greater than 6 months.

Intermodality Randomized Trials

A small number of randomized trials have compared different treatment modalities. All such trials have suffered major difficulties in the accrual of patients. Reed et al. [13] reported on a comparison between intubation, intubation plus external beam irradiation and laser plus external beam irradiation. Only 27 patients were randomized over a 4-year period. There was no significant difference in the improvement in swallowing between the groups, although the least morbid arm of the study was where laser therapy was followed by external beam irradiation. Only one patient in this group required further local therapy, suggesting that radiotherapy may have played a role in retarding tumour regrowth. The morbidity of Atkinson tube intubation was demonstrated with two out of ten tube-related perforations in the intubation only arm (one requiring laparotomy), one tumour perforation at the time of tube insertion and one patient with compression of the distal trachea requiring tracheostomy in the intubation plus radiotherapy arm.

Sander et al. [14] reported on 39 evaluable patients who were randomized between laser therapy and laser therapy plus brachytherapy. Brachytherapy used a HDR machine delivering 3 weekly treatments of 7 Gy at 1 cm. The mean age was 71 and Karnofsky score 55. Twenty-two patients had adenocarcinoma and 17 squamous cell carcinoma. Laser therapy resulted in complete patency. The first dysphagia-free interval was an average of 32 days in the laser alone group (20 patients) compared with 68 days in the laser plus brachytherapy group (19 patients). This difference was not statistically significant for the whole group, but was highly significant ($p = 0.001$) when the analysis was restricted to the 17 patients with squamous carcinoma. Oesophagitis was noted in four patients, all of whom received laser plus brachytherapy.

Conclusions

The heterogeneous patient mix in large non-randomized studies of the treatment of oesophageal cancer creates difficulties in assessing the benefits of therapy. Improvements in dysphagia may be obtained by endoluminal brachytherapy or external beam radiotherapy. In the presence of visceral metastases or poor performance status, the very limited survival of patients requires a treatment which is of limited duration and toxicity and produces rapid improvement. Intraluminal brachytherapy fulfils most of these requirements, although alternative treatments such as laser therapy and intubation are also effective.

There is a need to measure the symptomatic benefit and toxicity of short fractionation schedules of external beam radiotherapy.

For patients with incurable disease but of good performance status, or disease confined to the mediastinum, more aggressive therapy is likely to achieve symptomatic benefit of longer duration in the form of external beam irradiation combined with brachytherapy. This approach has the advantage of treating extra-oesophageal disease, although with a higher level of treatment-related toxicity. It is in this group of patients that the role of synchronous chemo/radiotherapy deserves further evaluation.

Stomach Cancer

The majority of studies evaluating the use of radiotherapy in patients with gastric cancer have concentrated on adjuvant radiotherapy. However, there has never been any clear evidence that the use of radiotherapy in these circumstances has been beneficial in improving survival. The role of palliative radiotherapy in patients with gastric cancer is limited. However, in selected patients with bleeding from the primary site which is difficult to manage by other means, short courses of radiotherapy in which a total dose of 20 Gy is given in five treatments using parallel opposed fields may be helpful.

In addition, patients who are symptomatic as a result of nodal disease in the region of the porta hepatis may similarly be helped by palliative radiotherapy. Such patients frequently have jaundice, but may also have lymphadenopathy. Radiotherapy may be very successful in relieving these symptoms without causing undue toxicity.

Pain may also be caused by extension of disease from the primary site. Again in selected patients the use of short fractionated regimens of radiotherapy can provide successful palliation.

Pancreatic Cancer

Most patients with pancreatic cancer present with jaundice, weight loss or pain. Interventional radiological techniques include the placement of plastic or metal mesh stents either at the time of ERCP or via the transhepatic route. Successful stenting alows the rapid palliation of the symptoms resulting from jaundice and remains the treatment of choice for patients with advanced or metastatic disease. The role of palliative radiotherapy remains poorly defined due to the lack of information about symptomatic response and the perceived requirement of high doses of radiation. The surrounding normal tissues, including the duodenum, kidneys, liver and spinal cord, present a considerable challenge to the radiotherapist to deliver radiotherapy safely and minimize acute toxicity.

It is disappointing that despite published literature documenting aggressive approaches, including high-dose external beam radiotherapy, synchronous chemo/radiotherapy and the use of intraoperative radiotherapy, the reported end-points remain overall survival and treatment-related toxicity with no assessment of quality of life or symptomatic benefit. This section will focus on the very few studies that have reported any useful information on symptomatic benefit.

Dobelbower et al. [15] reported on a selected group of 40 patients with locally extensive unresectable cancer of the pancreas. The diagnosis was confirmed at laparotomy and biliary bypass performed if indicated for jaundice. Patients with distant metastases or haematogenous spread to the liver were excluded. Thirty-three (82%) patients presented with jaundice, 32 (80%) with pain and 28 (70%) with weight loss. Fractionated radiotherapy was given to a total dose of 59–70 Gy over a 7–9-week period and five patients (12%) failed to complete treatment and a further six (15%) experienced significant nausea. The only symptomatic benefit from radiotherapy reported was relief of pain in 22 (69%) of patients.

Whittington et al. [16] reported on 104 patients with unresectable carcinoma of the pancreas. This study included 38 patients with stage IV disease, Karnofsky scores of less than 40 or tumours larger than 2500 cm^3. Forty-eight patients were treated with precision high-dose (PHD) radiotherapy and 18 patients with PHD radiotherapy and ^{125}I implantation. The median survival for the group treated with palliative radiotherapy was 5 months. The palliative benefit of radiotherapy was defined as a symptomatic response that continued until the final admission. The response of pain to radiotherapy was complete in five (45%) patients and partial in one (9%); jaundice was relieved in ten (67%) patients.

Haslam et al. [17] reported on 29 patients, of whom 23 were suitable for radical irradiation and six had non-localized disease who were treated for relief of symptoms only. Treatment delivered a total dose of 50.40–66.80 Gy over 6–14 weeks, with most patients receiving 60.00–61.00 Gy in 10 weeks. Fifteen patients also received synchronous 5-fluorouracil on an *ad hoc* basis. The median survival for the group treated with radical intent was 7.5 months. Of interest is the definition of palliation used by the authors. For example, good palliation was defined as at least two of the following: complete relief of pain for at least 4 weeks, weight gain not due to ascites, relief of obstructive symptoms and jaundice and a decrease in size of a palpable mass. Good palliation was seen in 45% of the patients, was fair in 24% and 31% were not benefited. Using a defined scoring system for acute toxicity, this was described as severe in 10% and moderate in 38% of patients.

Green et al. [18] reported on 20 patients who received radiotherapy for the main complaint of pain, of whom 11 had proven liver metastases. Eight patients had a biliary diversion procedure, and 12 received concomitant 5-fluorouracil. Out of 22 patients 17 had significant alleviation of pain. The radiation dose ranged from 6.00 Gy over 4 days to 50.00 Gy over 48 days. The average tumour dose for a favourable response was 14.40 Gy over 14 days. Three patients developed nausea during radiotherapy.

The authors treat patients with unresectable pancreatic cancer with palliative intent. For patients without evidence of metastases with good performance status and local disease up to a maximum diameter of 5–6 cm, an aggressive approach is used combining external beam radiotherapy (50–55 Gy in 25 fractions) with continuous infusion of 5-fluououracil and boluses of mitomycin C in the first and fifth week. Patients with poor performance status, local disease greater than 6 cm or with disseminated disease are considered for palliative radiotherapy, and are given 30 Gy in ten fractions using a three-field plan. Treatment is given with the intention of relieving symptoms, most commonly pain.

Conclusions

There is a great need to record prospectively symptoms, toxicity and quality-of-life measures when patients are treated with palliative radiotherapy. Until these data are recorded it will not be possible to conclude how worth while any improvement in survival of a few months has been. The very sparse data on pain relief are disappointing and radiotherapy has not been compared with, for example, invasive nerve blocks of the coeliac axis. There is ample scope for many research protocols to help define the palliative role of radiotherapy in incurable pancreatic cancer.

References

1. Bown SG (1991) Palliation of malignant dysphagia: surgery, radiotherapy, laser, intubation alone or in combination? Gut 32:841–844.
2. Albertsson M, Ewers SB, Widmark H, Hambraeus G, Lillo-Gil R, Ranstam J (1989) Evaluation of the palliative effect of radiotherapy for esophageal carcinoma. Acta Oncol 28:267–270.
3. Wara WM, Mauch PM, Thomas AN, Phillips TL (1976) Palliation for carcinoma of the esophagus. Radiology 121:717–720.
4. Rowland CG, Pagliero KM (1985) Intracavitary irradiation in palliation of carcinoma of oesophagus and cardia. Lancet 2:981–983.
5. Jager JJ, Pannebakker M, Rikjen J, deVos J, Vismans FJF (1992) Palliation in esophageal cancer with a single session of intraluminal irradiation. Radiother Oncol 25:134–136.
6. Fleischman EH, Kagan AR, Bellotti JE, Streeter OE, jr, Harvey JC (1990) Effective palliation for inoperable esophageal cancer using intensive intracavitary radiation. J Surg Oncol 44:234–237.
7. Harvey JC, Fleischman EH, Bellotti JE, Kagan AR (1993) Intracavitary radiation in the treatment of advanced esophageal carcinoma: a comparison of high dose rate vs. low dose rate brachytherapy. J Surg Oncol 52:101–104.
8. Brewster AE, Davidson SE, Makin WP, Stout R, Burt PA (1995) Intraluminal brachytherapy using the high dose rate microSelectron in the palliation of carcinoma of the oesophagus. Clin Oncol 7:102–105.
9. Pakisch B, Kohek P, Poier E et al. (1993) Iridium-192 high dose rate brachytherapy combined with external beam irradiation in non-resectable oesophageal cancer. Clin Oncol 5:154–158.
10. Sur RK, Singh DP, Sharma SC et al. (1992) Radiation therapy of esophageal cancer: role of high dose rate brachytherapy. Int J Radiat Oncol Biol Phys 22:1043–1046.
11. Flores AD, Nelems B, Evans K, Hay JH, Stoller J, Jackson SM (1989) Impact of new radiotherapy modalities on the surgical management of cancer of the esophagus and cardia. Int J Radiat Oncol Biol Phys 17:937–944.
12. Herskovic A, Martz K, al-Sarraf M et al. (1992) Combined chemotherapy and radiotherapy compared with radiotherapy alone in patients with cancer of the esophagus [see comments]. N Engl J Med 326:1593–1598.
13. Reed CE, Marsh WH, Carlson LS, Seymore CH, Kratz JM (1991) Prospective, randomized trial of palliative treatment for unresectable cancer of the esophagus. Ann Thorac Surg 51:552–555; discussion 556.
14. Sander R, Hagenmueller F, Sander C, Riess G, Classen M (1991) Laser versus laser plus afterloading with iridium-192 in the palliative treatment of malignant stenosis of the esophagus: a prospective, randomized, and controlled study. Gastrointest Endosc 37:433–440.

15. Dobelbower RR, Borgelt BB, Strubler KA et al. (1980) Precision radiotherapy for cancer of the pancreas: techniques and results. Int J Radiat Oncol Biol Phys 6:1127–1133.
16. Whittington R, Dobelbower RR, Mohiuddinn M (1981) Radiotherapy of unresectable pancreatic carcinoma: a six year experience with 104 patients. Int J Radiat Oncol Biol Phys 7:1639–1644.
17. Haslam JB, Cavanaugh PJ, Stroup SL (1973) Radiation therapy in the treatment of irresectable adenocarcinoma of the pancreas. Cancer 32:1341–1345.
18. Green N, Beron E, Melbye RW et al. (1973) Carcinoma of the pancreas – palliative radiotherapy. Am J Roentgenol Radium Ther Nucl Med 117:620–622.

9 – *Part 2:* Non-Curative Radiotherapy for Lower Gastrointestinal Tract Cancer

D.J. Sebag-Montefiore and S.J. Arnott

Introduction

As mentioned in the Introduction to Part 1 of this chapter, gastrointestinal tract malignancies account for nearly a quarter of deaths in the UK. For most patients surgery remains the treatment of choice as primary management. However, the disappointing results of surgery as a single modality of treatment have led to an evaluation of the use of both chemotherapy and radiotherapy in the adjuvant setting.

Unfortunately, in trying to assess the value of palliative radiotherapy for these patients, there is a lack of published documentary evidence to support its benefit. This is partly because many of the studies have attempted to evaluate radiotherapy as an alternative to surgery in curative treatment and have not accurately assessed symptom relief. In lower gastrointestinal malignancy this is the case for anal cancer, where chemo/radiotherapy has been so successful as a curative non-surgical treatment that very little information on palliative treatment is available, and this is further confounded by the fact that salvage treatment after chemo/radiotherapy for recurrence usually requires surgery.

The increasing use of adjuvant radiotherapy in patients with operable rectal cancer leaves two patient groups for assessing palliative benefit. In patients with fixed tumours the intention is to allow sufficient regression to allow surgery, whereas the greatest information is available in the palliative treatment of local recurrence.

In order to try to make a valid assessment of symptomatic benefit of radiotherapy, information from studies that have mainly reported on improvements in survival have not been included. Such studies have frequently failed to provide adequate information on symptomatic benefit and treatment-related toxicity. In those circumstances where there is a lack of published information, personal experience is described.

Rectal Cancer

The discussion of the non-curative treatment of rectal cancer will focus on patients who present with fixed inoperable disease and those presenting with local recurrence. There are numerous studies reporting the treatment of fixed inoperable tumours with preoperative radiotherapy. Unfortunately, these studies concentrate on the curative resection rate, local control and survival. There is very little information that has evaluated symptomatic benefit for those patients who remain unresectable. Patients are usually found to have developed local recurrence due to the development of local symptoms. Holm et al. [1] reported on 156 patients who developed local recurrence in the Stockholm I trial of 684 patients who were randomized between surgery with or without preoperative radiotherapy for resectable rectal cancer; 87% were symptomatic and 91% developed symptoms within 3 years of initial surgery. The local symptoms included pain in 62% of patients, 26% experienced micturition disturbances, 18% rectal or vaginal bleeding and 14% altered bowel habit. Only 12% of all local recurrences were macroscopically resectable despite laparotomy being performed on 46% of patients, emphasizing the importance of non-surgical treatment. The median survival was between 11 and 15 months and 3% of patients were alive at 3 years. One can conclude from this large study that nearly all patients who develop local recurrence present with distressing local symptoms and that half of these patients are likely to live at least 1 year, stressing the importance of assessing the symptomatic benefit and its duration when palliative radiotherapy is given.

Williams and Horwitz [2] reported, in 1956, detailed results using 1000 kV X-rays at St Bartholomew's Hospital to treat 189 cases of rectal cancer presenting between 1937 and 1954. A total of 128 (68%) patients had spread of disease beyond the rectum to neighbouring structures and/or involving regional lymph nodes and 27 (14%) patients had distant metastases. The aim in all cases was to deliver a radical dose of irradiation (60 Gy over 6–8 weeks). Symptomatic benefit was classified as complete, partial or no relief for the symptoms of pain, tenesmus, mucous discharge and bleeding. The greatest symptomatic relief was found for pain and was achieved in 90% of patients and was complete in 76%. Mucous discharge proved more difficult to relieve, and complete and partial relief was found in 41% and 26% of patients, respectively. The symptomatic benefits were achieved at the expense of acute toxicity, and approximately 50% of patients had their treatment interrupted or modified. The duration of symptomatic benefit was not stated. These authors clearly demonstrated that megavoltage radiation had a definite role in palliating the local symptoms of locally advanced rectal cancer.

Williams et al. [3] reported, in 1957, the results of treatment of local recurrence of rectal cancer using megavoltage X-rays, with useful information on the duration of symptom relief. A total of 82 patients were treated with radical radiotherapy over 6 weeks. Of a total of 74 evaluable patients, 19 had at least 10–12 months, 24 had at least 6 months and 41 had at least 3 months of relief.

Arnott [4] reported a pilot study of 55 patients with either local recurrence (38 patients) or inoperable disease (17 patients). The patients were treated with radiotherapy combined with 5-fluorouracil intravenously. Twenty patients received high-dose radiotherapy (50–55 Gy in 20 daily fractions and 35 patients received palliative radiotherapy (30–35 Gy in ten daily fractions). The symptomatic resolution of pain, mass and discharge was reported. Complete resolution of pain occurred in 29 (66%) patients and was partial in a further seven (16%). There was no apparent advantage for the high-dose schedule, as complete relief of pain was found in seven out of 14 patients compared with 22 out of 30 who were treated by the shorter regimen. There was little difference in the side-effects experienced between the high-dose and lower dose radiotherapy groups and most of the treatment-related toxicity appeared to relate to the different scheduling of the 5-fluorouracil.

Taylor et al. [5] studied the symptomatic benefit produced by radiotherapy for patients with recurrent (33 patients) and inoperable (41 patients) disease treated by radical radiotherapy and 145 patients treated by palliative radiotherapy, of whom 79/145 (54%) had synchronous distant metastases. Radical radiotherapy consisted of 45–55 Gy in 20 fractions or two courses of 30–35 Gy in ten fractions, and palliative radiotherapy consisted of 30–35 Gy in ten fractions. Complete relief of pain relief was found in 62% of radically treated and 30% of palliatively treated patients (Table 9.2.1). Although the total symptomatic response (partial + complete) was similar when radical and palliative were compared for pain, bleeding, discharge and diarrhoea, the group of patients who received radical radiotherapy appeared to derive more frequent complete relief of pain and diarrhoea. The duration of response was not stated.

Greater levels of acute toxicity were experienced when radical radiotherapy was given, with only 19% of radically treated patients avoiding acute toxicity compared with 61% of patients treated palliatively. Acute toxicity was described as generally mild and responsive to therapy. The 2-year survival for patients treated radically was 32% for patients with recurrent disease and 20% for patients with inoperable advanced disease compared with 10% of patients treated with palliative radiotherapy. A comparison of symptomatic benefit from the above studies is shown in Table 9.2.1.

Overgaard et al. [6] attempted to establish evidence of a dose-response relationship when radiotherapy was given in daily fractions of 2 Gy for symptom relief. A total of 113 patients were treated with radiotherapy, of whom 77 had recurrent disease and 18 primarily inoperable disease. Of the whole group, 25% had synchronous distant metastases. The total dose for palliative treatment was 23–45 Gy and 45–65 Gy for radical treatment. Subjective response was evaluable in 89 patients, ranging from 47% to 61% for three dose ranges below 55 Gy and were not significantly different. However, all 11 patients who received more than 56 Gy had a subjective response.

The clinical experience of the authors is that it is appropriate to treat patients who present with fixed tumours in the absence of metastatic disease with radical radiotherapy even if surgical excision is not a subsequent option. These patients appear to derive the maximal symptomatic benefit. Palliative radiotherapy using 30 Gy in ten fractions would be used for elderly, poor performance status patients and those with progressive metastatic disease.

Conclusions

There is a lack of published studies that have attempted to evaluate the palliative benefit of radiotherapy for patients with rectal cancer. The observations of Williams and colleagues [2, 3] were published over 40 years ago and contain more detail than the results published recently. Randomized trials have been very successful in defining the benefits of palliative treatment for patients with inoperable lung cancer and painful bony metastases and the comparison of short verses longer courses of radiotherapy. There is an urgent need to apply the same principles in order to define the palliative radiotherapy for local recurrence of rectal cancer and begin to address the optimal duration of treatment.

Table 9.2.1 Symptom relief following radiotherapy for recurrent rectal cancer

Reference	No.	Dose (Gy)	Pain		Tenesmus		Mucous		Bleeding	
			Complete	Partial	Complete	Partial	Complete	Partial	Complete	Partial
Williams and Horwitz [2]	189	60	49/102 (48%)	29/102 (28%)	36/66 (55%)	12/66 (18%)	47/116 (41%)	30/116 (26%)	103/135 (76%)	18/135 (13%)
Taylor et al. [5] (radical)	74	50–55	23/37 (62%)	11/37 (30%)	NR	NR	7/22 (32%)	12/22 (55%)	25/28 (89%)	–
Taylor et al. [5] (palliative)	145	30–35	27/73 (37%)	36/73 (49%)	NR	NR	17/50 (34%)	26/50 (52%)	29/46 (63%)	10/46 (22%)
Arnott [4]	55	30–55	29/44 (66%)	7/44 (16%)	NR	NR	4/15 (27%)	8/15 (53%)	NR	NR

Anal Cancer

There has been a radical change in recent years in the treatment of carcinoma of the anus. It is now clear that for most patients radiotherapy combined with chemotherapy is the treatment of choice in curative management. This treatment is so successful in producing local control that the role for palliative treatment is reduced. However, occasionally spread to the para-aortic lymph nodes occurs and this frequently is associated with considerable pain and neurological changes affecting the legs. These patients may successfully be managed using a technique of radiotherapy designed to encompass the para-aortic region, and is best combined with chemotherapy using mitomycin C and 5-fluorouracil. Doses of the order of 45 Gy in 25 fractions are necessary for these treatments to produce maximal symptomatic benefit. Mitomycin C in a dose of 10–12 $mg\,m^{-2}$ is given on the first day of treatment and 5-fluorouracil is given by continuous infusion in a dose of 1 $g\,m^{-2}$ each 24 h during the first 5 days of radiotherapy and also during the last 5 days of radiotherapy. In a number of patients, long-term control of such disease may be achieved.

Similarly, in selected patients who develop liver metastases, irradiation may be used in combination with chemotherapy for the treatment of the liver. In these circumstances the classic Nigro regimen may be used. Parallel opposed fields of radiotherapy are employed and midplane doses of 30 Gy delivered in 15 fractions are usually well tolerated. Again mitomycin C is given on the first day of treatment and 5-fluorouracil infusions are given during the first week of radiotherapy and also during the week following completion of the radiotherapy course. In a few patients, long-term control of liver metastases may be obtained. Complete eradication of disease sometimes occurs, with patients thereafter remaining completely disease free.

Local recurrence of disease is more difficult to treat if the patient has already received radiotherapy to the pelvis. However, implantation techniques can sometimes be helpful in which either iridium wires may be inserted into the anal canal, or into the anal margin if that is the site of recurrence. Doses in the order of 30 Gy expressed at the 85% isodose may be very helpful. Alternatively, equipment such as the microselectron may be used, in which a dose of 10 Gy given as a single treatment may prove effective. These patients frequently suffer from bleeding, discharge from the anus and pain. Implantation may be successful in relieving all of these symptoms.

Alternatively, electron therapy may be used if the recurrence is in the perianal region. If the patient has received previous radiotherapy, the doses should be limited to the order of 20 Gy in five fractions. In those patients who have been managed by surgery and have developed local recurrence, an attempt should be made to give radical radiotherapy combined with chemotherapy, as such patients may still be salvaged.

Conclusions

Primary synchronous chemo/radiotherapy is now established as the treatment of choice for anal cancer, with surgery reserved for local recurrence. This change in practice and the rarity of anal cancer means that there is very little information on the palliative benefit of radiotherapy. The limited scope for retreatment and the treatment of patients with recurrence who were initially managed by surgery have been described.

References

1. Holm T, Cedermark B, Rutqvist LE (1994) Local recurrence of rectal adenocarcinoma after "curative" surgery with and without preoperative radiotherapy. Br J Surg 81:452–455.
2. Williams IG, Horwitz H (1956) The primary treatment of adenocarcinoma of the rectum by high voltage roentgen rays (1000 kV). Am J Roentgenol 76:919–928.
3. Williams IG, Schulman IM, Todd IP (1957) The treatment of recurrent carcinoma of the rectum by supervoltage X-ray therapy. Br J Surg 44:506–508.
4. Arnott SJ (1975) The value of combined 5-fluorouracil and X-ray therapy in the palliation of locally recurrent and inoperable rectal carcinoma. Clin Radiol 26:177–182.
5. Taylor RE, Kerr GR, Arnott SJ (1987) External beam radiotherapy for rectal adenocarcinoma. Br J Surg 74:455–459.
6. Overgaard M, Overgaard J, Sell A (1984) Dose-response relationship for radiation therapy of recurrent, residual and primarily inoperable colorectal cancer. Radiother Oncol 1:217–225.

10 – Non-Curative Radiotherapy for Gynaecological Cancer

P.R. Blake

Introduction

Gynaecological cancer has an incidence of approximately 15 000 cases per annum in the UK, in comparison with 25 000 cases per annum of breast cancer. The three most common types of gynaecological cancer are carcinoma of the ovary, carcinoma of the cervix and carcinoma of the endometrium, with approximately equal incidences but very varying mortality rates. Although at 5 years only 20–30% of patients with ovarian cancer will be alive, the opposite is true of cancer of the endometrium and half of those patients diagnosed with cervical cancer will be alive. Overall, approximately 50% of patients with gynaecological cancer will be cured of their disease, but the other 50% will either develop local recurrence or metastasis, to which they will eventually succumb.

Worldwide the pattern of incidence of these three main types of gynaecological cancer is quite different. In particular, cancer of the cervix is extremely common in developing countries, where it is the most prevelant female cancer. Cancer of the cervix ranks second only after breast cancer in incidence in the female population worldwide, with an annual incidence of 500 000. In addition, the survival rate in developing countries from this disease is very low because of late presentation and inadequate treatment facilities and it therefore represents a major public health problem. In developed countries, ovarian cancer is becoming more common, with its associated poor prognosis. Equally, endometrial cancer also has an increasing incidence and, because it usually presents at an early stage, this tumour has a relatively good prognosis.

Therefore, gynaecological cancer is a major cause of death in women worldwide and cancer of the cervix particularly so.

There are other, rarer gynaecological tumours of the vagina and vulva and the very rare gestational trophoblastic tumours. Although the question of palliation for these small numbers of patients is paramount for the individual, it does not present the public health problem of providing palliation for patients with advanced carcinoma of the cervix.

Radiotherapy has an important place in the non-curative treatment of gynaecological cancer, particularly cancer of the cervix, vulva and vagina. Endometrial cancer presents less of a problem, as patients with this disease are usually suitable for curative treatment and the symptoms produced by ovarian cancer are, in general, not amenable to the localized treatment possible with

Table 10.1 Symptoms amenable to palliation by radiotherapy

Efficacy	Symptom	Source
Good	Pain	Primary pelvic or metastatic disease
	Bleeding	Pelvic tumour , vaginal, rectal or urethral Skin involvement or metastases
	Discharge	Pelvic tumour PV
Medium	Obstruction	Bowel, ureter or urethra
Poor	Incontinence	Urine or faeces
	Fistulae	Vesicovaginal, rectovaginal or enterovaginal
	Skin ulceration	Skin involvement

radiotherapy. However, there are exceptions to this rule for patients with particular symptoms, as will be detailed.

Local Problems Amenable to Palliation with Radiotherapy

As it is the symptoms that are treated in palliative therapy, rather than the specific disease, it is more appropriate for palliative therapy to be discussed by symptom rather than by disease type (Table 10.1). The symptoms are, of course, very dependent upon the site of disease.

Pain

Pain may be caused by either primary or recurrent tumour at any site. In gynaecological cancer, pain is commonly in the pelvis or the small of the back, but if there is sacral plexus involvement there may well be radiation of pain down the inner aspects of the thighs and into the back of the knee. A patient presenting with pain such as this requires both radiotherapy for the long-term control of the symptom and also analgesia for immediate relief.

Pain is usually best treated by irradiating the whole of the mass causing the symptom. Occasionally, pain may be made worse in the first few days of radiotherapy, if it is caused by pressure effects in a relatively enclosed space, as radiotherapy may cause initial oedema in the tumour. If this is the case, then prednisolone 10 mg t.d.s. may help as a co-analgesic for a few days. Either 20 Gy in five fractions over 5 days or 30 Gy in ten fractions over 12 days will usually produce good pain relief by the end of the first week of treatment. Larger masses are usually better treated by the longer course, as there is less normal tissue toxicity (mainly diarrhoea from irradiation of small bowel).

Pain control may be difficult to achieve when there is direct nerve involvement. Occasionally, patients are seen in whom, although the pain in the pelvis improves, the radiation of pain down the leg persists. Pain may also be produced from metastases in the para-aortic nodes eroding either posteriorly into the vertebral bodies or laterally into the psoas muscles, causing difficulty in walking. Again, localized disease such as this is readily amenable to palliation by radiotherapy.

An uncommon cause of pain in gynaecological cancer is gross involvement of the liver with metastases, causing stretching of the liver capsule, producing pain in the right upper quadrant of the abdomen and in the right shoulder. The liver is an organ that is quite sensitive to radiotherapy, but a short fractionated course of 20–30 Gy can be given, together with steroids, to help relieve liver capsule pain.

A common occurrence with cancer of the cervix or cancer of the ovary is ureteric obstruction, which can lead to hydroureter and hydronephrosis. As a general rule, this symptom does not cause pain unless the kidney becomes infected. Under these circumstances treatment with antibiotics should be instituted and consideration given to the use of a ureteric stent. However, this has to be considered carefully as, if hydronephrosis is a terminal event producing uraemia and eventual death, then it might not be appropriate to reverse this process in a patient who would otherwise die from more symptomatic or distressing problems, such as bowel obstruction or haemorrhage.

Bleeding

Any tumour that is active in the vagina or cervix can cause bleeding and, occasionally, this is the mode of death. However, in a large number of patients vaginal bleeding is a relatively chronic problem, with the passing of small quantities of serosanguineous fluid or occasional clots each day. Although this, in itself, is not life threatening it is a distressing symptom for the patient and can cause anaemia, requiring blood transfusion.

Traditionally, bleeding has been treated by a small number of large fractions of radiotherapy. However, there is no clear evidence that a regimen based on this is superior to one with a more standard fraction size. A regimen as detailed later in this chapter should be adequate (Table 10.2).

Bleeding usually stops quickly after radiotherapy is commenced and is often reduced within 2–3 days. However, it is occasionally persistent and thought may be given to intracavitary therapy in a patient where the bleeding tumour presents a surface against which the intracavitary applicator can be applied. Often this is not the case if there is craggy tumour at the vaginal vault, so the circumstances in which intracavitary therapy can be helpful are limited. Nevertheless, it is a technique to consider, especially in a patient who has previously received a radical dose of external beam radiotherapy, where it is inadvisable to treat with more external beam therapy if the patient may survive long enough to develop late effects from this re-irradiation. If an intracavitary applicator is used, then high dose-rate brachytherapy causes the least logistical problems for the patient, as it seldom takes more than a few minutes and can usually be performed on an outpatient basis. Where this is not available, low dose-rate brachytherapy using caesium sources will usually require admission for one or two nights.

Whenever brachytherapy is considered, it must be borne in mind that the

Table 10.2 Palliative radiotherapy regimens

Dose (Gy)	Fractions	Time (days	Field sizes (cm)
8–10	1	1	<6 × 6
20	5	5	<10 × 10
30	10	12	<15 × 15
45	25	33	>15 × 15

volume of tumour irradiated is very small indeed and the effective dose will probably only treat the top few millimetres of tumour, particularly if it is not possible to use an intrauterine tube. With thin plaques of tumour in the vagina this may be appropriate, but with larger tumours such superficial irradiation is unlikely to produce haemostasis for long.

Bleeding from skin metastases from carcinoma of the vulva is best approached with electron therapy or superficial X-rays. However, the dose should be conservative, as the vulval skin tolerates radiation badly (not more than 30 Gy in ten fractions over 12 days).

Discharge

Many tumours in the pelvis that produce vaginal discharge, if treated by radiotherapy, will regress and there will be an improvement in this symptom. However, the main cause for discharge is infection of necrotic tumour material and, although improvement may be noted in previously untreated disease, if necrosis is due to previous radiotherapy, the discharge is unlikely to be helped by additional palliative radiotherapy.

In all patients with a vaginal discharge, the smell and discomfort may be helped by appropriate use of antibiotics, especially metronidazole which is active against anaerobic bacteria. On occasions this may be given as a gel to be applied inside the vagina and this may avoid the systemic side-effects of the oral preparation.

Obstruction

Carcinoma of the ovary, in particular, can cause bowel obstruction. However, the ureters may also be blocked by this tumour as they may be by advanced carcinoma of the cervix or pelvic node disease from any gynaecological cancer. Occasionally, obstruction of the urethra is seen by vaginal tumours or by subendothelial metastases from carcinoma of the cervix or endometrium.

Bowel obstruction is not usually helped by radiotherapy. It is seldom possible to pinpoint the site of obstruction with sufficient accuracy to be able to irradiate this without damaging large quantities of surrounding dilated bowel. These patients are usually best managed conservatively or surgically, although those with obstruction in the rectum may benefit from palliative external beam therapy. Unfortunately, many of these patients will not present until symptoms are so severe that colostomy is needed.

Ureteric obstruction occurs as a late event in many patients with recurrent carcinoma of the cervix, and textbooks will quote that the differential diagnosis lies between recurrent tumour and radiation fibrosis. However, the author has yet to see a case of ureteric obstruction that is not associated with recurrent tumour. Therefore, this is a symptom which, in the short term, may be amenable to palliation with radiotherapy, although a more usual approach would be to introduce a ureteric stent. As mentioned earlier on the subject of pain, careful thought must be given to the relief of ureteric obstruction in patients with incurable disease, as to relieve this problem may only leave the patient to die from something worse, for instance haemorrhage or bowel obstruction. There is no place for the use of nephrostomies in the palliative treatment of a patient with ureteric obstruction, as these are symptomatic in themselves, require considerable attention and reduce the quality of the patient's life for those few extra weeks that the patient gains.

Urethral obstruction is uncommon but may be treated on an individual basis by either external beam therapy to the lower pelvis or an intracavitary insertion to treat the anterior half of the vagina. However, most patients will have this symptom managed by insertion of a suprapubic catheter.

Incontinence

Recurrent or advanced tumours causing incontinence of faeces and urine are relatively uncommon and radiotherapy has little part to play in the management of faecal incontinence. However, urinary incontinence due to distortion of the bladder base by tumour may be relieved by palliative external beam radiotherapy, although the management of this problem by either indwelling catheter or by a surgical approach involving urinary diversion should be given early consideration, as urinary incontinence is a particularly depressing and debilitating symptom.

Fistulae

Fistulae between the bowel and the vagina or the bladder and vagina will usually require a surgical approach for management. The role of radiotherapy for control of this particular symptom is minor and, indeed, radiotherapy may be thought to make the symptom worse in some cases. Worsening of flow through the fistula can be caused by tumour regression produced by the radiotherapy and, very rarely, by radionecrosis, although this would be an unusual problem to encounter in less than 6–12 months following treatment.

Occasionally, fistulae may open between the bowel and the skin, particularly if there has been tumour seeding into a laparotomy scar, usually in patients with carcinoma of the ovary. The author's experience of this problem is that localized radiotherapy can lead to drying up and closing of fistulae between the bowel and the skin, although consideration would usually be given to a surgical approach in the first instance.

Skin Ulceration

Skin ulceration is a particular problem for patients with carcinoma of the vulva, many of whom are elderly and unsuitable for radical surgery. There is no effective curative non-surgical treatment for this disease and, therefore, patients with advanced vulval tumours may present for palliation having had no previous therapy. This is an unusual situation in gynaecological oncology, where most tumours can be treated with radical intent in the first instance.

As the vulval skin is intolerant of large doses of radiotherapy, palliation has traditionally been a protracted course taking several weeks. However, a particular problem with this group of patients is that they tend to be elderly, be from lower socioeconomic groups and live alone in poor accommodation. Protracted periods in hospital can lead to institutionalization and difficulty in rehabilitation to their home environment. Therefore, if they are to be palliated by radiotherapy, the treatment course should be short.

The social problems of these patients has very much encouraged radiotherapists to try new regimens to reduce skin reaction and enable the patient to return home earlier. Techniques such as radiotherapy combined with chemotherapy [1] may be appropriate for younger patients with advanced primary or recurrent disease, whereas shorter courses of radiotherapy alone have been tried for more elderly patients. Experience has been gained with a 1-week course of 20 Gy in five fractions and 30 Gy in ten fractions over 2 weeks and also by using a twice daily fractionation of 45 Gy in 30 fractions over 3 weeks [2].

Both intracavitary and interstitial implants may have a place to play in recurrent vulval disease at the introitus, but more lateral tumours are not suitable for this sort of palliation.

Skin ulceration from metastases from gynaecological cancers may be treated by electron therapy.

Distant Problems

Lymph Nodes

Lymph node masses in the groins which are causing symptoms of pain, bleeding or obstruction of flexion of the hip can be treated by either electrons or cobalt irradiation. Pelvic and para-aortic node masses require treatment with higher energy X-rays from a linear accelerator. An unusual situation in gynaecological oncology is for there to be involvement of mediastinal lymph nodes causing superior vena caval obstruction. If this occurs, it must be treated as an emergency with dexamethasone 4 mg q.d.s. and radiotherapy to the mediastinum. Traditionally, large fraction sizes have been used but, as is the case for achieving haemostasis with radiotherapy, there is no clear evidence that large fraction sizes are really indicated. A regimen of 20 Gy in five fractions over 1 week would usually be effective in relieving this condition.

Node involvement in the left supraclavicular fossa is uncommon, but is seen in a small percentage of patients with recurrent or advanced gynaecological cancer. It is usually associated with para-aortic node involvement and may be particularly distressing to the patient because of its superficial nature, allowing it to be both palpated and seen. It may be the only external manifestation of a patient's disease and, therefore, carry a great emotional importance. For this reason supraclavicular fossa metastases should be treated at the earliest opportunity, even if asymptomatic. Electron therapy to deliver 30 Gy in ten fractions over 2 weeks is usually sufficient, as these patients most commonly have bulk disease elsewhere, limiting their life span.

Lung Metastases

Lung metastases from gynaecological tumours are usually multiple and, therefore, not amenable to treatment with radiotherapy. However, occasionally a solitary metastasis occurs which may produce symptoms of haemoptysis or cough. In these circumstances, palliative treatment is indicated and, as with primary bronchogenic carcinoma, this may well be treated with a parallel opposed pair to give a single fraction of 10 Gy or two fractions to give a total dose of 18 Gy. If the patient has no evidence of disease elsewhere and it is felt that long-term control of the metastasis is required, a more protracted course of 30 Gy in ten fractions over 2 weeks is indicated. There are no gynaecological tumours which produce isolated pulmonary metastases in which it is worth considering radical radiotherapy.

Bone Metastases

None of the gynaecological cancers commonly spread to bone, but it is an occasional event. The bones that are usually involved are those of the pelvis by direct spread, vertebral bodies by invasion from involved para-aortic nodes, and blood-borne metastases to the vertebral bodies, ribs, skull and long bones. For blood-borne metastases it would appear that a short course of radiotherapy or, indeed, a single fraction is as valuable as a protracted course [3]. The bones involved by direct invasion will be treated, as is appropriate for the adjacent mass of tumour and any other symptoms produced by that. An unusual situation is for a patient to present with spinal cord compression, which should be managed by immediate administration of steroids, assessment as to whether or not neurosurgical decompression is possible and, if not, by urgent radiotherapy.

Brain Metastases

As with bone metastases these are seen only uncommonly in gynaecological oncology and those that are seen usually arise in patients with carcinoma of the ovary. They can be palliated by treatment with steroids followed by cranial irradiation. Trials are under way to assess the value of single fraction radiotherapy to the brain for the control of metastatic disease in comparison with more protracted courses.

Skin Metastases

Skin metastases are uncommon from gynaecological cancer, but may occur by lymphatic permeation from vulval cancer or blood-borne spread from other tumours. If psychologically distressing to the patient or if symptomatic, they may be treated by superficial X-rays or electrons.

Ascites

Ascites is not a problem that can usually be dealt with by conventional radiotherapy. However, radiolabelled monclonal antibody therapy and radioisotope colloids have been used in an attempt to reduce the rate of accumulation

Table 10.3 Cervical cancer – strictures on treatment

	Response	Relapse-free survival	Overall survival	Safety	Convenience	Affordability
Primary (good prognosis)	+	+	+	+	–	–
Primary (bad prognosis)	+	+	–	+/–	+/–	+/–
Recurrence	+	–	–	–	+	+

of ascites in patients with carcinoma of the ovary. Neither of these therapies is very effective in this circumstance and neither is used routinely.

Occasionally, when there is ascites associated with large quantities of tumour and it is felt that continued tapping of the ascites would be deleterious to the patient, large-volume external beam radiotherapy may be attempted. A regimen that has been used has been 8 Gy in two fractions over 2 days, given to the whole abdominopelvic volume. Treatment needs to be covered by dexamethasone 4 mg q.d.s. and antiemetics. However, reduction in the rate of accumulation of ascites can be achieved for a few weeks with this therapy and it is worth considering if there is no further anti-tumour treatment available and if a LeVeen (peritoneovenous) shunt is felt to be inadvisable or has previously failed.

Doses and Techniques

When treating a patient to achieve palliation, rather than cure, the constraints on the treatment technique and dose delivered are different. First, rapid control of symptoms is usually required for palliation, whereas in curative treatment it may be accepted that control of symptoms takes longer if the ultimate chance of success is thereby made greater. Secondly, it is important that the treatment itself does not produce symptoms of its own that become a problem for the patient. Thirdly, the logistics of undergoing radiotherapy for a patient who is symptomatic from their disease should not be so severe as to pose a problem in themselves. Fourthly, in hard-pressed departments palliative therapy may be seen to have to take a second place to curative therapy and, therefore, to make less demand on limited resources (Table 10.3).

The effect of these constraints is largely to make palliative radiotherapy a treatment that is delivered by simple techniques in short courses to doses lower than those that would be given with curative intent.

External Beam Therapy

At most sites, simple techniques would be used, either a direct field or a parallel opposed pair. This may be modified in the event of the patient having had previous radiotherapy with curative intent, in order to avoid previously irradiated tissues. However, the consequences of re-irradiating parts of the body should be assessed in relation to the likely life expectancy of the patient, as re-irradiation with a simple technique may well be acceptable to a patient with a limited life span, because the late effects would be unlikely to occur in that short time. The techniques used should also be possible with the patient lying in a comfortable position that does not exacerbate their symptoms.

Using external beam therapy it would be common to use palliative doses that are approximately half of those that would be delivered with curative intent. In addition, in order to achieve rapid symptom control and to be economical with resources, it is not unusual to give rather larger fractions than would be the case for treatment given with curative intent. For instance, a regimen of 20 Gy in five fractions over 5 days or 30 Gy in ten fractions over 12 days might be used, depending on the volume of tissue irradiated. As a general rule, the larger the volume of tissue irradiated, the smaller the individual fractions have to be and the longer the treatment has to take. For a large volume, such as the para-aortic nodes, palliation may only be achieved by a protracted course of radiotherapy delivering 45 Gy in 25 fractions over 5 weeks, as the overlying small bowel tolerates large fraction sizes only poorly. Although the particular symptom being treated may dictate the dose and fractionation schedule, as a general rule palliative regimens are simple and are applicable to most symptoms at most sites (see Table 10.2).

Intracavitary Therapy

Intracavitary therapy is largely only useful for superficial tumour deposits causing symptoms in the cervix or vagina. These symptoms are usually those of bleeding or discharge, as pain is usually indicative of a more deeply infiltrating lesion which would require external beam therapy, rather than the very localized treatment possible with intracavitary therapy. With this type of treatment, reference must be made to previous treatment, as the high local dose can otherwise cause tissue necrosis and side-effects of considerable inconvenience to the patient, such as rectovaginal or vesicovaginal fistulae. However, it is still a useful technique, even in previously treated patients, for the prevention of bleeding and, ideally, should be delivered at high dose-rate using a remote afterloading mechanism. This usually allows the treatment to be given as an outpatient procedure and, in a previously untreated patient, bleeding from vaginal nodules may be controlled by five fractions of 5.5 Gy, given at 0.5 cm depth from the surface of the vaginal applicator, over 2½ weeks, treating twice weekly. The author has also found this to be a very satisfactory dose for the very rare vaginal melanomas which, unfortunately, always prove fatal but which cause severe local problems in terms of discharge and bleeding. These unpleasant symptoms may be controlled for a year or more by palliative regimens such as this.

Electron Therapy

Electrons are suitable for superficial deposits of tumour, particularly around the introitus, vulva and perineum, provided that the patient can be positioned to allow good access to the area. Some treatment machines have very awkward electron applicators that make apposition of the head of the collimator to the vulva quite difficult. The patient may have to be treated in the "knee-chest" position, which can be uncomfortable for the more elderly patient. Doses delivered with electrons are, again, similar to those for palliative treatment with external beam radiotherapy, being short courses of 1 or 2 weeks to give 20 Gy in five fractions or 30 Gy in ten fractions. Occasionally, a solitary metastasis in the introitus from carcinoma of the endometrium may be symptomatic. A tumour such as this can be treated with the intention of producing a more long-lasting palliation by using a longer course of radiotherapy, as the natural history of this disease can be very slow and it may be some considerable time, possibly even years, before there is further evidence of disease elsewhere. Nevertheless, the vulva is an area sensitive to radiation and the symptoms of recurrent or metastatic tumour should not be exchanged for those of radionecrosis of the skin. This largely limits the dose that can be given by external beam therapy in that area to 50 Gy in standard 2 Gy fractions, given daily.

Sites for Radiotherapy

The radiotherapy volumes used to treat symptoms will largely depend upon the symptom and its site. Ideally, tumour should be imaged by CT scan or ultrasound and treatment planned with a simulator. However, these facilities may not be available in hard-pressed departments or in developing countries and, in general, the volume is fairly standard for patients with pelvic tumours requiring palliation, this being the true pelvis incorporating the upper vagina. For patients with symptomatic disease in the perineum, vulva and lower vagina, the volume may best be treated by using electrons with a direct perineal field. Electrons may also be used to treat the umbilicus for patients with metastases from carcinoma of the ovary at that site ("Sister Joseph's nodule"). The liver capsule may require irradiation when this is stretched and causing pain by metastases. The whole abdomen may be treated in patients with end-stage ascites, and extra-abdominal sites for treatment will be dictated by the location of blood-borne metastases.

Measuring Outcome

In the past, radiotherapy studies have largely concentrated on the curative treatment of cancer and little attention has been paid to its role in palliation. More recently, in the UK, there have been studies on the palliation of bone metastases and of brain metastases by radiotherapy. To date there have been no studies on the use of radiotherapy for the palliation of gynaecological cancer and it may well be appropriate that this is considered, particularly for those patients where current palliative techniques are disappointing, for instance patients with carcinoma of the vulva.

Outcome measures must be related not only to the improvement in the symptom, but to the general wellbeing and quality of life of the patient and their ability to function independently in the community.

References

1. Whittaker SJ, Kirkbride P, Arnott SJ, Shepherd JH (1990) A pilot study of chemo-radiotherapy in advanced carcinoma of the vulva. Br J Obstet Gynaecol 97:436–442.
2. Harrington KJ, Lambert HE (1994) Current issues in the non-surgical management of primary vulvar squamous cell carcinoma. Clin Oncol 6:331–336.
3. Price P, Hoskin PJ, Easton D, Austin D, Palmer S, Yarnold JR (1988) Low dose single fraction radiotherapy in the treatment of metastatic bone pain: a pilot study. Radiother Oncol 12:297–300.

11 – Non-Curative Radiotherapy for Neurological Cancer

R. Barton, L. Brazil and Michael Brada

Introduction

Tumours in the central nervous system (CNS) include metastatic disease and primary tumours which range from highly malignant such as high-grade gliomas to curable tumours which include meningiomas, benign pituitary adenomas and cranial germ-cell tumours. Radiotherapy is the mainstay of primary therapy both in the curative and the palliative setting.

Brain tumours with rare exceptions do not metastasize outside the CNS and the aim of radiotherapy is to achieve local control either with radiation alone or in combination with surgery or chemotherapy. Despite the demonstrable failure of radiation as curative treatment in the more aggressive tumour types, it is generally given with radical intent to prolong survival. There has been little regard to the palliative benefit of radiation and the requirements of palliative treatment to be short, well tolerated and effective in relieving symptoms.

The difficulty in assessing the palliative efficacy of radiotherapy in neurological tumours is due to the complex neurological problems arising from the combination of damage to the CNS by the tumour and its treatment. The expression of such damage includes a whole range of neurological dysfunction, and epilepsy as well as psychosocial consequences. While it is possible to measure individual neurological deficit there is no good, easily applicable global scale which would encompass all the problems encountered. Over the years most studies have relied on functional scales such as the Karnofsky performance status (KPS) or the neurological performance status, which have not been fully validated in brain tumour patients. Most information on the potential palliative effectiveness of radiotherapy is based on these measures and will need to be re-evaluated with newer, more reliable functional and quality-of-life scales. This is particularly important when attempting to compare the efficacy of different palliative regimens where survival and disease control are not the primary end-points.

To evaluate the palliative efficacy of irradiation it is necessary to describe the whole range of problems encountered in brain tumour patients, and develop scales to be able to measure effectively a change in score. As in other malignant disease it is, however, difficult to distinguish the effects of treatment aimed at controlling the tumour from those of other palliative approaches aimed at reducing raised intracranial pressure, and treating epilepsy and other symptoms.

Table 11.1 Clinical features at diagnosis of cerebral glioma (From Thomas and McKeran [1], by permission, Edward Arnold, publisher)

Symptoms	Frequency (%)
Headache	71
Epilepsy	54
Mental change	52
Hemiparesis	43
Vomiting	32
Dysphasia	27
Impaired consciousness	25
Visual failure	18
Hemianaesthesia	14
Cranial nerve palsy	11

Problems Encountered in Brain Tumour Patients

Patients with brain tumours present with features of raised intracranial pressure, epilepsy and focal or general neurological dysfunction, with physical disability, communication and personality change. The relative frequency of symptoms in patients presenting with cerebral tumours has been described previously (Table 11.1). Such lists demonstrate the range of symptoms encountered, but do not give an accurate view of the severity and the range of disability and the effect on the patient and their carers. At the time of disease progression, the range and severity of deficit often increase and the majority of patients are disabled. The psychological effects of the diagnosis of brain tumour and the disability also have devastating psychosocial implications which relate to all interpersonal relationships and employment prospects, and any semblance of normal life is usually destroyed.

Measurement of Treatment Efficacy

It is difficult to apply the standard end-points of cancer therapy when assessing efficacy of brain tumour treatment. The possible end-points are listed in Table 11.2. Undoubtedly survival is relevant, but in the context of essentially palliative treatment perhaps not of primary importance. Tumour control/progression-free survival and tumour response are particularly difficult to measure in the CNS. Although new generation CT and MRI scanners and functional imaging with PET have revolutionized CNS imaging, the interpretation of imaging remains problematic.

MRI and CT scans have high sensitivity and accuracy in the initial diagnosis of brain tumour. X-ray or magnetic density and the enhancing characteristics of

Table 11.2 End-points of efficacy of brain tumour therapy

Quality of life
Functional status/neurological impairment
Functionally independent survival
Survival
Progression-free survival
Neurological deficit-free survival
Tumour response

tumour help to define tumour size, but such imaging properties do not necessarily reflect the overall tumour mass. They are an indirect measure, relying on radiological characteristics of tumour cells, cell density and the permeability of the tumour vasculature which is usually impaired in comparison with the blood–brain barrier of healthy CNS.

Response to treatment is reflected in changes in mass effect, usually with restoration of normal anatomical appearance. However, the use of corticosteroids alone may produce a similar effect. With few exceptions (e.g. germinoma or primary cerebral lymphoma which disappear following treatment), the assessment of size of lesion is not helpful, as changes in size or enhancing characteristics of glioma after treatment are usually not predictive of outcome. In addition, contrast enhancement and peri-tumour low density may be the result of surgery and subsequent alteration may simply represent resolution of post-surgical changes and are not a measure of success of therapy. Radiological assessment is therefore highly unreliable as a means of assessing efficacy of radiotherapy. Nevertheless, a reduction in mass effect and the size of the enhancing mass is usually accompanied by neurological improvement.

PET scanning may overcome some of the problems of radiological imaging as it provides a measure of tissue function in terms of oxygen uptake and metabolism, sugar metabolism or proliferative activity. Similar metabolic information may also be obtained from magnetic resonance spectroscopy. Assessments of early post-treatment changes and their relevance are only just emerging from present studies and their significance is not clear.

Function and Quality of Life

While it is possible to develop objective measures of neurological impairment and consequent disability, measures of handicap and quality of life are more individual, subjective and perhaps more relevant.

The assessment of palliative effectiveness of treatment by combining radiological response and clinical response is inadequate [2]. Clinical response is usually measured as a change detected on traditional neurological examination and may have no bearing on functional ability. Objective measures have only been developed in recent years and should include changes in functional status, cognitive funtion and overall quality of life.

The most frequently employed method of clinical measurement of physical function is the use of a physical grading system of power. This is an unreliable and subjective assessment without full validation. There is also no clear correlation between loss of power and disability. A more appropriate method of assessment of functional status is an index of activities of daily living (ADL), either by physical testing or through a questionnaire. One such scale, the verbally administered scale (Table 11.3), has been fully validated in patients following stroke and has been used as a measure of functional status in patients with glioma [3].

The Barthel Index (BI) is reliable, sensitive to change and easy to use. It also provides practical information which is useful in assessing rehabilitation needs. However, it is only of value in patients with physical disability which is sufficiently severe to influence ADL. It also suffers from a ceiling effect; it cannot detect changes in patients with mild physical impairment not affecting ADL. Such

Table 11.3 The Barthel ADL Index is based on the factors and scores shown

Bowels: 0 = incontinent 1 = occasional accident 2 = continent	Bladder: 0 = incontinent or catheterized and unable to manage 1 = occasional accident (maximum 1 × per 24 h 2 = continent (for over 7 days)
Grooming: 0 = needs help 1 = independent, face/hair/teeth/shaving	Toilet needs: 0 = dependent 1 = needs some help but can do something 2 = independent but with some difficulty 3 = normal
Feeding: 0 = unable 1 = needs help cutting, spreading butter, etc. 2 = independent but slow 3 = normal	Transfer: 0 = unable 1 = major help (1–2 people, physical) 2 = minor help (verbal or physical) 3 = independent but slow 4 = normal
Mobility: 0 = immobile 1 = wheelchair independent, including corners, etc. 2 = walks with help of 1 person (verbal or physical) 3 = independent but slower than before 4 = normal	Dressing: 0 = dependent 1 = needs help, but can do about half unaided 2 = independent but has difficulties 3 = normal
Stairs: 0 = unable 1 = needs help (verbal, physical, carrying aid) 2 = independent up and down but slow and with difficulty 3 = normal	Bathing 0 = dependent 1 = independent

patients can be subjected to more detailed tests of physical dysfunction using the Edinburgh Functional Index Test [4].

Cognitive function has a number of components which include IQ tests, memory, speech and language, visuo-perception and visuo-constructional abilities. A battery of psychological tests, although informative, are not practical for routine use. New, easy to administer, validated methods of assessment are needed to evaluate all brain tumour patients.

Quality-of-life measures have not been routinely applied to brain tumour patients. Performance status measurement with KPS has been used as a rather inadequate surrogate and more appropriate scales are needed. The EORTC core questionnaire QLQ-C30 with a brain tumour module has been developed and is being tested in prospective studies of brain tumour patients [5].

Conventional Radiotherapy of High-Grade Glioma

Radiotherapy is established as the principal treatment in patients with high-grade glioma. The addition of radiotherapy to best supportive care prolongs survival [6, 7] but the overall prognosis remains poor with median survival of 40–50 weeks and few patients surviving beyond 2 years.

Radiotherapy is conventionally given as external beam irradiation to the whole brain, the tumour and a margin or to a combination of both. It is delivered to a radical dose of 55–60 Gy over 6 weeks in 30 or more fractions at $\leqslant$ 2 Gy/fraction. The radical high dose approach to treatment has been reinforced by a MRC study which compared 60 Gy in 30 fractions against 45 Gy in 20 fractions [8]. The higher dose schedule resulted in a 3-month prolongation of median survival (12 vs. 9 months), and the 6-week 30-fraction high-dose regimen is therefore considered the standard. No additional survival benefit has been demonstrated by increasing the dose further to 70 Gy with conventional external beam radiotherapy [9].

The assessment of palliative effectiveness in terms of functional improvement and quality of life is difficult. The majority of radiotherapy trials have only recorded performance status at presentation and use the information for its prognostic value and not to assess palliation. Kristiansen et al. recorded the performance status before craniotomy in 118 patients who were randomized postoperatively between radiotherapy, radiotherapy with bleomycin and no further intervention [6]. A five-point scale was used, ranging from "full capacity for work" to "bedridden", and patients were reassessed at intervals after craniotomy. In all three groups performance status improved in the immediate postoperative period, but patients receiving radiotherapy maintained the improvement for longer, with 30% able to undertake some light work at 6 months compared to less than 10% of those receiving no radiotherapy.

Toxicity of Conventional Radiotherapy

Although the standard radiotherapy regimens are below the conventional radiation tolerance of neural tissue, the treatment is not entirely without toxicity. Transient early reactions to large-field irradiation include mild features of raised intracranial pressure with occasional worsening neurological deficit, presumed to be due to oedema within the tumour or the surrounding normal brain. Such transient symptoms usually occur in patients with unresected tumours and generally respond to corticosteroids. The most distressing complication of cranial irradiation is alopecia, starting in the second or third week of treatment. It is unavoidable and usually permanent in the regions of high-dose treatment. The transient effect of skin irradiation with erythema is not common, but irradiation of the external auditory meati and the middle ear may result in secretory otitis media.

Late radiation damage with demyelination and necrosis is uncommon with conventional doses and fractionation. It is considered to be due to depletion of oligodendrocytes and endothelial cells and the damage manifests as progressive focal or global features indistinguishable from tumour recurrence or progression, unless patients are subjected to reoperation. Such an aggressive approach with repeat surgery is reserved for young and fit patients and the resected lesions usually show a combination of necrosis and recurrent tumour.

Lower doses of radiation which do not cause necrosis may result in neurological disturbance without identifiable structural defect. This has been identified in children who may suffer intellectual impairment following whole-brain irradiation, particularly if this is given under the age of 4 years. Adults surviving radical radiotherapy for brain tumours have also been reported to develop neuropsychological impairment, but it is difficult to distinguish damage caused by tumour from that caused by surgery and subsequent radiotherapy. The frequency and severity of cognitive impairment following standard localized brain irradiation of high-grade glioma has not been documented.

Alternatives to Conventional Radiotherapy

Assuming that the limitation to conventional radiotherapy is damage to normal brain outside the high-dose volume, techniques have been developed to deliver radiation to small volumes with high precision either using stereotactic external beam radiotherapy (SRT) [10] or with interstitial brachytherapy (IRT) with implanted radiation sources [11]. The aim of these techniques is to give a higher tumour dose without increasing the dose to surrounding normal brain, thereby improving the therapeutic ratio. Patients with primary high-grade glioma have been treated with SRT or IRT boost. Although the survival results in phase II studies appear superior to conventionally treated patients [12], this may be entirely due to patient selection [13], and we are awaiting the results of randomized studies of IRT and SRT boost which are currently in progress. Even if survival is marginally improved using such techniques, the treatment is accompanied by a high incidence of necrosis at the irradiation site, requiring reoperation.

A conventional 6-week course of radiotherapy is considered optimal in terms of survival benefit, but the short overall life expectancy means that it is essentially a palliative treatment. In this respect it lacks the attributes of palliative therapy of convenience, lack of toxicity, simplicity and short duration. Based on known prognostic factors for survival, which include age, performance status and tumour histology, it is possible to separate patients into individual prognostic groups [14, 15]. One approach to improve the acceptability of radiotherapy and maintain the principle of high-dose irradiation is to reduce the treatment time. This can be achieved with accelerated radiotherapy, where the same high dose is given over a shorter time by using multiple fractions per day. A total of 156 patients with high-grade glioma were treated at the Royal Marsden Hospital to a dose of 55 Gy in 32–36 (usually 34) fractions twice daily over a period of 3 weeks (update of [16]). The median survival of 10 months is comparable to that achieved in a matched cohort treated in conventional manner [16]. The shorter treatment time was acceptable to patients and staff and did not result in any obvious increase in early toxicity. However, the logistics of twice daily treatment is difficult both for the patient and the running of the department. The palliative effectiveness of such a regimen has not been formally assessed, but in patients where BI measurements were made prior to and 1–3 months after treatment, 62% had stable or improved functional status.

For the poor prognostic group of severely disabled and elderly patients with high-grade glioma, an aggressive 3-week course of intensive radiotherapy is too onerous. A reasonable option is a hypofractionated course of irradiation, as used in the treatment of brain metastases. Two regimens have been examined in phase II studies [17, 18]. At the Royal Marsden Hospital 60 patients were treated to a dose of 30 Gy in six fractions over 2 weeks (update of [18]). The median survival of 6 months was comparable to similar patients subjected to radical radiotherapy. The treatment was also reasonably effective as palliative therapy, with three-quarters of surviving patients showing improvement or stabilization of functional status 1–3 months after treatment. Such altered fractionation regimens provide reasonable alternatives for what is essentially palliative radiotherapy. Their overall efficacy in comparison to other approaches has to be evaluated in future randomized studies; in poor prognosis patients the control group should include supportive care alone and in good prognosis patients, standard high-dose radiotherapy.

Recurrent High-Grade Glioma

With few exceptions, patients with high-grade glioma develop recurrent disease. Treatment at recurrence should be for palliative purposes alone. However, the perception, particularly in the eyes of the patient and the carer, too often is that the priority should be prolongation of survival. Prognosis of patients with recurrent high-grade glioma from the time of recurrence is not known. The only information available is based on patients sufficiently fit to be considered for further active treatment. The patients are highly selected in terms of age, performance status and general medical fitness. Nevertheless, such studies indicate that prognostic factors at recurrence are the same as those at presentation [19], with median survival measured in months.

Many treatments vie for the position of most effective therapy at the time of recurrence. The lack of consensus on the best approach merely indicates the poor effectiveness of the majority of treatment approaches. Because of the poor prognosis, recurrent glioma is often considered the "testing ground" for the most innovative treatment approaches. This has often led to the mistaken perception of "breakthrough" in the treatment of glioma and sometimes unsubstantiated claims of the efficacy of such novel treatments.

Conventional re-irradiation of the original tumour site has little value. Large tumour volumes are rarely re-irradiated, partly due to the poor efficacy and partly because of the fear of necrosis after high cumulative radiation doses. Radical attempts at retreatment are reserved for small tumours and include reoperation [20] and high-dose localized irradiation. The latter can be achieved with interstitial radiotherapy or with stereotactically guided external beam radiotherapy.

Interstitial brachytherapy has been claimed as the most effective treatment in recurrent glioma [11]. In the series reported from San Francisco, high-activity ^{125}I sources were implanted directly into the tumour and patients received doses ranging from 50 to 150 Gy (median 70 Gy). The median survival after treatment was 54 weeks for recurrent glioblastoma and 81 weeks for anaplastic astrocytoma [21]. Late side-effects were common, with half the patients requiring resection for necrosis. In these patients viable tumour was often found within the necrotic tissue. The "quality of survival" was assessed with KPS and steroid dependency. While the majority of patients (97%) were steroid dependent at the time of treatment at 18 months and 36 months, 67% and 53% of patients respectively remained steroid dependent. There was a small decrease in mean KPS, from 87 to 79 and to 76 over the same period. Functional status was therefore preserved in a selected group of long-term survivors, but less than half survived beyond 18 months. The individual changes in quality of life and functional ability are not reported. The treatment is highly interventional, as initial radiotherapy is an invasive procedure and more than half the patients require reoperation.

The Royal Marsden Hospital group reported patients with recurrent glioma treated with fractionated SRT on a dose escalation protocol [22]. The median survival was 10 months and the majority of patients retained a functional ability and symptom profile comparable to pretreatment levels. The results of a recent update of 30 patients with recurrent high-grade glioma treated with SRT are similar and only two patients needed reoperation for necrosis. While SRT remains a palliative treatment similar in efficacy to IRT, it is a non-invasive, well-tolerated treatment with little toxicity which can be carried out in an outpatient setting.

There are many phase II studies of single agent and combination chemotherapy. They report radiological/clinical responses in 20–40% of patients. The overall response correlates with prognosis as fit, young patients have a higher response rate than poorer prognosis patients [19]. Nitrosoureas are currently the most effective agents (BCNU or CCNU), but there are no randomized studies comparing single agent with combination chemotherapy in recurrent tumours. New agents such as other nitrosourea derivatives or temozolomide (dacarbazine derivative) are undergoing large phase II trials.

While the palliative efficacy of treatment for recurrent disease is very poorly documented, it can be broadly stated that "response" to therapy is associated with stabilization or improvement in neurological status. However, patients with severe disability rarely have full recovery and the duration of improvement is also short-lasting. It is therefore entirely reasonable that patients with severe disability are offered supportive care alone, with attention to the considerable support needed by their carers who often have to deal with someone not only with physical but also cognitive impairment and personality change.

Low-Grade Gliomas

Low-grade gliomas include the entities of surgically curable pilocytic astrocytomas usually occurring in the posterior fossa in children, and the indolent but infiltrative and progressive low-grade astrocytomas (defined as astrocytomas on the WHO grading system) as well as oligodendrogliomas, mixed oligoastrocytomas and ependymomas. Such tumours in adults occur primarily in the cerebral hemisphere and while by histological appearance and relatively slow growth are considered benign, the overall results are poor as they eventually progress, transform to higher grade and become untreatable. The reported 5- and 10-year survival rates of patients with astrocytoma are in the region of 50% and 20%, respectively, and as in high-grade tumours age and performance status are the most important prognostic factors for survival [23].

Pilocytic astrocytomas can be cured by surgery. While this is generally true for childhood tumours, a similar strategy should be adopted for hemispheric pilocytic astrocytomas in adults. There is retrospective data to suggest that radiotherapy improves survival in patients with incompletely excised tumours [24].

The role of surgery and radiotherapy in astrocytomas and oligodendrogliomas is poorly defined. In general, it is recommended that patients with suspected low-grade tumours should have histological confirmation of the diagnosis, although the behaviour of histologically unverified presumed gliomas is similar to the histologically verified counterparts [25]. A number of retrospective studies suggest that radiotherapy confers a survival advantage [23]. Randomized studies comparing immediate versus delayed radiotherapy are currently under way and will provide information on the efficacy of radiotherapy. Nevertheless, in patients with unresectable tumours irradiation often reduces the size of the tumour mass, with improvement in symptoms including focal neurological deficit and frequency of seizures which are a common feature of low-grade gliomas. While the general impression is that radiotherapy is a useful palliative tool in patients with low-grade glioma, there are no large prospective studies which document the effect of radiation on quality of life and functional ability.

The radiotherapy technique for low-grade gliomas is similar to that used for high-grade tumours, with radiation confined to the region of abnormality on imaging, presumed to represent tumour, and a small margin. The conventional treatment is given in daily fractions to doses of 55–60 Gy over a period of 6 weeks. Treatment to higher doses and the use of unconventional fractionation may result in higher late normal tissue toxicity which, in these patients, is currently not considered acceptable. Small apparently localized low-grade tumours have been treated with IRT [26], with excellent resolution of tumour on imaging. However, there is as yet no proof of superior efficacy of this treatment approach compared to conventional treatment, as survival results are comparable to similar patients selected using the same criteria.

One of the unacceptable side-effects of irradiation, particularly in younger age groups with longer survival expectancy, is permanent alopecia. Newer techniques of irradiation allow for scalp shielding which improves the cosmetic outcome without compromising tumour control.

The majority of low-grade gliomas recur and at the time of relapse 30–60% transform to high-grade tumours. The overall treatment approach is similar to recurrent high-grade gliomas. However, the prognosis even at the time of recurrence is better than in patients with high-grade tumours *ab initio*.

Brain Metastases

Brain metastases develop in 10–15% of patients with malignancy. While the highest risk of metastatic disease in the brain is associated with tumours such as small cell lung cancer, the high incidence of breast and non-small cell lung cancer means that these represent the largest proportion of patients with brain metastases.

Brain metastases usually develop in the context of systemic metastatic cancer and the treatment is essentially palliative. Corticosteroids improve symptoms in up to 60% of patients and this may be sufficient treatment in the face of extensive metastatic disease. Survival is determined by performance status, the control of primary tumour, age and the extent of metastatic disease at the time of radiotherapy for brain metastases [27].

Radiotherapy provides effective palliation and can produce neurological improvement in up to 70% of patients [28]. However, the long-term results in terms of symptom and tumour control are disappointing, with an overall median survival of 4 months and 1-year survival < 20%. Comparison of various radiotherapy schedules in large randomized studies suggest that a short 1-week regimen is as effective as longer more intensive treatment [28] in terms of survival, improvement of neurological deficit, time to progression of neurological symptoms and the frequency of intracranial failure, which is the cause of death in up to half of the patients. Newer palliative whole-brain radiotherapy regimens are even shorter and on current evidence 18 Gy in three fractions is as effective as more protracted regimens [29].

Selected patients with solitary brain metastases have a better outcome, with median survival of 9–12 months [30, 31]. On current evidence, surgery combined with whole-brain irradiation is considered the treatment of choice, but this approach is only appropriate for patients with absent or static systemic disease [32]. Localized irradiation in the form of radiosurgery/SRT [10] appears equally as effective as surgical excision and is gaining popularity, particularly in the palliative setting, where patients can be spared invasive neurosurgical procedures. Following one or two fractions of radiosurgery the majority of patients show functional improvement accompanied by radiological resolution of tumour. The prognosis both in terms of tumour control and survival is similar to that achieved with surgery, with the activity and extent of systemic disease the major determinants of survival [33].

In summary, whole-brain irradiation together with corticosteroids remains the accepted palliative treatment for patients with multiple brain metastases and this approach provides functional improvement in over two-thirds of patients. However, a large proportion of patients will relapse with disease in the brain and the median survival is only of the order of 4–6 months. Patients with solitary metastases may be treated effectively with either surgery or more recently SRT/radiosurgery. However, invasive treatment should be reserved only for patients with static or absent systemic disease.

Spinal Cord Compression

Spinal cord compression is a common complication of cancer, occurring overall in approximately 5% of patients who die with metastatic disease. In adults, at least 50% arise from carcinomas of the breast, prostate or lung, usually in the setting of disseminated disease. Cord compression is usually caused by extradural tumour either in the vertebral bodies, the paravertebral space or, more rarely, the extradural space itself. Meningeal or intramedullary disease is rare. The thoracic spine is affected most commonly, at a rate out of proportion to the number of thoracic vertebrae, possibly reflecting high local blood flow.

Clinical manifestations of spinal cord compression include back or neck pain, limb weakness, sensory disturbance and loss of sphincter control. Pain is the initial symptom in 95% of adults, and this may precede other symptoms or neurological signs by days or months [34, 35]. It may be localized to the involved site or be referred in a dermatomal or specifically radicular pattern and is not usually relieved by rest.

Models of spinal cord compression show that it begins with compression of the vertebral venous plexus, resulting in cord oedema, venous haemorrhage, ischaemia and finally infarction [36], suggesting that early diagnosis is important if the lesion is to be reversible.

The investigation of choice in suspected spinal cord compression is an MRI scan of the vertebral column. If not available, the diagnosis can be made on myelography, with CT. Plain radiographs reveal the site of vertebral metastases in 85% of cases and this, along with clinical signs consistent with spinal cord compression, may be enough for emergency treatment. The initial treatment for spinal cord compression consists of analgesia and corticosteroids [37], given prior to a definitive diagnosis.

A proportion of patients undergo surgery. When combined with postoperative radiotherapy it is effective both in pain relief and in allowing patients to maintain or gain the ability to walk; 58% of those able to walk at presentation are able to do so after treatment [38]. The majority of patients with metastatic spinal cord compression have bone disease. Vertebral body resection is the definitive procedure in patients who have limited disease and a relatively long life expectancy. Laminectomy is less traumatic, but produces only a temporary relief of pressure and should be considered only for posterior lesions causing anterior compression. Most neurosurgery centres will consider, for decompressive surgery, patients who have a rapid onset of symptoms with a good premorbid performance status, those in whom neurological deterioration continues in spite of radiotherapy or those in whom the diagnosis of malignancy has not been made.

Radiotherapy is the mainstay of treatment for patients presenting with spinal cord compression due to known malignancy (except tumours known to be chemosensitive). A review of 70 cases of breast cancer developing cord compression showed that all ambulant and 65% non-ambulant patients treated with radiotherapy alone were able to walk after treatment. In addition, 71% of those treated with radiotherapy alone reported an improvement in pain, 62% in sphincter control and 55% in sensory symptoms [39]. The reported benefit of radiotherapy depends in part on the definition of the patient groups. Some differentiate between those who are able to walk, those who are weak (paraparetic) and those who have no residual power (paraplegic). When defined in this way < 5% of the paraplegic patients are able to walk after treatment [38]. The histology of the primary tumour also has a bearing on the likely outcome of treatment. Patients with myeloma, lymphoma or carcinoma of the breast have a higher initial response rate (60–80%) than patients with melanoma, carcinoma of the lung or prostate cancer (20–50%) [38].

The dose and fractionation of radiotherapy vary between centres and radiotherapists, and there are no randomized studies examining this issue. Doses range from relatively high, such as 30 Gy in ten fractions over 2 weeks, to shorter fractionation regimens, of 20 Gy in five fractions, or to a single 8–10 Gy fraction which may be adequate in paraplegic patients where the emphasis is pain relief rather than the return of function. Dose/fractionation regimens should be compared in randomized controlled trials which should assess walking and general functional ability, pain relief and quality of life. Treatment may not affect survival and it may be appropriate to express results in terms of the proportion of remaining life for which symptoms are improved.

In summary, the best treatment for spinal cord compression has not been defined, but most patients will receive corticosteroids and radiotherapy with a selected few also undergoing surgery and, where appropriate, chemotherapy or hormonal therapy. The most important criterion for identifying those who will benefit from vigorous treatment is their ability to walk at the start of treatment. This, along with the extent of disease and histology, allows a reasoned plan of approach for each individual.

Conclusions

Radiotherapy is the mainstay of non-curative treatment in patients with glioma, brain metastases and spinal cord compression. It may prolong survival and in the majority of patients improve functional status.

However, more vigorous assessment of palliative efficacy in terms of improvement in neurological function and quality of life is needed. New radiotherapy approaches aim to reduce treatment intensity in poor prognosis patients and increase it with high-precision techniques in the favourable prognosis patients.

The correct management of patients with brain tumours cannot be considered simply as treatment with radiotherapy, surgery or other treatment modalities. Patients with CNS tumours usually have major neurological deficit with physical disability as well as cognitive impairment, communication difficulties and personality change. Any active treatment should include rehabilitation managed by a multidisciplinary rehabilitation team. The diagnosis of brain tumour, the neurological consequences and the poor overall prognosis have a devastating psychological effect on the patient, family and friends, and all require sympathetic and practical support which cannot be derived from radiation alone.

References

1. Thomas DGT, McKeran RO (1990) Clinical manifestations of brain tumours. In: Thomas DGT (ed) Neuro-oncology – primary malignant brain tumours. Edward Arnold, London, 141–147.
2. MacDonald DR, Cascino TL, Schold SCJ, Cairncross G (1990) Response criteria for phase II studies of supratentorial malignant glioma. J Clin Oncol 8:1277–1280.
3. Brazil LC, Thomas R, Laing R et al. (1997) Verbally administered Barthel Index as functional assessment in brain tumour patients. J Neuro-oncol 34, 187–192.
4. Grant R, Slattery J, Gregor A, Whittle IR (1994) Recording neurological impairment in clinical trials of glioma. J Neuro-oncol 19:37–49.
5. Osoba D, Aaronson NK, Muller M et al. (1996) The development and psychometric validation of a brain cancer quality-of-life questionnaire for use in combination with general cancer-specific questionnaires. Qual Life Res 5:139–150.
6. Kristiansen K, Hagen S, Kollevold T et al. (1981) Combined modality therapy of operated astrocytomas grade III and IV. Confirmation of the value of postoperative irradiation and lack of potentiation of bleomycin on survival time: a prospective multicenter trial of the Scandinavian Glioblastoma Study Group. Cancer 47:649–652.
7. Walker MD, Alexander E, Hunt WE et al. (1978) Evaluation of BCNU and/or radiotherapy in the treatment of anaplastic gliomas. J Neurosurg 49:333–343.
8. Bleehen NM, Stenning SP and on behalf of the Medical Research Council Brain Tumour Working Party (1991) A Medical Research Council trial of two radiotherapy doses in the treatment of grades 3 and 4 astrocytoma. Br J Cancer 64:769–774.
9. Chang CH, Horton J, Schoenfeld D et al. (1983) Comparison of postoperative

radiotherapy and combined postoperative radiotherapy and chemotherapy in the multidisciplinary management of malignant gliomas. Cancer 52:997–1007.
10. Brada M, Laing R (1994) Radiosurgery/stereotactic external beam radiotherapy for malignant brain tumours: the Royal Marsden experience. In: Wiestler OD, Schlegel U, Schramm J (eds) Molecular neuro-oncology and its impact on the clinical management of brain tumours. Springer-Verlag, Berlin, pp 91–103.
11. Sneed PK, Larson DA, Gutin PH (1994) Brachytherapy and hyperthermia for malignant astrocytomas. Semin Oncol 21:186–197.
12. Loeffler J, Alexander E III. (1991) Stereotactic radiosurgery for malignant gliomas. Second International Neuro-oncology Conference, London.
13. Curran WJ, Scott CB, Weinstein AS et al. (1993) Survival comparison of radiosurgery-eligible and -ineligible malignant glioma patients treated with hyperfractionated radiation therapy and carmustine: a report of Radiation Therapy Oncology Group 83–02. J Clin Oncol 11:857–862.
14. Curran WJ, Scott CB, Horton J et al. (1993) Recursive partitioning analysis of prognostic factors in three radiation therapy oncology group malignant glioma trials. J Natl Cancer Inst 85:704–710.
15. MRC Brain Tumour Working Party (1990) Prognostic factors for high-grade malignant glioma: development of a prognostic index. J Neuro-oncol 9:47–55.
16. Brada M (1995) Central nervous system tumours. In: Horwich A (ed) Oncology – a multidisciplinary textbook. Chapman and Hall, London, pp 395–416.
17. Bauman GS, Gaspar LE, Fisher BJ et al. (1994) A prospective study of short-course radiotherapy in poor prognosis glioblastoma multiforme. Int J Radiat Oncol Biol Phys 29:835–839.
18. Thomas R, James N, Guerrero D et al. (1994) Hypofractionated radiotherapy as palliative treatment in poor prognosis patients with high grade glioma. Radiother Oncol 33:113–116.
19. Rajan B, Ross GM, Lim CC et al. (1994) Survival in patients with recurrent glioma as a measure of treatment efficacy: prognostic factors following nitrosourea chemotherapy. Eur J Cancer 30A:1809–1815.
20. Moser RP (1988) Surgery for glioma relapse: factors that influence a favourable outcome. Cancer 62:381–390.
21. Leibel SA, Gutin PH, Wara WM et al. (1989) Survival and quality of life after interstitial implantation of removable high-activity Iodine-125 sources for the treatment of patients with recurrent malignant gliomas. Int J Radiat Oncol Biol Phys 17:1129–1139.
22. Laing RW, Warrington AP, Graham J et al. (1993) Efficacy and toxicity of fractionated stereotactic radiotherapy in the treatment of recurrent gliomas (phase I/II study). Radiother Oncol 27:22–39.
23. Vecht CJ, Haaxma-Reiche H, Noordijk EM et al. (1993) Treatment of single brain metastasis: radiotherapy alone or combined with neurosurgery? Ann Neurol 33:583–590.
24. Shaw EG, Daumas-Duport C, Scheithauer BW et al. (1989) Radiation therapy in the management of low-grade supratentorial astrocytomas. J Neurosurg 70:853–861.
25. Rajan B, Pickuth D, Ashley S et al. (1994) The management of histologically unverified presumed cerebral gliomas with radiotherapy. Int J Radiat Oncol Biol Phys 28:405–413.
26. Ostertag C, Warnke P (1991) Interstitial radiotherapy for brain tumours. Br J Neurosurg 5:421–436.
27. Diener-West M, Dobbins TW, Phillips TL, Nelson DF (1989) Identification of an optimal subgroup for treatment evaluation of patients with brain metastases using RTOG study 7916. Int J Radiat Oncol Biol Phys 16:669–673.
28. Borgelt B, Gelber R, Kramer S et al. (1980) The palliation of brain metastases: final results of the first two studies by the radiation therapy oncology group. Int J Radiat Oncol Biol Phys 6:1–9.

29. Haie-Meder C, Pallae-Cosset B, Laplanche A et al. (1993) Results of a randomized clinical trial comparing two radiation schedules in the palliative treatment of brain metastases. Radiother Oncol 26:111–116.
30. Patchell R, Tibbs P, Walsh J et al. (1990) A randomised trial of surgery in the treatment of single metastases to the brain. N Engl J Med 322:494–500.
31. Smalley SR, Laws ER, O'Tallon JR, Shaw EG, Schray MF (1992) Resection for solitary brain metastases. J Neurosurg 77:531–540.
32. Noordijk EM, Vecht CJ, Haaxma-Reiche H et al. (1994) The choice of treatment of single brain metastasis should be based on extracranial tumour activity and age. Int J Radiat Oncol Biol Phys 29:711–717.
33. Engenhart R, Kimmig BN, Hover KH et al. (1993) Long-term follow-up for brain metastases treated by percutaneous stereotactic single high-dose irradiation. Cancer 71:1353–1361.
34. Byrne TN (1992) Spinal cord compression from epidural metastases. N Engl J Med 327:614–619.
35. Helweg-Larsen S, Sorensen PS (1994) Symptoms and signs in metastatic spinal cord compression: a study of progression from first symptom until diagnosis in 153 patients. Eur J Cancer 3:396–398.
36. Kato AM Ushio Y, Hayakawa T et al. (1985) Circulatory disturbance of the spinal cord with epidural neoplasm in rats. J Neurosurg 63:260–265.
37. Sorensen PS, Helweg-Larsen S, Mouridsen H, Hansen HH (1994) Effect of high-dose dexamethasone in carcinomatous metastatic spinal cord compression treated with radiotherapy: a randomised trial. Eur J Cancer 1:22–27.
38. Gilbert RW, Kim J-H and Posner JB (1978) Epidural spinal cord compression from metastatic tumour: diagnosis and treatment. Ann Neurol 3:40–51.
39. Hill ME, Richards MA, Gregory WM, Smith P, Rubens RD (1993) Spinal cord compression in breast cancer: a review of 70 cases. Br J Cancer 68:969–973.

12 – Non-Curative Treatment for Head and Neck Cancer

Gillian M. Sadler and Jeffrey S. Tobias

Introduction

Even with the most aggressive initial multi-modality treatment possible, a large proportion of patients treated for head and neck cancer are not cured of their disease. Early glottic tumours are the exception, with 5-year survival figures in excess of 85% for T_1 lesions. For many subsites cure is not possible in the majority of patients, who so frequently present with advanced disease, are often relatively unfit and functionally older than their chronological age would suggest. Overall about 60% of patients will develop local recurrence, and distant metastases will occur in 20–30% [1]. For those with recurrence in the primary site or a nodal recurrence without evidence of more distant dissemination of disease, salvage surgery may be possible. For many patients, however, even at the first evidence of disease recurrence, the only appropriate treatment options are palliative.

The quality of life for these patients with uncontrolled disease is likely to be very poor. They face fundamental problems in such basic functions as maintenance of nutrition and communication, as well as pain and the social isolation often caused by visible disfigurement. This may be due to the tumour mass itself in the case of advanced local disease in sites such as the maxillary antrum or oral cavity, to enlarged and maybe fungating neck nodes, or to surgical treatment. Although reconstructive techniques employed in major head and neck surgery have improved immeasurably in recent years, extensive resections are still likely to lead to visible disfigurement. Following palliative surgical treatment there is often a poor quality of life associated with a worsening perception of medical care [2]. Many of these patients will have been dependent on cigarettes and alcohol for many years. Advice to try to cut down or discontinue these habits is often given to patients about to undergo radiotherapy, as continuing during treatment will make mucosal side-effects far worse. Progression of disease may also cause difficulty in partaking in these habits. Both situations may lead to difficulties due to withdrawal, adding to the other problems experienced, and further eroding quality of life.

A recent review of palliative care for these patients in Japan [3] makes sober reading, with nearly half having uncontrolled pain. In the fortnight before death under 30% were able to eat, and less than a quarter of the group of 52 patients evaluated were able to speak. It seems clear that even if cure cannot be anticipated, there is great scope for thoughtful treatment with palliative intent to improve quality of life. Unfortunately there is little documented evidence helping us towards the best way of achieving these aims. Attempts have been made to validate various quality-of-life assessments for this particular patient group [4], which have found that the most discriminating factors involve the quality of speech, the ability to eat, the perceived level of energy and psychological wellbeing.

Radiotherapy

Palliative radiotherapy is employed as both the initial modality of treatment for patients presenting with advanced, surgically incurable tumours, and for palliation in those with progressive disease despite initial aggressive treatment.

In the former situation, radiotherapy avoids often mutilating surgery and the associated functional and psychological disability [2]. In order to secure local control, and so palliate symptoms, however, high doses are required. In many other situations good palliation can be achieved by merely reducing the bulk of tumour rather than eradicting it. With head and neck tumours, due to tumour occurring in positions where relatively small tumour bulk may interfere considerably with function, and the typically short doubling times observed, this is often not the case. Palliation is, therefore, usually attempted by using radical treatment methods, aiming to clear tumour as completely as possible from the sites being treated. This may initially seem contrary to the usual principles of palliative radiotherapy, in which a small number of fractions are used to enable treatment to be completed as quickly as possible, and with the minimum of treatment-related morbidity. Clinical experience, however, shows that regimens such as 20 Gy in five fractions over 1 week do not give long-lasting symptom relief, due to persisting tumour which then regrows rapidly. Following this type of treatment it would often be difficult to give any further radiotherapy, as large fractions have been used, and further treatment runs an unacceptable risk of excessive normal tissue morbidity.

In centres routinely treating at 2 Gy per fraction it is not uncommon for patients to be treated over 6½ weeks, in order to achieve a "radical" tumour dose – though still recognizing that this is treatment with essentially palliative intent. As for all patients receiving > 60 Gy to the head and neck, this may be associated with considerable mucositis, with patients often needing hospitalization for nutritional support, skin and mouth care, and analgesia. Although the acute reaction will settle in due course, we need to be sure that patient survival is likely to be long enough to warrant a period approaching perhaps 3 months in which their treatment and its side-effects are likely to be as troublesome as the disease bulk and symptoms being palliated. Our clinical impression is that in patients with a good performance status this is often the case, and that the associated local control may allow for a good quality of life for a considerable period, despite problems with xerostomia and taste disturbances which may persist after the acute reaction has settled [5].

It can be very difficult to decide whether this sort of approach is justified in the presence of gross local disease which may prove impossible to control with radiotherapy, and will undoubtedly recur even if this is achieved in the short term. Both a prediction of radiosensitivity and rapid palliation of painful local disease can be achieved with the use of neo-adjuvant chemotherapy. We commonly use a combination of cis- or carboplatin and 5-fluorouracil (5-FU). Cisplatin 100 mg m^{-2} is given over 4 h after prehydration on day 1, followed by 5-FU 1000 mg m^{-2} over 24 h on days 1–5. This is given for two cycles, each of 21 days, with radiotherapy planning occurring at the time of the second cycle. If the volume to be irradiated includes the auditory nerve, we substitute carboplatin (5 × AUC) for the cisplatin, to avoid ototoxicity. If there is no response to chemotherapy the tumour is unlikely to be radiosensitive [6] and embarking on a long course of radiotherapy with its associated morbidity is unlikely to have much to offer.

Patients with an initially poor performance status may also be unsuitable for conventional protracted treatment. In these situations accelerated treatment schedules may be more appropriate. Regimens such as 40 Gy in 15 fractions over 3 weeks are often used and adequate local control often achieved. There are few recent randomized series to suggest what might be the optimum treatment schedule in this situation, although a series reported in the early 1980s suggested that there was little to choose between these two regimens [7].

Weissberg and colleagues [7] randomized a series of surgically unresectable patients between a "conventional" fractionation of 60–70 Gy at 2 Gy per fraction and an accelerated schedule of 44 Gy at 4 Gy per fraction over 2–3 weeks. None of the patients had disease beyond the head and neck. Cord doses were limited to 44 Gy in the conventional arm and 28 Gy with the higher dose per fraction treatment arm. In all, 26 out of 31 patients receiving 2 Gy per fraction and 30 of 33 patients receiving 4 Gy per fraction completed treatment as prescribed. The acute reactions occurred earlier in the accelerated group but were of similar severity as in the conventional group. There was no noticeable difference in late effects in the 10% of patients, in each group, who achieved a long survival. Overall control rates and palliation of tumour-related symptoms were equivalent.

Re-irradiation of Recurrent Disease

There are more published data regarding re-irradiation of recurrent disease [8–11]. Reported series approach this difficult problem in several different ways. However it is tackled the problems remain the same: namely to palliate these patients' symptoms without causing radiation-induced myelitis or major tissue necrosis. External beam radiotherapy and brachytherapy have been used as single or combined modalities of treatment, and there were also trials of neutron therapy in the 1970s and early 1980s [9, 10].

Two series reported in the mid-late 1980s addressed the problem of re-irradiation for recurrent squamous cell carcinoma after previous radical radiotherapy [8, 9]; both found a dose reponse with regard to local control. Kramara et al. reports local control rates of 64% in patients re-treated with more than 50 Gy, as opposed to only 17% in those receiving a smaller dose. Pomp's series of 55 patients [9], all of whom had relapsed after radical radiotherapy with or without chemotherapy and surgery, were retreated with a mean dose of 46 Gy (range 18–84 Gy). They had initially been treated to doses of between 30 Gy and 80 Gy (mean 46 Gy). Total doses ranged from 70 to 154 Gy. Median survival was 10 months, in keeping with other studies, although a surprisingly large proportion of patients (20%) survived a further 5 years. Patients with recurrent nasopharyngeal tumours did better than those with disease at other sites, with 5-year survival figures of up to 55%. Overall local control at 3 months was 53%, and 33% at the last follow-up prior to publication. Twenty-three patients (42%), however, suffered from late complications.

Patients who have previously been irradiated to a radical dose may be thought unsuitable for further radiotherapy due to unacceptable late morbidity, such as trismus from temporomandibular joint dysfunction, a dry mouth, and osteonecrosis. Palliative chemotherapy is often used instead, avoiding the potential complications of further irradiation. These also include soft-tissue fibrosis and, even more importantly, the development of radiation myelopathy. Myelopathy is the most feared adverse effect of radiotherapy in this region – with good reason. Treatment of head and neck tumours may mean that the cervical region of the spinal cord is included in the high-dose treatment volume. It is vital to keep this structure within "tolerance" to avoid late damage, as this may present with the devastating development of quadriplegia. Most studies show an average survival of only 5–12 months following either local recurrence for which further radical salvage treatment is not possible, or the development of metastases [12, 13]. Bearing this in mind, and the time-course for developing late radiation damage, it may be the case that we are perhaps a little over-cautious at times when discounting further radiotherapy.

Brachytherapy

Retreatment using interstitial radiotherapy as a single modality or in combination with further external beam treatment seems to cause fewer late complications with similar control rates. Vikram et al. [10] reported on 124 patients treated at the Memorial Sloan Kettering Institute with permanent ^{125}I implants for palliative intent. The patients were treated betwee 1965 and 1975. A total of 120 patients had previously had radical surgery and 121 had been irradiated. The majority of patients had more than one lesion, in which case the largest or most symptomatic lesion was implanted, and 20% of patients had distant metastases at the time of treatment.

In all, there was an objective response rate of 89% in the implanted lesions. Of the 71% in which a complete response (CR) occurred, 21% subsequently recurred at 1–15 months. Of the lesions in which a partial response (PR) was noted (18% of the total), 55% progressed before death. Smaller lesions showed a better response, with a CR achieved in 82% of lesions smaller than 3 cm, against only 31% in those greater than 6 cm. In 64% of instances the implanted tumour remained controlled until the time of death. This was achieved with a relatively low complication rate, although it is difficult to compare with series of external beam retreatment, as complications are not reported in directly comparable ways. Vikram et al. report a serious complication rate of 5.5%, with ulceration in 9% of patients.

Schmid's group [11] reported, in 1987, on a small group of 19 patients treated with a combination of external beam radiotherapy and interstitial treatment using ^{192}Ir. Thirteen of these patients had recurrent disease following initial treatment of radical intent, with the remaining six presenting with disease felt to be too large for surgery. This latter group were treated with a combination of 50 Gy external beam radiotherapy followed by an implant. Patients with recurrent disease were treated with initial "low-dose" external beam treatment - of 30–60 Gy - and then an implant, or with the implant as the sole modality. All implants were undertaken using after-loaded ^{192}Ir, to give a dose of between 10 and 50 Gy. In some cases this was given as a single fraction, but in others the brachytherapy was fractionated. Acute effects were tolerable and there were no reported late sequelae. (There was no response in one patient, and two died of metastatic disease.) At a median of 42 months, five of the 19 patients were alive without evidence of disease, and two had died of unrelated causes without evidence of their head and neck cancer relapsing. A further seven patients initially responded but then went on to recur locally.

If it is technically possible to use implants to treat recurrent disease, this this may well be worth while in terms of palliation, without causing as much morbidity as further treatment using external beam radiotherapy as a single modality, due to the high doses required to obtain local control. Unfortunately, the site and extent of disease frequently makes this approach impractical.

Neutrons

As mentioned previously, the role of neutron beam therapy was also investigated in the 1970s and early 1980s. Although initial results appeared encouraging, this has largely been abandoned at present since there is no clear benefit demonstrable over megavoltage photon irradiation [14], although the incidence of serious late effects is clearly higher. Although Errington and Catteral [15] found a high CR rate of 82% in a small group of 28 patients re-treated with neutrons following previous conventional irradiation (and a median survival of 20 months), there was also a 46% incidence of necrosis of some sort, reported as major in almost half of these cases. In 15 of the 23 patients in whom a CR occurred, it was maintained for over a year.

Chemotherapy

Response rates to chemotherapy are often quoted with the assumption that response is synonymous with palliation [16]. Unfortunately, as yet, hard evidence is not really available to support this claim although many current studies include quality-of-life assessments. Our clinical impression that this is the case needs to be confirmed. There is encouraging evidence from other sites that chemotherapy can lead to an improvement in quality of life in the palliative situation [17].

Choice of Agents

In the late 1970s and early 1980s single agent methotrexate was considered the standard treatment for palliative chemotherapy. Its reported response rate is around 30% [13], similar to other single agents considered "active" in this situation (Table 12.1). Clearly this leaves the majority of patients effectively untreated, despite undergoing treatment aimed at palliating their symptoms in their last few months of life. Worse still, many patients will be exposed to toxicity

Table 12.1 Response rates with high and low dose methotrexate compared with other single agent treatments

Drug	Total response rate (%)
Methotrexate (low dose)	30–40
Methotrexate (high dose)	40–50
Cisplatin	30
Bleomycin	20–30
Vinblastine	25
5-FU	15
Cyclophosphamide	35
Doxorubicin	20
Hydroxyurea	30

with no benefit. The toxicity associated with this is generally regarded as acceptable – but no doubt it is more so for the responding 30%! Some of the side-effects, when using this antifolate antimetabolite, can be ameliorated by the use of folinic acid rescue, but the principal symptomatic one is of mucositis. This is likely to be particularly troublesome in a group of patients who often have intra-oral symptoms that we are trying to palliate. As with other cytotoxics given in the palliative setting, care should also be taken to avoid excessive myelosuppression. High-dose methotrexate is not generally considered to be more effective in head and neck cancer, but does have considerably greater toxicity associated with its use. When used as a single agent, a dose of 60–100 mg m^{-2} every 21 days is often used, as this can be administered as a bolus or short infusion, so is also suitable for outpatient use.

During the last decade attempts to improve response rates have led to the introduction of chemotherapy using more toxic, but hopefully more effective, single agents – in particular cisplatin – or combinations of drugs (Table 12.2). Reports from uncontrolled studies suggest that combinations of cytotoxic agents appear to have higher response rates, with figures of up to 80% being reported [13, 18]. A number of studies have been published comparing these regimens with single agent methotrexate in a randomized manner, but most have found no significant difference. This is perhaps not surprising, as most centres only see relatively small numbers of patients. The majority of responding patients obtain partial rather than complete responses, and so may still be left with considerable amounts of viable tumour at the end of chemotherapy. This may well be

Table 12.2 Response rates with combination treatment regimens

Drugs	Total response rate (%)
Cisplatin, 5-FU	80
Cisplatin, bleomycin	50
Cisplatin, bleomycin, methotrexate	60
Bleomycin, methotrexate, cyclophosphamide, 5-FU	45
Vincristine, bleomycin, methotrexate, 5-FU, doxorubicin, hydrocortisone	67
Methotrexate, bleomycin, vinblastine	75
Methotrexate, 5-FU	50

symptomatic, and progress rapidly at the end of treatment. It is not, therefore, surprising that most responses are of short duration, lasting only a few weeks to months.

Cisplatin was developed after the fortuitous observation by Rosenberg, in 1965, that passing an electrical current through platinum electrodes could inhibit cell division of *E. coli* [18]. Subsequent testing, first in murine tumour models and then in patients with advanced malignancies, demonstrated its activity in many solid tumours. Initial problems of severe nephrotoxicity were overcome with the realization of the importance of adequate hydration. Cisplatin was first used in head and neck tumours by the National Cancer Institute in the mid-1970s. Initially it was used as a neo-adjuvant therapy prior to surgery and radiotherapy, in combination with bleomycin. In this Contracts Program study [19], only one cycle of chemotherapy was given, so assessing response caused considerable problems. Even so, some patients were noted to have entered a complete remission prior to the standard part of their treatment.

Since that time, regimens in which there is greater chance of observing response have been developed as, no matter how active a drug is, this is easier to do adequately if more than one cycle of treatment is given. Cisplatin has become a widely used drug in the treatment of advanced head and neck cancer, after recognition of the relatively high response rates seen. As with other agents, there are many more partial than complete responses and both are more common in patients naive to chemotherapy when compared to those that have been pre-treated. In recent years it has been widely used in combination with fluorouracil, as response rates are certainly higher than when used as a single agent.

A review of the available evidence in 1991 [20], however, by Clarke and Dreyfuss suggested that cisplatin had not supplanted the role of methotrexate. Nilsco [12] had previously suggested that there was no clearly superior regimen to palliate recurrent squamous cell carcinomas of the head and neck. Most regimens gave response rates of between 30% and 60% and, as with cisplatin, previously untreated patients were more likely to respond. More recently, a meta-analysis of all the studies published between 1980 and 1992 looking at palliative chemotherapy in locally recurrent or metastatic head and neck cancer has been performed by Browman and Cronin [21]. This analysed the data from 15 studies. The chemotherapies employed were grouped as below for analysis of the results:

1. Single agent methotrexate (MTX) vs. all other therapies.
2. Single agents vs. combinations.
3. Single agent MTX vs. combinations.
4. Single agent MTX vs. single agent cisplatin (CP).
5. CP containing regimens vs. other.
6. CP and 5-FU vs. single agents.
7. CP and 5-FU vs. other combinations.

Only one study provided a statistically significant difference between treatment arms. This favoured the combination of cisplatin and 5-FU. When the meta-analysis was performed, however, it became apparent that single agent methotrexate was significantly worse in terms of response rate than other treatments. There was a non-significant trend in favour of single agent cisplatin compared with single agent methotrexate. Combinations of cytotoxic drugs gave significantly higher response rates than single agents (including single agent cisplatin), but a clearly superior combination could not be determined. Among combinations, however, there was a trend in favour of cisplatin + 5-FU (CI 59–1.49).

For overall survival, there appeared little to choose between the treatment groups. All reported survival times were short, with means of around 5 months. Three of the trials did report a statistically significant difference between the treatment arms, and in each case this was in favour of treatments including cisplatin. Unfortunately, the clinical significance of this appears highly questionable, as in each trial the gain in life was less than 1 month, and these very modest increases in recorded survival were gained at the expense of increased toxicity, in particular nausea and vomiting. Admittedly the earlier studies analysed would have been carried out before $5HT_3$ antagonists were available. It is probable that with their routine use in platinum-containing regimens, the number of patients experiencing moderate or severe nausea and vomiting would now be far fewer. Nevertheless in-patient admission is still usually required despite this, to ensure adequate hydration.

The erosion of time at home is often a major consideration for patients who realize that the treatment they are about to undertake is only aimed at relieving symptoms, and that their survival is limited. This may be felt to argue against the use of cisplatin in favour of outpatient regimens. The situation is made more complex, however, by evidence in favour of cisplatin actually increasing time at home [22], although there is little increase in overall survival. It may be that the higher response rates (many of which will be PRs) are reflected in amelioration of the symptoms that would otherwise have necessitated hospital admission. If this is the case, then chemotherapy with an equivalent response rate but which can be given on an outpatient basis may be preferable even to this. Carboplatin has been suggested to fill this role [23]. It seems to be as effective as cisplatin, in combination with 5-FU, but less toxic. The reduction in nausea, vomiting and appetite suppression often allows better nutrition, offering potential for improved quality of life over that gained by cisplatin. It is of course more expensive. Outpatient administration may offset additional drug costs, but in any event many of these patients require admission for symptom management at the time when palliative chemotherapy is undertaken.

Combinations of vincristine, methotrexate with folinic acid rescue, bleomycin and 5-FU (VBMF) have been widely used, sometimes with the addition of doxorubicin and hydroxyurea. VBMF is one of the regimens used in ongoing studies assessing the role of chemotherapy in initial radical management of advanced head and neck tumours [24]. In this situation it may have the potential for improving survival when given concurrently with radical radiotherapy. VBMF with or without adriamycin and hydroxyurea was used for palliation in the 1970s by O'Connor and others [25] and their initial reports suggested an important role, with response rates of up to 75% in previously unirradiated patients. Response rates of 50% were reported in those previously treated with radical radiotherapy. These figures are made difficult to interpret alongside more recent studies, however, as they excluded patients dying before achieving a PR, those that only received one cycle and those switched to alternative regimens.

Tannock et al. [26] subsequently reported on this regimen and found it to be far less useful. Out of 57 patients treated, responses were only observed in six. The remissions were only of short duration, as seen with all other regimens, and they experienced one toxic and three other sudden deaths. Like most other reports in the literature this remains a little difficult to interpret, as patients achieving less than 50% reduction in their disease bulk will not be counted as responders. It may be that patients missed by these criteria actually have lesser responses that improve their symptoms. Until studies are available with rigorous assessment of the actual palliation achieved, rather than crude measures of tumour regression, this remains a problem in trying to interpret virtually all the available data, from the point of view of symptom control.

In our institution we frequently use VBMF (vincristine 1.4 mg m^{-2} – max of 2 mg, bleomycin 30 mg, methotrexate 100 mg m^{-2}, 5-FU 500 mg with folinic acid rescue 15 mg p.o. × 6 starting at 24 h both as neo-adjuvant and palliative treatment. When combined simultaneously with radical radiotherapy, there is no doubt it increases the degree of acute toxicity. As a single modality, however, it appears to be fairly well tolerated by most patients preferring to avoid hospital admission. As the drugs are all given by bolus injection, it can easily be given in an outpatient setting. Our clinical impression is that the response rate appears similar to, but perhaps slightly less than that of cisplatin and fluorouracil, but for patients unwilling to be admitted to hospital this appears to be a satisfactory trade-off.

Chemotherapy has also been used in combination with hyperthermia in patients who failed conventional treatment for recurrent disease [27]. Responses were seen in about one-third of a small group of 14 patients. Although this does not seem to be any better than the response rates described with conventional palliative chemotherapy, it is of interest that three of five patients who had already failed single agent methotrexate went on to respond to a combination of methotrexate and radiofrequency hyperthermia. Patients received metronidazole in addition to the chemotherapy, which was more often with multiple agents. As in other studies using hyperthermia, ensuring adequate, uniform heating was a considerable technical problem, restricting the number of patients felt to be suitable for treatment. Another problem described was the number of patients developing burns. Although only described as superficial, these occurred in six out of the 14 patients, which was a higher than expected incidence. This is not a technique that has come into routine clinical use for patients with advanced head and neck cancer.

Chemo/radiotherapy

Combinations of chemotherapy with radiotherapy are far more widely employed. This approach has often been used in patients with good performance status, aiming at long-term palliation of locoregional recurrence [28, 29]. Both Gandia and Weppelman's groups combined radiotherapy with concurrent 5-FU and hydroxyurea.

Gandia's group gave 5-FU 800 mg m^{-2} i.v. and hydroxyurea 1–1.5 g p.o. daily for 5 days, simultaneously with 2 Gy per fraction daily for 5 days on alternate weeks, with the aim of exploiting the radiosensitizing properties of the chemotherapy. The total number of courses given depended both on the previous radiotherapy details and the patients' tolerance to treatment. Usually between 40 and 60 Gy were given, provided that the soft-tissue dose remained below 110 Gy and the cord dose below 50 Gy.

Weppelman et al. used 5-FU 300 mg m^{-2} i.v. and hydroxyurea 1.5–2 g p.o. daily for 5 days with radiotherapy. Initially 40 Gy was given in 2 Gy fractions. Treatment was daily, for 5 days during weeks 1, 3, 5 and 7, so that up to four fortnightly courses were given. Later they changed the irradiation to 1.2 Gy b.d. on treatment days, so that a total of 48 Gy was given. This was found to be tolerated better and gave an equivalent response rate.

Both groups' regimens were reported as giving good palliation to responding patients, although exactly how this was assessed is unclear. Gandia reports a 55% response rate, lasting an average of 16 months in the 40% of patients who obtained a CR. Overall survival of both groups is probably similar at around 1 year, with Gandia reporting a median survival of 11 months as compared to Weppelman's 56% 1-year survival figures. This latter was despite three deaths during treatment. Significant haemotological toxicity was noted, despite good mucosal tolerance.

Unusual Tumour Types

Although the great majority of head and neck tumours are squamous cell carcinomas, other histological types are also encountered. These may cause special problems in management, although the general aims of palliation for patients with incurable disease will be identical. The site of tumour and its recurrence may also have a bearing on both management and outcome.

Melanoma

About 20% of all malignant melanomas occur in the head and neck region. The great majority of these arise from the skin, and should be treated along the same lines as other cutaneous melanomas. A small number (less than 5% of the total) originate from mucosal surfaces, and most of these are in the nose or paranasal sinuses. Even with radical surgery the outlook is poor, with 5-year survival in the order of 25%. Many patients will, therefore, need to be considered for palliative treatment at some stage.

Presentation is often late, and surgery may not be possible in all cases. With these advanced tumours it may be difficult to irradiate adequately, due to the presence of sensitive normal structures such as brain or spinal cord. Melanoma has often been regarded as radioresistant, although modern treatment techniques are gradually dispelling this view. There is some evidence to suggest that larger than usual fraction size may improve results: 24 Gy in three fractions over 3 weeks has been shown to be effective [30], but will exceed brain and cord tolerance. If falling within the treatment area, these organs should be shielded out for the final fraction, if at all possible.

Palliation with chemotherapy for mucosal melanomas is not often successful. In view of the poor response rates, if it is to be attempted at all, there is probably little advantage in aggressive DTIC containing regimens over the much simpler and better tolerated vindesine 5 mg given every 2–3 weeks.

Sarcoma

Head and neck sarcomas occur very rarely in adults. Rhabdomyosarcomas account for about 5% of childhood tumours, and about one-third of these arise in the head and neck. Patients requiring palliative treatment will usually already have undergone extensive multimodality treatment. This will invariably have included chemotherapy, used due to the high incidence of micrometastases at presentation, as well as surgery and/or radiotherapy. Planning of palliative treatments, therefore, has many of the same problems as when dealing with adult patients with the much commoner carcinomas. There are often additional difficulties due to the young age of patients who may not fully understand the treatment, but are all too well aware of its toxicity.

Palliative chemotherapy often employs oral etoposide which avoids the need for hospital admission and is often well tolerated.

Adenoid Cystic Tumour

These slow-growing malignant tumours of salivary glands (both major and minor) show a great propensity for perineural invasion. The natural history is usually long, with patients commonly dying of metastatic disease 10–20 years after initial presentation. The combination of these factors often makes energetic attempts at obtaining local control justified, even in cases where surgical resection is known to be incomplete and radiotherapy unlikely to be curative. High-dose radiotherapy is often employed to try to prevent the development of pain due to perineural invasion, as this is so often difficult to treat satisfactorily with analgesics. Shrinkage of residual or recurrent disease after radiotherapy will be very slow, and may take many months.

Nasopharyngeal Carcinoma

Although much less common in the Western world than in the Far East, nasopharyngeal carcinoma still presents particular management problems. It is often locally advanced with bilateral cervical lymphadenopathy at presentation. Initial rates of local control are good with radical radiotherapy, but in view of the large tumour bulk, it is perhaps not surprising that many patients go on to relapse. Surgical salvage is not usually possible, particularly as there is so often evidence of skull base involvement with bone erosion and cranial nerve palsies.

Even in these situations, this group of patients can be expected to survive for longer than similar patients with primaries at other head and neck sites. Relatively aggressive palliation is therefore often undertaken. Response rates to platinum-containing regimens are around 70%, though likely to be lower in patients that have been exposed to induction chemotherapy. Consideration should also be given to further local radiotherapy, if the risk of severe late effects is not too great.

Perhaps related to the fact that survival with recurrent disease is often of a relatively lengthy duration, patients with nasopharyngeal carcinoma also seem to be at greater risk of developing disseminated disease with bony metastases. Short courses of local radiotherapy usually give good symptomatic relief.

Lymphoma

Lymphomas may occur within the head and neck region, particularly in relationship to Waldeyer's ring. Radical treatment will usually be undertaken for high-grade disease, but in cases where this is unsuccessful similar methods of palliation are used as for lymphomas in other sites. There are usually fewer problems in planning palliative radiotherapy than when undertaking treatment for other histological types of head and neck malignancy. As in other sites, lymphomas are highly radiosensitive, allowing relatively low doses to be used. This means that morbidity of treatment is correspondingly slight.

Standard palliative chemotherapy may be used if disease is not easily encompassable within a single radiation field. For patients already failing regimens such as CHOP, combinations such as ImMVP16 (ifosfamide, methotrexate, etoposide) may be useful.

Conclusions

Successful palliative treatment for patients with head and neck malignancies is often very demanding, requiring great care and expertise from all involved in their care. This is due to many factors, including the patients' often poor performance status, difficulties in communication and nutrition due to disease, and the depression often associated with these isolating functional disabilities. Technically it can be very difficult, particularly when further radiotherapy is employed. Although we have reason to believe that this will often improve quality of life, it is vital that it is planned with the utmost care, to avoid serious late morbidity. Further research is urgently required, aimed at confirming our clinical impressions of good-quality palliation through active treatment, as we must recognize that there is often a considerable price to pay in terms of morbidity.

It would seem that the strategies most likely to result in tumour response and, so one would hope, palliation, currently involve the use of platinum-containing combination chemotherapy and/or local radiotherapy. If tumours are suitable for implantation, this may well provide a very good compromise between giving a high dose to obtain local control of tumour and at the same time avoiding excessive late morbidity. Unfortunately this is only appropriate in the minority of patients. The poor quality of life and extremely unpleasant symptoms experienced by patients with advanced head and neck cancer mean that it is vital that we put great efforts into adequately palliating those that cannot be cured, and closely audit the results of these efforts.

References

1. Hong WK, Bromer R (1983) Chemotherapy in head and neck cancer. N Engl J Med 308:75–79.
2. Brugere J, Louvard N (1986) Quality of life in head and neck cancers. Bull Cancer Paris 73(5):634–640.
3. Sakai T, Mineta H, Mizuta, Nozue M (1992) Evaluation of terminal care for head and neck cancer patients. Nippon Jibiinkok Gakkai Kaiho 95(3):324–328.
4. Rathmell AJ, Ash DV, Howes M, Nicholls RJ (1991) Assessing quality of life in patients treated for advanced head and neck cancer. Clin Oncol 3(1):10–16.
5. Brewin TB (1982) Appetite perversion and taste changes triggered or abolished by radiotherapy. Clin Radiol 33:471–475.
6. Tobias JS (1992) Current role of chemotherapy in head and neck cancer. Drugs 43:333–345.

7. Weissberg JB, Son YH, Percarpio B, Fischer JJ (1982) Randomized trial of conventional versus high fractional dose radiation therapy in the treatment of advanced head and neck cancer. Int J Radiat Oncol Biol Phys 8(2):179–185.
8. Kramara A, Eschvege F, Richard JM, Langois SD et al. (1985) Re-irradiation of head and neck cancer. Radiother Oncol 3:27–33.
9. Pomp J, Levendag PC, van Putten WL (1988) Re-irradiation of recurrent tumours in the head and neck. Am J Clin Oncol 11:543–549.
10. Vikram B, Hilaris BS, Anderson L, Strong EW (1983) Permanent iodine-125 implants in head and neck cancer. Cancer 51(7):1310–1314.
11. Schmid AP, Vinzenz K, Pavelka R, Karcher H, Dobrowsky W (1987) Interstitial radiotherapy with Ir-192 as a palliative treatment modality in head and neck cancer. J Craniomaxillofac Surg 16(6):365–368.
12. Nilsco AN (1986) Chemotherapy of head and neck cancer. Clin Oncol 5(3):575–594.
13. DeVita VT, Hellman S, Rosenberg SA (1985) Cancer: Principles and practice of oncology, 4 ed. Lippincott-Raven, Philadelphia, p 582.
14. Skolyszewski J, Koreniowski S (1988) Re-irradiation of recurrent head and neck cancer with fast neutrons. Br J Radiol 61:527–528.
15. Errington RG, Catteral M (1986) Re-irradiation of advanced tumours of the head and neck with fast neutrons. Int J Radiat Oncol Biol Phys 12:191–195.
16. Vokes EE, Weichselbaum RR, Lippman SM et al. (1993) Medical progress: head and neck cancer. N Engl J Med 328:184–194.
17. Coates A, Gebski V, Bishop J et al. (1987) Improving the quality of life during chemotherapy for advanced breast cancer. N Engl J Med 317:1490–1495.
18. Rosenberg B (1985) Fundamental studies with cisplatin. Cancer 55:2303–2316.
19. Head and Neck Contracts Program (USA) (1987) Adjuvant chemotherapy for advanced head and neck squamous cell carcinoma. Cancer 60:301–311.
20. Clark JR, Dreyfuss AI (1991) The role of cisplatin in treatment regimens for squamous carcinomas of the head and neck. Semin Oncol 18:34–48.
21. Browman GP, Cronin L (1993) Standard chemotherapy in squamous cell head and neck cancer: what we have learned from randomized trials. Semin Oncol 21(3):311–319.
22. Morton RP, Stell PM (1984) Cytotoxic chemotherapy for patients with terminal squamous carcinoma – does it influence survival? Clin Otolaryngol 9(3):175–180.
23. Aisner J, Sinibaldi V, Eisenberger M (1992) Carboplatin in the treatment of squamous cell head and neck cancers. Semin Oncol 19(1 suppl 2):60–65.
24. UKCCR Head and Neck Collaborative Group UKHAN 1 A trial of chemotherapy with radiotherapy in the treatment of advanced squamous carcinoma of the head and neck. CRC Clinical Trials Office, London.
25. O'Connor AD, Clifford P, Dalley VM et al. (1979) Advanced head and neck cancer treated by combined radiotherapy and VBM cytotoxic regimen: 4 year results. Clin Otolaryngol 4:325–337.
26. Tannock I, Sutherland D, Osoba D (1982) Failure of short course multiple drug chemotherapy to benefit patients with recurrent metastatic head and neck cancer. Cancer 49:1358–1361.
27. Moffat FL, Rotstein LE, Calhoun K, Langer JC, Makowka L, Ambus U et al. (1984) Palliation of advanced head and neck cancer with radiofrequency hyperthermia and cytotoxic chemotherapy. Can J Surg 27(1):38–41.
28. Gandia D, Wibault P, Guillot T, Bensmaine A, Armand JP et al. (1993) Simultaneous chemoradiotherapy as salvage treatment in loco-regional recurrence of head and neck cancer. Head Neck 15(1):8–15.
29. Weppelman B, Wheeler RH, Peters GE, Kim RY, Spencer SA et al. (1992) Treatment of recurrent head and neck cancer with 5-fluorouracyl, hydroxyurea and re-irradiation. Int J Radiat Oncol Biol Phys 22(5):1051–1056.
30. Harwood AR, Cummings BJ (1982) Radiotherapy for mucosal melanomas. Int J Radiat Oncol Biol Phys 8:1121–1126.

Section 3

Non-Curative Chemotherapy

13 – Non-Curative Chemotherapy for Breast Cancer

A. Jones

Introduction

There are 30 000 new cases of breast cancer per annum in the UK and approximately 15 000 deaths per annum. This means that some 40% of women diagnosed with breast cancer will die of their disease, usually because of the development of distant metastases. During the course of metastatic breast cancer a woman may be exposed to a variety of treatments, including local treatments for specific problems such as radiotherapy and surgery, and systemic treatment such as hormone manipulation and chemotherapy. If all treatments were without toxicity, they would be likely to be considered "worth while" even if objective benefit was only experienced by some of the patients. In practice, not all patients benefit from all treatments and this, together with the economic costs involved, make the question of how worth while is non-curative treatment for breast cancer harder to answer.

It is important to recognize that the natural history of metastatic breast cancer is extremely variable, ranging from a few months to many years. In one series, the median survival of 250 patients with untreated breast carcinoma diagnosed at the Middlesex Hospital between 1859 and 1934 was 31 months [1]. This variability reflects inherent biological differences between the disease in different patients. Retrospective studies indicate that conventional chemotherapy in metastatic breast cancer does not have a major impact on survival, although it is likely that some patients, especially those who present with rapidly progressive visceral disease and who respond to treatment, do have their lives prolonged by a few months [2]. Chemotherapy in patients with more indolent disease may have little effect on survival and its value has to be measured in terms of symptom control. If the value of non-curative treatment is assessed by survival, it is important to measure this from an agreed fixed point, i.e. the initial development of metastases rather than the time of first chemotherapy, to assess survival of the whole breast cancer population. If currently available non-curative treatments have only a minor effect on survival, the value of treatment has to be assessed by other parameters.

It is frequently stated that treatment for advanced breast cancer is palliative rather than curative in intent. The body of literature regarding treatment of advanced breast cancer, however, report clinical trials which use the classical end-points defined by objective response rates (complete and partial remission), recurrence free and overall survival [3]. When chemotherapy was introduced in advanced breast cancer no randomized trials were undertaken to assess the impact of chemotherapy compared with best supportive care alone on quality of life, and such studies are now inappropriate for ethical reasons given the high response rates associated with chemotherapy. Although objective responses to treatment may be associated with an improvement in disease-related symptoms [4], any such benefit has to be weighed against the toxicity of the treatment itself and therefore response rate alone is not necessarily a valid surrogate end-point for effective palliation. In this context, failure to achieve an objective response rate (either complete or partial remission) on active therapy, but the continuation of stable disease rather than disease progression, may be associated with a useful reduction in symptoms. This is probably due to a reduction in tumour volume of less than 50%, i.e. not a true partial response. This is particularly seen with hormonal therapy in patients with breast cancer. For example, although only 30% of patients achieve an objective response with tamoxifen, a further 20% have stable disease for a median of 15–18 months. This may provide useful palliation of disease-related symptoms and should be regarded as worth while.

Extrapolation of the results of clinical trials may not be appropriate for the majority of patients with advanced breast cancer in the community, as selection factors which allow patients entry into trials may be restrictive. Patients selected for trials may have superior performance status and other pretreatment factors. In addition, resources may differ between smaller hospitals and major centres. Patients entered into clinical trials may have a superior prognosis compared with those who are not [5]. In practice, the objective response rate is likely to fall, with more patients treated out of trials, and this makes the issue of judging the effective palliation even more vexed.

Breast cancer differs from other malignancies both in its natural history and the pattern of metastatic disease and also in the range of treatment options available. Unlike other cancers, these include hormone therapy, which is very effective for many patients, as well as chemotherapy. In general, systemic treatment is given to patients with pre-symptomatic and symptomatic progressive disease, and local treatments are reserved for specific problems, e.g. spinal cord compression, brain metastases and incipient fracture of long bones. In the UK, most patients with metastatic breast cancer receive a trial of hormone therapy first and cytotoxic chemotherapy is reserved for those patients with rapidly progressive visceral disease (e.g. liver and lymphangitis) and those who fail on hormone therapy.

Health Economics

The benefit, or otherwise, of non-curative treatment for breast cancer can be judged in a number of ways. Response and survival have been discussed. The other parameters include quality of life (discussed later), the patient's perception of the benefit and also the resource and cost implications for the Health Service. The high prevalence and often long time-course of breast cancer makes major demands on health care resources.

There is little information available on the use of hospital resources and resulting costs of treating any advanced cancer. Routine audit of the results of non-curative treatment is costly and is rarely practised, but is essential if we are to have reliable data for assessing quality of practice. Most economic studies focus on cost, particularly of individual drugs, as this is the easiest parameter to quantify. More sophisticated costing estimates involving in-patient stays (which are likely to be the major component of costs), investigations, as well as drug costs and other treatment modalities, involve assumptions which can be subject to criticism [6, 7]. Standard costs outside drug costs are not readily available in the UK, but the tests to assess objective response, e.g. detailed X-rays and scans, may be both time consuming and costly [8]. One retrospective analysis in the UK examined the records of 50 patients with advanced breast cancer who died between 1988 and 1990, and costed their treatment, including investigations, in-patient stays, drugs and radiotherapy costs [9]. In this study, the median duration of advanced disease was 17 months and the median in-patient stay 32 days, accounting for 56% of total costs. Cytotoxic drugs accounted for only 9% of total costs and radiotherapy 8%. The implication of this study is that the major component of the total cost of managing advanced breast cancer is due to the time spent as an in-patient. The actual economic costs of standard treatment are relatively low and if chemotherapy or other treatments help to keep patients out of hospital then clearly this would be considered "worth while" in economic terms and indeed in terms of patient preference [10].

Another study in the UK constructed a model using local unit costs and serum tumour markers as a measure of response [11]. In this model, early discontinuation of therapy based on tumour markers (when no change would be made by standard UICC criteria) was projected to save substantial sums of money. While this is only a model, the authors argue for careful analysis of costs incurred in breast cancer treatment in a randomized trial.

High-dose chemotherapy with autologous bone marrow or stem cell support may only be appropriate for a small number of women with metastatic disease and the costs of this procedure are high. Using a decision analysis model based on a Markov process, Hillman et al. [12] assessed the efficacy and cost effectiveness of standard dose and high-dose chemotherapy and concluded that high-dose treatment provided substantial benefit, but this benefit was dependent on whether the risk of recurrence was constant or decreased with time and that the costs involved may be untenable, especially if the risk of recurrence was constant. Although long-term follow-up suggests that a small number of women become long-term survivors, there are insufficient data for cost–benefit ratios to be assessed and these need to be part of ongoing randomized trials.

Hormone Therapy

Most women with advanced breast cancer are given a trial of endocrine therapy as initial treatment for metastatic disease unless they have life-threatening or symptomatic visceral disease (e.g. lung/liver) which necessitates the more rapid objective response which may be achieved by chemotherapy. Hormonal therapy is the main modality of treatment for a mean of 14 months in women with breast cancer [7]. Endocrine treatment yields response rates of approximately 30%, with a median response duration of 15 months. The time to objective response is usually 2–3 months. Postmenopausal status, a prolonged disease-free interval, bone and soft-tissue metastases and the presence of oestrogen receptors on the primary tumour are all associated with a higher likelihood of response.

Tamoxifen can be used in both pre- and postmenopausal women and is generally well tolerated with vasomotor side-effects (hot flushes) and gynaecological side-effects (menstrual irregularity, vaginal discharge) in 15% of women. Severe depression has been reported in approximately 1%. Following progression after tamoxifen, second- and third-line endocrine therapy can be used either with progestogens in pre- and postmenopausal women or with aromatase inhibitors only in postmenopausal women. In general, drugs in these classes can be given orally and are well tolerated, with little difference in response or quality of life when measured [13], although dose-related side-effects of progestins were shown to impair quality of life at higher doses without any objective improvement in survival [14].

At present there are no convincing data to suggest that combinations of endocrine treatment or endocrine treatment in combination with chemotherapy are superior in terms of survival (although response rates may be higher).

Chemotherapy

A variety of cytotoxic drugs have single agent activity in breast cancer. In general, combination regimens achieve higher response rates of 40–60% than single agent treatment and are used more commonly. Most responses are partial, with a complete response of only around 10% and median duration of response around 10 months. More intensive combination regimens have been used with higher objective response rates, including more complete responses [15], but there is no evidence that higher response rates translate into improved survival. The possible exception to this is with the use of high-dose chemotherapy with bone marrow or peripheral blood stem cell support in women with newly diagnosed metastatic disease and an expected poor prognosis. In single arm studies, 5-year survival for these patients is 25% compared with 5% for historical controls [16]. These results need confirmation in prospective randomized trials, even if it is confirmed that the substantial majority of patients thus treated do not benefit and such therapy is only applicable to a minority of women with advanced breast cancer.

The median duration of response following chemotherapy is 6–12 months. While an objective response may be associated with improvement in symptoms [4], it is important to note that the outcome for patients treated outside trials may be considerably inferior in terms of response. In one study of 758 consecutive patients receiving chemotherapy for advanced breast cancer, both in and out of clinical trials, the response rate to first-line chemotherapy was only 34%, with a median duration of response of 7.8 months, median time to progression 3.7 months and median survival of 7.9 months [17]. In this study, one-third of the patients received two or more chemotherapy regimens, with a fall in response rate to only 16%, with median time to progression of 2.3 months for second- and third-line chemotherapy. This study, together with the high-dose study, raises interesting questions about the value of non-curative treatment for breast cancer. First, can we select patients more likely to respond, and secondly, do patients who do not have an objective response benefit from non-curative treatment either in terms of quality of life or (less likely) prolonged survival?

The patient's performance status before treatment is not always recorded, but in breast cancer, as with other cancers, this has considerable prognostic significance [18, 19]. A short disease-free interval following primary treatment and the presence of liver metastases, or abnormal liver function tests, are also associated with a poorer prognosis [17–20]. Most studies have shown that patients with more than two metastatic sites have inferior survival [17–20]. Some studies suggest that prior adjuvant chemotherapy predicts for inferior response and/or survival after chemotherapy for metastatic disease [18–20], but this is not confirmed in other randomized studies [17, 21, 22]. This may in part reflect differences in disease-free interval between adjuvant chemotherapy and the development of metastatic disease.

In multivariate analysis, young age appears to be an adverse prognostic factor, with significantly shorter survival in patients aged under 35 years in one large study of 1168 patients [23], and poorer survival in women aged under 45 years in another long-term follow-up study [24]. Older women with breast cancer may be offered chemotherapy, but older patients are poorly represented in clinical trials and less data are available. In the study of consecutive patients in a single unit by Gregory et al. [17], advanced age was associated with inferior survival. Another study designed to determine the effect of age in treatment outcome found response rates of 40%, 31% and 29% to chemotherapy for the age groups less than 50, 50–69 and $\geqslant 70$ years respectively, but no difference in time to progression or survival [25]. Older women who have become resistant to hormone therapy should not be excluded from chemotherapy on the basis of age alone.

Given these prognostic variables, can we select patients who should not receive chemotherapy? While we can identify groups with higher and lower probabilities of response, we cannot exclude a reasonable chance of a worthwhile response in an individual patient. In practice, most patients are offered first-line chemotherapy, but treatment should only be continued after two or three cycles if there is evidence of both an objective and subjective benefit. Twenty-five per cent of patients respond within 3 months and virtually all responses have occurred within 2–5 months [26].

There is no consensus on a "best" drug regimen, although randomized studies indicate that doxorubicin-containing regimens yield 10–20% higher response rates than combination regimens with doxorubicin [27]. Newer drugs such as paclitaxel and docetaxel have response rates equivalent to doxorubicin and evidence of activity in patients resistant to doxorubicin and its analogue. It has not been shown that the use of these drugs improves survival, and decisions about appropriate palliative chemotherapy must weigh response against toxicity.

Modern antiemetic regimens using $5HT_3$ receptor antagonists mean that most chemotherapy for advanced breast cancer is well tolerated and can be given safely in the outpatient setting, with improved quality of life as measured by the Rotterdam Symptom Checklist or Functional Living Index List [28]. In one study evaluating palliative chemotherapy given in hospital or at home, hospital-administered chemotherapy was perceived as more distressing, particularly in terms of anxiety and depression [10]. The practicalities of home-based chemotherapy may limit this approach, but outpatient as opposed to in-patient treatment is preferable both from patients' perspective and in economic terms. Scalp cooling may reduce the risk of alopecia, with doxorubicin-containing regimens thereby lessening another unpleasant side-effect.

Relatively few randomized studies have included quality of life as an outcome measure [29–32] and still less in phase II trials of new drugs. While a patient's perception of whether chemotherapy is worth while or not may not entirely correlate with quality of life, the use of quality-of-life measures probably does give a more realistic estimate of benefit. Quality of life is a multidimensional concept incorporating physical activities of daily living, psychological disturbance, social interactions (including family and professional), sexual aspects (including appearance and cosmetic problems) and economic aspects. These dimensions may interact. These should be measured by simple instruments validated for stage of disease and cultural context. Quality-of-life instruments should also allow comparison of treatment regimens which may have different qualitative and quantitative toxicity. The choice of quality-of-life instruments is outside the remit of this chapter, but a number of methods are available and validated in patients with breast cancer, including linear analogue self-assessment (LASA), which are easy to use [29, 33], the EORTC-Q30 questionnaire [34] and the FACTB questionnaire, which are designed for use in cancer clinical trials. These instruments have site-specific modules, e.g. for breast cancer.

In clinical trials in breast cancer, with patients in whom quality of life was an end-point, compliance with the EORTC and breast cancer chemotherapy questionnaires was high at 95%, indicating that quality-of-life data can be collected given appropriate resources. Out of the trial setting, this level of compliance is likely to fall and there are few data on quality-of-life assessments in non-trial patients.

In one study examining the effect of dose on quality of life using two different dose levels of CMF, patients receiving the higher dose level had a trend towards better symptom relief and general wellbeing despite greater objective nausea and vomiting [30]. This improvement was associated with higher response rates (30% vs. 11%), emphasizing the need for using adequate doses of chemotherapy if the decision is made to use cytotoxic drugs. Other studies have also indicated that nausea and vomiting were not powerful independent predictors of variation in quality of life in breast cancer patients, although they are ranked high on the list of important toxicities as perceived by patients [29, 35].

Using LASA, Coates and colleagues demonstrated no difference in response, survival or quality of life between a regimen containing doxorubicin and cyclophosphamide (AC) and another regimen generally accepted as less toxic (cyclophosphamide, methotrexate, 5-fluorouracil and prednisolone [CMFP]), although there was more objective toxicity with vomiting and alopecia with AC as measured by standard WHO criteria. This study also addressed the question of intermittent therapy (stopping after three cycles) vs. continuous therapy (continuing until disease progression), in the hope that the intervals of freedom from cytotoxic therapy would contribute to improved quality of life. Intermittent therapy had an inferior response rate (33% vs. 49%) and inferior quality of life compared with continuous therapy [29].

In another randomized clinical trial comparing intermittent and continuous chemotherapy, baseline quality-of-life scores measured by LASA and quality of life index at the start of chemotherapy were significant predictors of subsequent survival [36]. Changes in score for mood, pain and quality of life from the end of the first three cycles also predicted a better outcome independent of other recorded prognostic factors.

Special Sites

Bone Disease

Bone is the site of first recurrence in up to 40% of patients with relapsed breast cancer and is present in some 60–70% of patients with advanced disease. Bone metastases are a major cause of morbidity due to the pain, risk of pathological fracture, hypercalcaemia and neurological complications and may lead to prolonged hospitalization and the use of health care resources [9]. Patients with bone-only metastases may survive in excess of 5 years and it is important that these patients have optimal management to maintain a good quality of life.

Radiotherapy for localized painful lesions and systemic therapy for widespread disease remains the mainstay of treatment. Bone metastases are frequently reported to respond less well to systemic treatment than soft-tissue or visceral disease, however this may only reflect inadequacy of current methods for assessment of response. Recalcification is only seen in 10–20% of patients, but pain relief is more common.

A major factor in the development of bone metastases is enhanced numbers of active osteoclasts leading to bone resorption. Bisphosphonates are pyrophosphate analogues resistant to endogenous phosphatases which are potent inhibitors of osteoclastic bone resorption. These drugs are effective treatment for hypercalcaemia of malignancy, itself a problem in some 30% of women with advanced breast cancer. There has been a considerable interest in the potential role of bisphosphonates in the palliation of bone metastases. A number of randomized trials have been published suggesting that bisphosphonates reduce the incidence of skeletal morbidity in patients with metastatic bone disease, as measured by the rate of vertebral fracture, the development of hypercalcaemia and fracture at other axial sites [37, 38]. The benefit of treatment was dose dependent and also depended on compliance, which was only 70% in those studies which assessed it. Although there was no effect on survival in these studies the reduction in skeletal morbidity is a worth while aim. A number of new oral bisphosphonates have become available and these preparations should be evaluated for efficacy and compliance. Bisphosphonates may be a useful adjunct to treatment in patients with bone-only disease, although at risk of developing bone disease. However, clearly more research is necessary to define optimal schedules and which patients actually benefit from bisphosphonates as their widespread use in all women with metastatic breast cancer would have major cost implications.

Bone metastases may cause pathological fracture of long bones and spinal cord compression. Although relatively uncommon these complications are major sources of morbidity. Fractures and cord compression occur in patients known to have bone disease and should be anticipated. Prophylactic surgical pinning may maintain mobility. Most patients who develop spinal cord compression have warning symptoms for at least a week before diagnosis and early decompressive surgery and/or radiotherapy can prevent paraplegia and will restore mobility in 45% of patients [39]. This is true even with cervical spine metastases in whom average post-operative survival after stabilization was 12 months [40].

Brain Metastases

Although brain metastases are rare as the site of first relapse, the incidence during the course of metastatic breast cancer is reported between 6 and 39% [41]. The overall prognosis with brain metastases is considered poor with a median survival of some 16 weeks with two-thirds of deaths due to neurological factors, however 20% of patients do survive more than 1 year. Useful palliation may be achieved by radiotherapy using short schedules with only a few fractions for patients with multiple metastases and this is worth while both in terms of symptom relief and reducing in-patient stays. Patients with a solitary brain metastasis may live longer and surgery may be necessary in the absence of disease elsewhere to exclude a primary brain tumour. When other prognostic factors are controlled for, there has been no difference demonstrated between surgery and radiotherapy as treatment of a solitary metastasis.

Conclusions

The prevalence and long natural history of breast cancer make the disease a major cause of morbidity and mortality. The assessment of how worth while treatments are could be made with respect to survival, relief of symptoms, toxicity of treatment, quality of life and health economics. Current treatment has little impact on survival, although some women with aggressive disease may have their lives prolonged. Both hormonal and endocrine treatment can relieve symptoms caused by metastatic breast cancer. As there are few side-effects associated with hormone treatment, most women should be offered this as first-line therapy unless clinical factors (e.g. aggressive disease) dictate otherwise. The toxicity of standard dose chemotherapy is low, provided that it is expertly administered, and as we cannot determine reliably women who would not benefit, despite a plethora of prognostic factors, it is worth while to consider most women with metastatic disease for a trial of chemotherapy. The response rates for second- and third-line chemotherapy are much lower and decisions about whether treatment is appropriate should be made on an individual basis.

Quality-of-life instruments have been validated in breast cancer and may give a more accurate perspective of benefit of treatment from the patient's point of view, although even these instruments are designed by health care professionals and perhaps assessment of the patient's view on whether treatment is worth while or not should be sought and may yield interesting answers [42]. Finally, we cannot ignore health economics in relation to any common disease, although for breast cancer it would appear that the morbidity from the disease process is the major component of cost rather than the treatment *per se*.

References

1. Bloom HGJ (1968) Survival of women with untreated breast cancer past and present. In: Forest APM, Kunkler PB (eds). Prognostic factors in breast cancer. ENS Livingstone, Edinburgh, pp 3–19.
2. Powles TJ, Smith IE, Ford HT et al. (1980) Failure of chemotherapy to prolong survival in a group of patients with metastatic breast cancer. Lancet i:580–582.

3. Hayward JL, Carbone PP, Heuson JC, Kumaoka S, Segeloff A, Rubens RD (1978) Assessment of response to therapy in advanced breast cancer. Br J Cancer 38:201–205.
4. Baum M, Priestman T, West R, Jones E (1980) A comparison of subjective responses in a trial comparing endocrine with cytotoxic treatment in advanced carcinoma of the breast. The 2nd EORTC Breast Cancer Working Conference, pp 223–226
5. Maher E (1992) The use of palliative radiotherapy in the management of breast cancer. Eur J Cancer 28:707–710.
6. Hurley SF, Huggins RM, Synder RD, Bishop JF (1992) The cost of breast cancer recurrences. Br J Cancer 65:449–455.
7. de Koning HV, van Inveld BM, de Haes JCJM et al. (1992) Advanced breast cancer and its prevention by screening. Br J Cancer 65:950–955.
8. Rees GJ (1985) Cost-effectiveness in oncology. Lancet 2:1405–1408.
9. Richards MA, Braysher S, Gregory WM, Rubens RD (1993) Advanced breast cancer: use of resources and cost implications. Br J Cancer 67:856–860.
10. Payne SA (1992) A study of quality of life in cancer patients receiving palliative chemotherapy. Soc Sci Med 35:1505–1509.
11. Robertson JFR, Whynes DK, Dixon A, Blamey RW (1995) Potential for cost economics in guiding therapy in patients with metastatic breast cancer. Br J Cancer 72:174–177.
12. Hillman BE, Smith TJ, Desch CE (1992) Efficacy and cost-effectiveness of autologous bone marrow transplantation in metastatic breast cancer: estimates using decision analysis while awaiting clinical trial results. J Am Med Assoc 267:2055–2061.
13. Hultborn R, Terje I, Holmberg E et al. (1992) Second line endocrine treatment of advanced breast cancer: a randomised crossover study of medroxyprogesterone acetate and aminoglutethemide. Ann Oncol suppl 5:75.
14. Kornblith AB, Hollis DR, Zuckerman E, Lyss AP, Kinnelas GP, Cooper MR et al. (1993) Effect of megestrol acetate on quality of life in a dose response trial in women with advanced breast cancer. J Clin Oncol 11:2081–2089.
15. Jones AL, Smith IE, O'Brien MER et al. (1994) Phase II study of continuous infusion fluorouracil with epirubicin and cisplatin in patients with metastatic and locally advanced breast cancer: an active new regimen. J Clin Oncol 12:1259–1265.
16. Dunphy FR, Spitzer G (1990) Long term complete remission of stage IV breast cancer after high dose chemotherapy and autologous bone marrow transplantation. Am J Clin Oncol 13:364–366.
17. Gregory WM, Smith P, Richards MA, Twelves CJ, Knight RK, Rubens RD (1993) Chemotherapy of advanced breast cancer: outcome and prognostic features. Br J Cancer 68(5):68–75.
18. Swenerton KD, Legha SS, Smith T, Hotobagyi G, Gehan EA, Yapp H, Gutterman JU, Blumenschein GR (1979) Prognostic factors in metastatic breast cancer treated with combination chemotherapy. Cancer Res 39:1552–1562.
19. Namer M, Mercier M, Hurteloup P, Bonnerterre J, Bastif P (1990) Prognostic factors of metastasised breast cancer patients. Breast Cancer Res Treat 16:60–65.
20. Falkson G, Gelman R, Ralkson CI, Glick J, Harris J (1991) Factors predicting the response, time to treatment failure, and survival in women with metastatic breast cancer treated with DAVTH: a prospective Eastern Co-operative Oncology Group study. J Clin Oncol 9:2153–2161.
21. Valagussa P, Tancina G, Bonadonna G (1986) Salvage treatment of patients suffering relapse after adjuvant chemotherapy. Cancer 58:1411–1417.
22. Kardinel CG, Perry MC, Korzun AH et al. (1988) Responses to chemotherapy or chemo-hormonal therapy in advanced breast cancer patients treated previously with adjuvant chemotherapy. A subset analysis of the CALBG study 8081. Cancer 61:415–419.
23. Falkson G, Gelman RS, Pretorios FJ (1986) Age as a prognostic factor in recurrent breast cancer. J Clin Oncol 4:663–671.

24. Falkson G, Gelman RS, Leone L et al. (1990) Survival of premenopausal women with metastatic breast cancer. Longterm follow-up of Easter Co-operative Oncology Group and cancer and leukaemia group B studies. Cancer 66:1621–1629.
25. Kristman K, Muss HB, Case LD, Stanley V (1992) Chemotherapy of metastatic breast cancer in the elderly: the Piedmont Oncology Association experience. J Am Med Assoc 268:57–62.
26. Pronzato P, Bertelli G, Gardin G, Rubergoti A, Conti PF, Rosso R (1993) Analysis of time to response in chemotherapy in 316 metastatic breast cancer patients. Oncology 50:460–465.
27. Ahern RP, Smith IE, Ebbs SR (1993) Chemotherapy and survival in advanced breast cancer: the inclusion of doxorubicin in Cooper type regimens. Br J Cancer 67:801–805.
28. Clavel M, Soukop M, Greenstreet VL (1993) Improved control of emesis and quality of life with ondansetron in breast cancer. Oncology 50:180–185.
29. Coates A, Gebski V, Bishop J, Jeal P, Woods R, Schnieder R et al. (1987) Improving the quality of life during chemotherapy for advanced breast cancer: a comparison of intermittent and continuous treatment strategies. N Engl J Med 317:1490–1495.
30. Tannock I, Boyd N, Deboer G, Erlichman C, Fine S, Larocque G et al. (1988) A randomised trial of two doses of cyclophosphamide, methotrexate and fluorouracil chemotherapy for patients with metastatic breast cancer. J Clin Oncol 6:1377–1387.
31. Fraser S, Dobbs H, Ebbs S, Fallowfield L, Bates T, Baum M (1993) Combination or mild single agent chemotherapy for advanced breast cancer? CMF versus epirubicin measuring quality of life. Br J Cancer 67:402–406.
32. Richards M, Hopwood P, Ramirez A, Twelves C, Ferguson J, Gregory W, Swindall R et al. (1992) Doxorubicin in advanced breast cancer: influence of schedule on response, survival and quality of life. Eur J Cancer 28A:1023–1028.
33. Bliss JM, Robertson B, Selby PJ et al. (1992) The impact of nausea and vomiting upon quality of life measures. Br J Cancer 19:514–522.
34. Aaronson MK, Ahmedzai S, Bergman B, Bullinger M, Karl A, Duez NJ et al. (1993) The European Organisation for Research and Treatment of Cancer QLQ-C30: a quality of life instrument for use in international clinical trials in oncology. J Natl Cancer Inst 85:372–374.
35. Bliss JM, Selby PJ, Robertson B, Powles TJ (1992) A method for assessing the quality of life of cancer patients: replication of the factor structure. Br J Cancer 65:961–966.
36. Coates A, Gebski V, Signorini D, Murray P, McNeill D, Burn M, Forbes JF (1992) Prognostic value of quality of life scores during chemotherapy for advanced breast cancer. J Clin Oncol 10:1833–1838.
37. Van Holten Verzantvoort ATM, Kroon HM, Vijvoeto LN, Kleton FG, Beex LVAN, Blijhan G, et al. (1993) Palliative pamidronate treatment in patients with bone metastases and breast cancer. J Clin Oncol 11:491–498.
38. Patterson AH, Palls TJ, Karness JA, McClosky E, Hanson J, Ashley S (1993) Double-blind control trial of oral clodronate in patients with bone metastases in breast cancer. J Clin Oncol 11:59–65.
39. Hill ME, Richards MA, Gregory WM, Smith P, Rubens RD (1993) Spinal cord compression in breast cancer, a review of 70 cases. Br J Cancer 68:969–974.
40. Jonnson B, Jonnson H, Karlstrom G, Sjostrom L (1994) Surgery of cervical spine metastases: a retrospective study. Eur Spine J 3:76–83.
41. Glass JP, Foley KM (1987) Brain metastases in patients with breast cancer. In: Harris JR, Holliman S, Henderson IC, Kinne DW (eds) Breast disease. Lippincott, Philadelphia, pp 480–488.
42. Slevin ML, Stubbs L, Plant HJ, Wilson P, Gregory WM, Arms PJ, Downer SM (1990) Attitudes to chemotherapy: comparing views of patients with cancer with those of doctors, nurses and general public. Br Med J 300:1458–1460.

14 – Non-Curative Chemotherapy for Small Cell Lung Cancer

C.M. McLean and R.C.F. Leonard

Introduction

Lung cancer is a major cause of mortality and morbidity in the community. There are 40 000 new cases per annum in the UK and the disease accounts for 16% of all cancer deaths. Approximately 25% of all lung cancer cases are of the small cell pathological subtype. It is now recognized that small cell lung cancer (SCLC) is a systemic disease and that at the time of presentation most patients have dissemination, whether metastases are clinically apparent or not. The tumour is relatively chemosensitive but, despite a 60–70% complete clinical response rate to combination chemotherapy, only 15–20% of patients with seemingly limited disease are alive 2 years after diagnosis. Patients with extensive disease at presentation rarely live longer than 12 months. Overall, 2–3% of patients are alive at 5 years and can be considered cured of their disease. In essence, therefore, the treatment intent for patients, even with apparently limited disease, is the palliation of symptoms.

Over the last 20 years a greater understanding of the natural history of SCLC has developed and the emphasis in treatment has changed from surgery and radiotherapy towards a primary role for chemotherapy. All patients have a substantial chance of symptomatic improvement provided by an optimal chemotherapeutic response, chemotherapy now being considered as first-line treatment. Extensive research over the last 25 years has been performed into both single agent and combination chemotherapy. Comparison of different regimens, optimal duration of treatment and intensification of treatment are all issues that continue to attract investigation. In more recent studies, however, investigators have attempted to evaluate the impact of treatment on the quality of life of their patients as well as achieving the therapeutic goal of obtaining long-term disease-free survival with the lowest possible morbidity.

Quality of Life in Patients with SCLC

Evaluating the merits of cancer treatments, particularly those treatments given with palliative intent, is a complex process. In a disease such as SCLC, where chemotherapy may be toxic and to date has resulted in only modest prolongation of survival, the assessment of quality of life as an outcome measure, in both routine clinical practice and in clinical trials, is paramount. There is a plethora of tests of quality of life, but many of them are difficult to score, complicated, lengthy and measure quality of life at one specific point in time. Many tests may be applicable for patients with chronic debilitating illnesses, but equally many are inappropriate for cancer patients undergoing often mutilating and distressing treatment. In such patients a satisfactory instrument for assessment which is both reliable and valid has yet to be developed. The EORTC questionnaire [1], for example, contains 47 questions that seek to measure key dimensions, including symptoms of disease, side-effects of treatment, physical functioning, psychological distress, social interaction, sexuality, body image and satisfaction with medical care. It cannot be administered frequently. By comparison, the Spitzer QL index [2] assesses only five variables, including physical activity, daily living, perception of own health, support from family and friends and outlook on life. It has the attraction of being simple, easy and quick to administer, but does not do justice to the different aspects of quality of life and does not reflect change over time.

Geddes et al. [3] recognized that, for patients receiving chemotherapy for SCLC, many of the available tests were suboptimal, particularly as they did not reflect changes over time. They devised the use of a self-administered daily diary card which was aimed at giving information more responsive to short-term changes in wellbeing. The questions were designed to cover three categories: symptoms related to the treatment (nausea, vomiting and appetite), symptoms related to the disease (pain, etc.) and a general assessment of wellbeing (mood, sleep and activity). They reported that the diary card was easy to use and sensitive to day-to-day changes. Compliance was good (68%) and patient and research nurse assessments were in reasonable agreement. The diary card demonstrated worsening of nausea, mood and general wellbeing as the treatment continued. Physical variables such as pain, sleep and activity were largely unaffected.

Staging

SCLC is conventionally staged anatomically, with the result of classifying patients into two categories, "limited" or "extensive" disease. Such staging is based on the identification of sites of tumour involvement. Limited stage disease is defined as tumour confirmed to one hemi-thorax and the regional lymph nodes, whereas extensive stage disease is defined as disease beyond these bounds. Anatomical staging allows the selection of individual patients considered for local radical treatment. It has failed, however, adequately to predict outcome, the median survival for limited disease being longer than extensive disease by only a few months. The use of invasive diagnostic procedures to determine disease extent is undoubtedly for many patients an unnecessary extra burden. With isotopic bone scans costing between £80 and £120 and CT scans between £150 and £200, the tests certainly increase the cost of medical care. The identification of simple inexpensive indices of prognosis which correlate with outcome in terms of disease-free survival or overall survival is therefore needed. Such indicators may replace invasive expensive tests in the more appropriate formulation of a treatment strategy and at the same time minimize the risk and discomfort to the patient.

To this end a number of studies [4–6] have investigated retrospectively a series of clinical, haematological and biochemical tests with respect to their predictive power and their ability to reflect disease burden. Univariate analyses in these studies have consistently demonstrated that prognosis is worse with deteriorating performance status, increasing age and reduced serum albumin. In addition, the importance of decreased plasma sodium, elevated alkaline phosphatase and alanine transaminase, and haemoglobin concentration, have also been identified. Serum lactate dehydrogenase levels in particular carry powerful prognostic significance. The presence of liver infiltration as defined by an abnormal scan and the confirmation of bone marrow involvement are recognized as important independent predictors, but on the basis of multivariate analysis it has been found that a prognostic index can be effectively obtained by the combination of clinical performance status scored with two or three simple biochemical tests, so that these more invasive tests can be excluded.

The reports of some studies, however, have not been entirely consistent and as a result an overview has been performed analysing the information on almost 4000 patients [7]. The overview concluded that in the short term (the 6 months after starting treatment) there were three groups of variables that were of importance for prognostic prediction. The first group, which were of primary importance, consisted of performance status, alkaline phosphatase and disease stage. The second group comprised age, sex, plasma sodium, gamma glutamyl transferase, albumin, urea and chloride, but the improvement in the prediction of survival obtained by their inclusion was reported as small. The third group, lactate dehydrogenase and aspartate aminotransferase, were potentially important prognostic factors, but the relatively small number of patients for whom these measurements were available prevented any definitive conclusions about their role. The overview based the prognostic index on survival up to 6 months. Thereafter, however, variables such as treatment response, current performance status and tumour progression were more useful predictors of long survival that the initial variables. At presentation, disease stage appears to be the most important predictor of long-term survival.

Richardson and colleagues have defined the cost savings associated with the use of an algorithm designed to allow the discontinuation of a sequential staging system, once a site of metastatic disease has been identified [8]. The rationale of sequential staging in SCLC is based on the concept that, in clinical practice, the identification of *all* sites of metastatic disease does not influence the choice of therapy. The purpose of staging is to identify patients with limited stage disease who may benefit from more intensive treatment with or without chest irradiation. They assumed that all patients had undergone initial assessment with clinical history and examination, routine blood tests (full blood count, urea and electrolytes, liver function tests), chest X-ray and histological diagnosis. Of the remaining five diagnostic procedures - isotope bone scan, CT scan of abdomen, cranial CT, bone marrow aspirate, and pulmonary function with chest CT (classed as a single indicator for chest irradiation) - 120 permutations were evaluated with regard to cost. These authors found little difference between the costs of the least expensive 24 permutations, but demonstrated that major savings could be made on the discontinuation of the algorithm. The main objection to sequential staging is the potential to prolong the time to complete staging, but Richardson and colleagues reported that 94% of patients with extensive disease were accurately staged within the first two steps of the algorithm. They concluded that the application of such an algorithm for staging SCLC could save one-third of the initial evaluation costs. Patients were also spared the burden of numerous investigations.

The use of a prognostic index or a staging algorithm allows the selection of patients for different treatment strategies, such as the evaluation of dose escalation in the good-risk population or the investigation of new chemotherapeutic agents in an untreated population of patients with poor-risk disease.

Single Agent Chemotherapy

A number of chemotherapy agents have been shown to produce response rates of at least 30% or more, including etoposide, doxorubicin, cyclophosphamide, ifosfamide, methotrexate and carboplatin. Given the availability of proven, active chemotherapy regimens, there has arisen the dilemma of how and when to test novel agents and regimens in this disease. One of the major problems in investigating new drugs is whether it is ethical to enrol untreated patients at the expense of delaying proven active first-line therapy, potentially compromising the patient's quality of life or survival. Conversely, there is little doubt that testing new treatments in patients who have failed conventional treatment substantially reduces the potential efficacy of the new treatment and enhances the risk of it being rejected inappropriately. One of the best examples of this phenomenon is the evaluation of etoposide, which, when administered as a single agent to previously treated patients with SCLC, produces a response rate of only 10% [9]. However, when administered to an untreated population of patients the response rate is as high as 80%.

Several authors have claimed that initial treatment with an investigational agent does not compromise survival in extensive stage disease, provided that an early crossover to standard therapy is undertaken. The National Cancer Institute of Canada Clinical Trials Group, in their first study [10], examined single agent epirubicin. Patients were assessed after the first cycle of treatment and those who demonstrated tumour regression continued epirubicin treatment. After the second cycle, patients who had fulfilled the criteria of partial remission (> 50% decrease of measurable disease) continued to receive the drug. If there was no response or progressive disease the patients changed to standard therapy. The response rate to single agent epirubicin was 50%. Treatment failures received etoposide/cisplatin and the overall response rate for the study was 62.5%, with a median length of survival of 8.3 months. This programme of new agent investigation continues to be active and may be a valuable method of assessing new drugs without apparent jeopardy to the patients.

Cullen et al., however, have shown that investigational agents used initially can compromise survival if "inactive" [11]. Cullen has therefore formulated guidelines to allow studies of new agents to continue ethically. Using an expected response rate for standard combination chemotherapy in extensive SCLC of 67% (2/3) he had demonstrated that as few as three patients are required to assess the efficacy of the agent. If all three patients are non-responders, the new agent can be quickly abandoned [12].

Etoposide has been shown to be one of the most active agents in the management of SCLC. It is reasonably effective and well tolerated in the management of elderly patients and those with extensive disease. The overall response rate of as much as 84%, however, depends on the schedule of drug administration and characteristics of the treated population. The selected route appears to have little impact on the response rate. However, Slevin et al. [13]

demonstrated that the scheduling of the drug had profound effects on the efficacy. In a randomized trial of previously untreated patients with SCLC, the response rate with 500 mg m^{-2} i.v. infused over 24 h was 10% as opposed to 80% when the drug was given as five infusions of 100 mg m^{-2} i.v. in 2 h on 5 consecutive days.

Etoposide given by the oral route has been shown to have approximately 50% bioavailability with much interpatient variation. The activity and toxicity of orally administered etoposide was investigated by Smit et al. [14]. The study showed a response rate of 71% in patients over the age of 70 years given a total dose of 800 mg m^{-2} over 5 days every 4 weeks. The median survival for patients with limited disease was 16 (range 6–32) months and for patients with extensive disease it was 9 (range 4–17) months, thus rivalling responses achieved with commonly used intravenous combination regimens. These authors reported minimal toxicity and the fact that no patient required hospitalization.

A study at St Bartholomew's Hospital and Homerton Hospital compared two different schedules of chronic oral etoposide [15]. A total of 67 patients with either extensive stage disease or limited disease were enrolled. The first 40 patients received 50 mg oral etoposide twice daily for 14 days every 21 days, and the subsequent 27 patients received 50 mg once daily for 21 days, repeated every 28 days. The response rates were 80% with the twice daily regimen and 50% with the once daily schedule. The medial remission duration and survival rates were amost identical for both groups.

Prolonged cyclical oral etoposide appears to be as effective as standard combination regimens for elderly patients or those medically unfit. When compared to intravenous combination chemotherapy it offers a more convenient, less toxic, less expensive, outpatient treatment option to patients with responsive but otherwise incurable disease.

Combination Chemotherapy

Despite the high response rates seen with single agent etoposide, combination chemotherapy has become the standard therapy in both extensive and limited SCLC. Optimum regimens should achieve an overall response rate of 85–95% in limited stage disease, with a complete response rate of 50–60% and a median survival of 12–16 months. Combination chemotherapy in extensive disease can achieve overall response rates of 75–85%, complete responses of 15–25% and a median survival of 7–11 months. This represents a four-fold improvement in survival over patients who receive no treatment. Although many combination regimens give similar results, perhaps the most commonly used regimen has been cyclophosphamide, adriamycin and vincristine (CAV). The CAV regimen combination with prophylactic CNS irradiation and chest radiotherapy was begun in 1974 at Indiana University and with minimum follow-up of 5 years, 15% of patients with limited disease remained disease free at the latest report, presumed cured. However, many small cell lung patients are elderly and suffer from varying degrees of neuropathy, pulmonary and heart disease. The CAV regimen is associated with frequent neurological and cardiac toxicity. The discovery that etoposide is one of the most active drugs in SCLC has therefore led to its incorporation into a number of first-line combination chemotherapy regimens,

Table 14.1 Commonly used effective combination chemotherapy regimens

Regimen	Drugs	Dosage/schedule
CAV	Cyclophosphamide	$1000\,mg\,m^{-2}$ i.v. day 1
	Adriamycin	$45\,mg\,m^{-2}$ i.v. day 1
	Vincristine	$2\,mg\,m^{-2}$ i.v. day 1
		Repeated every 3 weeks
ACE	Cyclophosphamide	$1000\,mg\,m^{-2}$ i.v. day 1
	Adriamycin	$45\,mg\,m^{-2}$ i.v. day 1
	Etoposide	$50\,mg\,m^{-2}$ i.v. days 1–5
		Repeated every 3 weeks
CAVE	Cyclophosphamide	$1000\,mg\,m^{-2}$ i.v. day 1
	Adriamycin	$50\,mg\,m^{-2}$ i.v. day 1
	Vincristine	$1.5\,mg\,m^{-2}$ i.v. day 1
	Etoposide	$50\,mg\,m^{-2}$ i.v. day 1
		Repeated every 3 weeks
EP	Etoposide	$100\,mg\,m^{-2}$ i.v. days 1–3
	Cisplatin	$25\,mg\,m^{-2}$ i.v. days 1–3
		Repeated every 3 weeks

and reviews of multicentre trials demonstrate that it can be added to or replace adriamycin or vincristine without loss of activity. Two controlled trials keeping CAV doses identical have compared CAV plus etoposide (CAVE) with CAV alone [16, 17]. The response rates were significantly greater with CAVE, but no difference in survival was observed. The toxicity of CAVE was greater than CAV alone. The replacement of vincristine by etoposide, however, as in the ACE (Adriamycin, cyclophosphamide and etoposide) regimen, has been shown to be as active as any other regimen in SCLC and to eliminate the toxicities of vincristine [18].

Second-line chemotherapy has been largely unsuccessful, with modest response rates of brief duration and median survival after relapse of only 2–3 months. Cisplatin and etoposide as single agents show unimpressive activity in CAV failures, but in combination there appears to be remarkable synergy and numerous published studies report reproducible 50% objective response rates [19]. The combination of cisplatin and etoposide has become one of the standard salvage therapies for CAV failures, but it has however had, at best, only a modest effect on palliation of symptoms and overall survival.

The most commonly used and effective regimens are given in Table 14.1.

Treatment Duration

Chemotherapy for SCLC was initially administered for prolonged periods, often until disease progression or death. The toxicity was considerable, probably resulting in poor quality of life. Two important trials in the UK, one by the CRC [20] and one by the MRC [21], have attempted to address the question of optimum duration of treatment. The CRC trial was of a complex design with two randomizations. The aims of the study were to determine the optimum duration of initial therapy and to ascertain if there was any added benefit of different chemotherapy for relapsed disease. A total of 610 patients with both limited and extensive disease (approx. ratio 1:3, respectively) were randomized to either four or eight courses of chemotherapy (cyclophosphamide, vincristine and etoposide) and also randomized on disease progression to receive either second-line chemotherapy (methotrexate and adriamycin) or supportive treatment only There was no significant difference in the response rates for the four or eight courses, 61% vs. 63% respectively. However it was noted that 50% of all those allocated to eight cycles failed to complete all the treatment. In subgroup analysis it was observed that 99 patients who achieved a complete response (CR) with initial therapy obtained a longer survival (42 weeks) with prolonged chemotherapy than those who did not (30 weeks). Treatment at relapse could not be given to 47% of those patients who had previously received eight cycles, compared with 37.5% of patients who received only four cycles, and the response rate was higher in this latter group (25.6% vs. 18.7%). The study concluded that stopping chemotherapy after four cycles with no further relapse therapy is associated with an inferior survival. There is a clear advantage for second-line therapy in those previously receiving short-course chemotherapy. In contrast, for those patients receiving eight cycles of initial treatment who relapse, further chemotherapy does not improve survival compared with symptomatic treatment alone.

The MRC study randomized patients between six or 12 cycles of a four-drug regimen (etoposide, cyclophosphamide, methotrexate and vincristine, 3-weekly). In common with the CRC study, both limited and extensive disease patients were included. However, those patients with limited disease (74%) received chest irradiation between the second and third cycles of chemotherapy. Patients achieving a CR or a partial response (PR) at six cycles were allocated to a further six cycles given at 4-weekly intervals or no further treatment. No difference in survival was observed. The study reported that the prolonged chemotherapy was associated with additional toxicity and poorer quality of life, as assessed intermittently by clinicians and daily by patients.

An EORTC trial [22] randomized patients to either five or 12 cycles of cyclophosphamide, adriamycin and etoposide and demonstrated no difference in survival regardless of disease extent or response to chemotherapy. A quality-of-life questionnaire was included, but the problem of having the questionnaire translated into several different languages, together with evaluation of the questionnaire, prevented a definitive conclusion. Many patients in the prolonged arm did not complete seven or more treatments or required dose reduction or delay in chemotherapy because of toxicity. In common with the CRC trial they found that the response rate to further chemotherapy on relapse was greater in those patients who had had the short-course chemotherapy.

The general conclusion from these studies is that prolonged chemotherapy neither improves the duration of survival nor the quality of life. There is possibly a subpopulation of patients who may benefit from prolonged therapy, but as yet there is no means of identifying such a group in advance. The current recommendation therefore is to treat responding patients with 4–6 cycles of combination chemotherapy. This approach does not compromise survival and minimizes the toxicity and expense of treatment.

Planned vs. "As Required" Chemotherapy

Prolonged treatment in patients with SCLC is associated with a corresponding reduction in quality of life attributable to the chemotherapy toxicity rather than the disease. The study by Geddes et al. [3], in which the use of a diary card for the assessment of quality-of-life measures was being evaluated, demonstrated an unequivocal deterioration in quality of life with extended chemotherapy. This observation has led to the philosophy of treating SCLC only when the disease progresses or symptoms occur. Chemotherapy on relapse appears to be effective after short courses of chemotherapy. This finding prompted a randomized trial of planned vs. "as required" (AR) chemotherapy [23]. Three hundred patients with untreated limited and extensive SCLC were randomized to receive either regular "planned" chemotherapy, given 3-weekly, or AR chemotherapy for tumour-related symptoms or radiological evidence of progression, following one cycle of cyclophosphamide, vincristine and etoposide. All patients kept a diary card recording changes in sleep patterns, mood, activity and general wellbeing. Despite the fact that the median treatment-free interval in the AR group was 6 weeks and 50% less chemotherapy was given (with a corresponding reduction in treatment-related nausea and vomiting), these patients reported more adverse symptoms with respect to sleep patterns, mood and general wellbeing. This perhaps surprising finding can be explained on both a psychological and physical basis. Psychologically, patients were thought to perceive the concept of AR chemotherapy as a failure of curative intent and that each required course of treatment reinforced the idea of progression of disease. Physically, it appears that the chemotherapy alleviated the symptoms of cancer when given regularly, albeit at the expense of some toxicity. The study concluded that for most patients regular chemotherapy is an effective and useful palliative treatment.

Non-Cross-Resistant Regimen

Despite the sensitivity of SCLC to initial treatment with cytotoxic drugs, the majority of patients relapse and their disease is usually resistant to further chemotherapy with the same drugs. The emergence of drug-resistant clones within tumours, as discussed by Goldie et al. [24], led to the proposal that two effective non-cross resistant regimens, A and B, could have superior results when given in alternation sequence ABABAB than in sequential sequence AAABBB. This hypothesis was tested by the National Cancer Institute of Canada and showed an improved survival for CAV alternating with etoposide/cisplatin (EP) compared with CAV alone [25]. The actual increase in median survival was, however, only 20% (6 weeks). The sequential programme was not tested in this study and therefore the trial could not distinguish whether the superiority of the cyclic alternating treatment was due to the alternating strategy or to the fact that EP was superior to CAV. Two subsequent studies [26, 27] have addressed this question. The US study randomized patients with extensive disease to either 12 weeks of EP, 18 weeks of CAV or the 18 weeks of alternation of these two regimens. There was no significant difference in the outcome in terms of complete response or median survival. There was, however, a non-significant improvement in the response duration in the alternating group, but at the expense of greater toxicity. The Japanese study demonstrated that the alternating regimen yielded a better survival compared with EP or CAV alone for patients with limited disease and suggested that the administration of the alternating programme may be more effective in patients with lesser tumour burden.

However, the general conclusion of these studies was that the alternating chemotherapy strategy should not be considered as standard treatment for patients with SCLC.

Dose Intensity

Dose intensification has been used to improve the outcome of several malignant diseases, including SCLC. Methods for intensifying the dose have included escalation of the administered drug or increasing the dose rate by shortening the intervals between treatments. The latter method of treatment was used with the weekly CODE regimen (cisplatin/oncovin/doxorubicin/etoposide) reported by Murray et al. [28]. The treatment was delivered at intervals of 1 week, rather than the more conventionsl 3-week spacing, such that the total dosage in the CODE regimen was delivered in approximately half the overall time of the standard regimen (9 vs. 18 weeks). To reduce bone marrow toxicity, the protocol was designed to alternate myelosuppressive treatment with non-myelosuppressive treatment. Supportive drugs included gastroprotective agents, prophylactic antibiotics and corticosteroids. A response rate of 94% and a CR rate of 40% was achieved. All patients had extensive disease and the median survival of 61 weeks was reported to be far superior to previous conventional chemotherapy. Toxicity, however, was significant with leucopenia occurring in the majority of patients, resulting in arguably unacceptable constitutional debility.

Increased drug dosage in randomized trials for both CAV and etoposide regimens have been reported. Johnson et al. [29] randomized 298 patients with extensive disease to either conventional dose CAV (cyclophosphamide 100 mg m^{-2}, adriamycin 40 mg m^{-2} and vincristine 1 mg m^{-2}) or high-dose CAV (cyclo. 1200 mg m^{-2}, adria. 70 mg m^{-2}, vinc. 1 mg m^{-2}). No advantage over conventional doses of the same agents, either in terms of overall survival or response rates, was observed. There was, however, a significant increase in haematological toxicity in the high-dose arm, such that even if there had been a small increase in response rate this would have been offset by the greater toxicity. A trial of EP in high dosage likewise failed to improve the outlook for these patients [30].

Dose Intensity with Haemopoietic Factors

Myelosuppression is the dose-limiting toxicity for most chemotherapeutic agents active in SCLC, resulting in both bacterial and fungal infection. Anaemia and thrombocytopenia can be treated by transfusion, but no effective method, until recently, existed to restore granulocyte and monocyte levels. Current standard therapy for patients presenting with fever in association with neutropenia includes hospitalization, with immediate treatment with empirically selected broad-spectrum antibiotics. The mortality for neutropenic sepsis among patients with disseminated infection is 10%. Colony-stimulating factors have been available for clinical investigation for some years. Granulocyte colony-stimulating factor (G-CSF) and granulocyte macrophage-stimulating factor (GM-CSF) have been shown to enhance both the production of mature myeloid elements and the function of these effector cells. This hastened haematological reconstitution could substantially reduce mortality, morbidity and expense of intensive chemotherapy. Several studies have demonstrated that G-CSF and GM-CSF shorten the duration of neutropenia after chemotherapy. In two randomized studies [31, 32] the patients were treated with cyclophosphamide, doxorubicin and etoposide and then randomized between G-CSF and placebo on the first cycle.

There was a reduction in febrile neutropenia and hospital admission in both trials. Although the trials were not designed to demonstrate any overall difference in outcome, no difference in response or survival was seen. The toxicity related to neutropenia was shown to be less with the use of G-CSF. G-CSF related toxicity was also minimal and included mild to moderate medullary bone pain. Side-effects seen with other cytokines, such as malaise, arthralgia, myalgia, fluid retention, hypotension and dyspnoea, were not associated with G-CSF. Crawford et al. [31] reported that the incidence of fever with neutropenia, antibiotic use and hospitalization were all reduced by approximately 50% in the G-CSF group, suggesting that there may also be a substantial economic impact. Criticisms of this trial, however, included the fact that higher than usual doses of myelosuppressive agents were used (cyclophosphamide 1000 mg m^{-2} day 1, doxorubicin 50 mg day 1, etoposide 120 mg m^{-2} days 1–3) and that the particular diligence with which temperatures were measured resulted in a higher incidence of neutropenia fever.

The cost impact of the treatment with G-CSF has been assessed by Nichols et al. [33]. The records of 137 consecutive, unselected patients were reviewed. The cost and therapeutic outcomes were assessed for each of the two models of G-CSF use: (1) pre-emptive – with all courses of chemotherapy; (2) reactive – with all cycles of chemotherapy following a neutropenic fever. Assessment for dose reduction only and no G-CSF was also made. Therapeutic outcomes such as neutropenic septic death, response rates and survival were all comparable. The incidence of febrile neutropenic events (18%) was significantly different to the incidence reported by Crawford and colleagues (77%). As a consequence of this low incidence of neutropenic fever and hospitalization, the study concluded that the routine use of G-CSF in SCLC patients treated with standard dose chemotherapy appeared to be expensive and was not associated with an obvious therapeutic benefit or cost saving. Without evidence of improvement in therapeutic outcome, reduction in therapy-related deaths or cost reduction, the only justification for pre-emptive use of G-CSF would be improved quality of life. Quality of life has not been formally assessed in any of these trials.

These trials have, however, prompted pilot studies to determine whether CSFs would allow dose intensification of chemotherapy in an attempt to improve the response rates in SCLC without the corresponding toxicity. Fukuoka et al. [34] compared the CODE regimen alone with CODE + 50 $\mu g\ m^{-2}$ G-CSF given daily on non-treatment days. The value of G-CSF in allowing administration of higher doses has yet to be answered, particularly since the value of greater dose intensity in SCLC remains questionable. The total dose delivered in the G-CSF arm was 85% predicted, compared with 76% predicted in the control arm. The trial was randomized and showed that the CR was similar in both arms, but the median length of survival in the G-CSF arm was 59 weeks compared to 35 weeks in the control arm. However, the response and survival rates in the G-CSF group were not superior to those achieved by Murray et al. [28] for CODE given with prednisolone and prophylactic antibiotics.

Dose Intensification with Autologous Bone Marrow Transplantation

The use of conventional doses of chemotherapy in patients with SCLC has resulted in only modest improvements in survival, promoting almost a decade of research into high-dose chemotherapy followed by autologous bone marrow transplant (ABMT). Unfortunately, most of the trials have been small and diverse, some focusing on limited disease patients and some including those with extensive disease as well [35]. High-dose therapy with ABMT has been investigated as initial induction treatment, as intensification following standard dose chemotherapy and as salvage on relapse.

The studies of high-dose induction chemotherapy have generally been disappointing. Most investigators recognize the need to determine subgroups of patients likely to benefit from intensification. These patients include those with early disease, better performance status and those who have responded well to standard dose induction. There has been only one randomized trial of high-dose therapy vs. conventional therapy [36]. Patients received five induction cycles, which included three cycles of methotrexate, cyclophosphamide and vincristine, followed by prophylactic cranial irradiation and then two cycles of cisplatin and etoposide. Patients who were sensitive to induction chemotherapy were than randomized to one additional course of cyclophosphamide $750\,mg\,m^{-2}$ i.v., etoposide $60\,mg\,m^{-2}$ i.v. and BCNU $600\,mg\,m^{-2}$ orally (conventional dosage) or to intensification with cyclophosphamide $6\,g\,m^{-2}$ i.v., BCNU $300\,mg\,m^{-2}$ i.v. and etoposide $500\,mg\,m^{-2}$ i.v., followed by ABMT. A significant proportion of patients had extensive disease and had only achieved a PR at the time of intensification. Although there was a significant conversion of patients from PR to CR (39–79%), no statistical difference in overall survival was observed. Toxicity was high; all patients experienced nausea and vomiting during the administration of cytotoxics. Four of 23 patients undergoing ABMT died during aplasia in the 4–12 days after the procedure.

Chemotherapy for Brain Metastases

The CNS has hitherto been considered a sanctuary site for metastatic tumour cells and, due to the presumed lack of penetrance of cytostatic agents into parenchymatous brain metastases, corticosteroids and radiotherapy have been the treatment of choice for decades. The prognosis for patients with SCLC who present with brain metastases initially is very different from those who relapse with intracranial disease. The latter indicates a very poor prognosis, whereas those patients with brain metastases as the only sign of dissemination at presentation have survival curves comparable to those of patients with limited disease [37]. During the last decade, several reports about the effect of systemic chemotherapy on brain metastases in SCLC have been published. There now appears to be adequate evidence that chemotherapy has a pronounced initial effect on such disease, and that first-line cranial irradiation may be deemed unnecessary. Intracranial and extracranial response rates appear to be similar. It remains unclear, however, what the role for consolidation cranial irradiation is, and what additional toxicity it would inflict on patients who are aleady burdened by the toxicity of systemic treatment [38].

Patients who develop brain metastases during or immediately after chemotherapy are probably resistant to further cytostatic agents, and second-line treatment is generally ineffective. For those patients, standard whole-brain irradiation and corticosteroids remain the most effective modes of palliation.

Frequently, brain metastases develop after prophylactic cranial irradiation (PCI) or therapeutic cranial irradiation. On the basis of favourable responses after high-dose cyclophosphamide, etoposide and ABMT, the EORTC Lung Cancer Cooperative Group performed a phase II study of high-dose etoposide ($1.5\,g\,m^{-2}$) in patients who had relapsed or progressive intracranial disease following cranial irradiation [39]. Twenty-eight patients were entered and the study produced a response rate of 43%. However, five patients died during neutropenic-related septicaemia, and it was felt that for palliative purposes the regimen was too toxic in heavily pretreated patients.

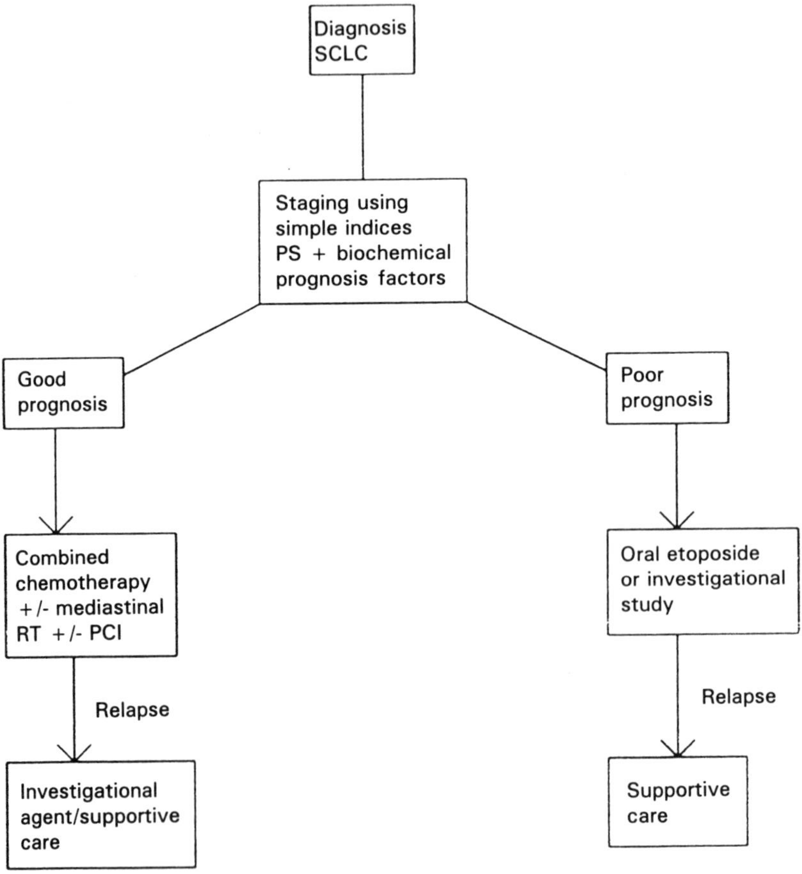

Figure 14.1 Chemotherapy in the palliation of small cell lung cancer

Conclusions

The following conclusions can be drawn concerning the place of chemotherapy in the palliation of SCLC (Figure 14.1):

1. Chemotherapy used judiciously, selectively and according to the patient's perceived tolerance and prognosis can provide effective palliation by improving the patient's symptoms, health status, quality of life and survival.
2. Selection of patients for the various drug regimens is critical. It is easy to overtreat and reduce the patient's quality of life or even cause serious morbidity and early death. Conversely, it is easy to underestimate the value of therapy and to undertreat to the patient's detriment in respect of quality of life and possibly survival.
3. Routinely, it is the practice to treat patients with multi-agent intravenous chemotherapy. The optimum duration is not clear or even necessarily uniform, but a reasonable guideline would be to treat for about 4–5 months, which in most patients would be a little beyond the time of best measurable response.
4. Despite the foregoing, oral etoposide, given in the appropriate schedule, is sufficiently active and well tolerated to be recommended as primary therapy for many patients with extensive disease. This would particularly apply to patients who are unfit and who are best managed at home rather than in hospital.
5. Despite the general enthusiasm for examining prognostic factors for outcome, the collaborative research of the last 5 years has failed significantly to influence the practice of clinicians. This is inefficient use of practical research which should have resulted in the reduction in the use of expensive and uncomfortable staging procedures.
6. There has been little progress in the management of this disease over a decade, despite occasional useful observation such as the recognition of the activity of etoposide. Trials therefore have to be encouraged in all aspects of management. Current questions remaining are appropriateness of PCI and the place of dose-intensive therapy. The latter was examined some 10 years ago in a series of small and poorly controlled trials which basically gave negative answers. However, with the availability of growth factors and safer transplantation methods the question might be readdressed with careful attention to the design of induction and high-dose therapy.
7. In the last decade several papers have appeared in the scientific and medical press concerning the potential application of peptide hormonal growth factors in the control of SCLC, itself a potential paradigm for the control of other cancers by biological and biosynthetic peptides. This area of research is at the very beginning of clinical application and may yet find a place in the routine palliative management of disease in the next decade.

References

1. Linssen AG (1981) The development of the complaint questionnaire at the Netherlands Cancer Institute. Proceedings of the First Workshop EORTC Study Group on Quality of Life, Amsterdam (internal publication).
2. Spitzer WD, Dobson AJ, Hall J et al. (1981) Measuring quality of life of lung cancer patients. J Chronic Dis 35:585–597.
3. Geddes DM, Dones L, Hill E et al. (1990) Quality of life during chemotherapy for small cell lung cancer. An assessment and use of a daily diary card in a randomised trial. Eur J Cancer 26:484–492.
4. Osterlind K, Anderson PK (1986) Prognostic factors in small cell lung cancer: multivariate model based on 778 patients treated with chemotherapy with or without radiation. Cancer Res 46:4189–4194.
5. Souhami RL, Bradbury I, Geddes DM et al. (1985) Prognostic significance of laboratory parameters measured at diagnosis in small cell lung cancer. Cancer Res 45:2878–2882.
6. Vincent MD, Ashley SE, Smith IE (1987) Prognostic factors in small cell lung cancer. A simple prognostic index is better than conventional staging. Eur J Cancer Clin Oncol 23:1589–1598.
7. Rawson R, Peto R (1990) An overview of prognostic factors in small cell lung cancer. A report from the sub-committee for the management of lung cancer of the UK Coordinating Committee on Cancer Research. Br J Cancer 61(4):597–604.
8. Richardson GE, Venzon DJ, Phelps R et al. (1993) Application of an algorithm for staging small cell lung cancer can save one third of the initial evaluation costs. Arch Intern Med 153:329–337.
9. Issell BF, Einhorn LH, Comis RL et al. (1985) Multicentre trial of etoposide in refractory small cell lung cancer. Cancer Treat Rep 69:127–128.
10. Blackstein M, Eisenhauer EA, Wierzbicki R, Yoshida S (1990) Epirubicin in extensive small cell lung cancer: a phase II study in previously untreated patients. A National Cancer Institute of Canada Clinical Trials Group study. J Clin Oncol 8:385–389.
11. Cullen MH, Smith ST, Benfield GFA et al. (1987) Testing drugs may prejudice treatment: A phase II study of oral idarubicin in extensive disease small cell lung cancer. Cancer Treat Rep 71:1227–1230.
12. Cullen M. (1988) Evaluating new drugs as first treatment in patients with small cell carcinoma. Guidelines for an ethical approach with implications of other chemotherapy-sensitive tumours. J Clin Oncol 6:1356–1357.
13. Slevin MC, Clarke PI, Joel SP (1989) A randomised trial to evaluate the effects of schedule on the activity of etoposide in small cell lung cancer. J Clin Oncol 7:1333–1340.
14. Smit EF, Carney DN, Harford P (1989) A phase II study of oral etoposide in elderly patients with small lung cancer. Thorax 44:631–633.
15. Clark P, Cottier B, Joel S (1991) Two prolonged schedules of single agent oral etoposide of differing duration and dose with untreated SCLC. Proc Am Soc Clin Oncol 10:286 (abstr).
16. Jett JR, Everson L, Therneau TM et al. (1990) Treatment of limited stage small cell lung cancer with cyclophosphamide, doxorubicin and vincristine with or without etoposide. A randomised trial of North Central Cancer Treatment Group. J Clin Oncol 8:33–39.
17. Messieh AA, Schweicker JM, Lipton et al. (1987) Addition of etoposide to cyclophosphamide, doxorubicin and vincristine for remission induction and survival in patients with small cell lung cancer. Cancer Treat Rep 71:61–66.
18. Bunn PA, Greco AF, Einhorn L (1986) Cyclophosphamide, doxorubicin and etoposide as first line therapy in the treatment of small cell lung cancer. Semin Oncol 13(3):45–53.

19. Einhorn LH (1986) Cisplatin and VP-16 in small cell lung cancer. Semin Oncol 13(3):3–4.
20. Spiro SG, Souhami RL, Geddes DM et al. (1989) Duration of chemotherapy in small cell lung cancer. A CRC trial. Br J Cancer 59:578–583.
21. Bleehan NM, Fayers PM, Girling DJ, Stephens RJ (1989) Controlled trials of 12 vs 6 courses of chemotherapy in the treatment of small cell lung cancer. Report to the Medical Research Council and its Lung Cancer Working Party. Br J Cancer 59:584–590.
22. Giaccone G, Dalesio O, McVie G et al. (EORTC) (1993) Maintenance chemotherapy in small cell lung cancer. Long term results of a randomised trial. J Clin Oncol 11:1230–1240.
23. Earl HM, Rudd RM, Spiro SG et al. (1991) A randomised trial of planned vs as required chemotherapy in small cell lung cancer: a CRC trial. Br J Cancer 64(3):566–572.
24. Goldie GH, Coldman AJ, Gudauskas GA (1982) Rationale for the use of alternating non-cross resistant chemotherapy. Cancer Treat Rep 66:439–449.
25. Evans WK, Feld R, Murray N (1987) Superiority of alternating non cross resistant chemotherapy in extensive SCLC. A multicentre randomised trial by the NCI Canada. Ann Intern Med 107:451–458.
26. Fukuoka M, Furuse K, Saijo N et al. (1991) Randomised trial of cyclophosphamide, doxorubicin and vincristine vs cisplatin and etoposide vs alternation of these regimens in small cell lung cancer. J Natl Cancer Inst 83:855–861.
27. Roth BJ, Johnson DH, Einhorn LH (1992) Randomised study of cyclophosphamide, doxorubicin and vincristine vs etoposide and cisplatin vs alternation of these 2 regimens in extensive small cell lung cancer. A phase III trial of the South Eastern Cancer Study Group. J Clin Oncol 10:282–291.
28. Murray N, Shan A, Osoba D (1991) Intensive weekly chemotherapy for the treatment of extensive small cell lung cancer. J Clin Oncol 9:1632–1638.
29. Johnson DH, Einhorn LH, Birch R et al. (1987) A randomised comparison of high dose vs conventional dose cyclophosphamide, doxorubicin and vincristine for extensive stage small cell lung cancer. A phase III trial of the South Eastern Cancer Study Group. J Clin Oncol 5:1731–1738.
30. Idhe DC, Mulshine JL, Kramer BS et al. (1991) Randomised trial of high vs standard dose etoposide (VP-16) and cisplatin in extensive small cell lung cancer. Proc Am Soc Clin Oncol 10:240 (abstr).
31. Crawford J, Ozer H, Stoller R et al. (1991) Reduction by granulocyte colony stimulating factor of fever and neutropenia induced by chemotherapy in patients with SCLC. N Engl J Med 325:164–170.
32. Trillet V (1991) Recombinant human granulocyte colony stimulating factor with chemotherapy for small cell lung cancer. Results of a randomised European multicentre trial. Third International Congress on Neoadjuvant Chemotherapy, Paris, Feb 6–9, p55.
33. Nichols CR, Fox EP, Roth BJ et al. (1994) Incidence of neutropenic fever in patients with standard dose chemotherapy for small cell lung cancer and the cost impact of treatment with granulocyte colony-stimulating factor. J Clin Oncol 13:1245–1250.
34. Fukuoka M, Takada M, Masuda N et al. (1992) Dose intensive weekly chemotherapy with or without G-CSF in extensive stage small cell lung cancer. Proc Am Soc Clin Oncol 11:29 (abstr).
35. Leonard RCF (1989) Small cell lung cancer. Guest Editorial. Br J Cancer 59:487–490.
36. Humblet Y, Symann M, Bosey A et al. (1987) Late intensification chemotherapy with autologous bone marrow transplantation in selected SCLC: a randomised study. J Clin Oncol 5:1864–1873.
37. Hazel GA van, Scott M, Eagan RT (1983) The effect of CNS metastases on the survival of patients with small cell lung cancer. Cancer 51:933–937.

38. Kristensen CA, Kristjansen PEG, Hansen HH (1992) Systemic chemotherapy of brain metastases from small cell lung cancer. A review. J Clin Oncol 10:1498–1502.
39. Postmus PE, Haaxma-Reiche H, Sleijfer DT et al. EORTC Lung Cancer Cooperative Group (1989) High dose etoposide for brain metastases in small cell lung cancer. Br J Cancer 59:254–256.

15 – Non-Curative Chemotherapy for Non-Small Cell Lung Carcinoma

Michael H. Cullen

Introduction

Changes in smoking habits in the UK and other Western communities are resulting in a decline in the incidence of lung cancer among men in recent years. In women it is still increasing (for the same reason). In many parts of the developing world tobacco consumption is growing, and an epidemic of lung cancer, similar to the one which affected Europe and North America in the second half of this century, will doubtless follow. There is little evidence that political intervention, on the scale required, will significantly influence these trends. So lung cancer is destined to remain the biggest cancer problem worldwide for the foreseeable future, with moe than half a million new cases diagnosed annually [1]. Approximately 80% of these tumours are of non-small cell histological type, including squamous, adeno- and large cell carcinomas.

Surgery and Radiotherapy in NSCLC

The only curative modality in non-small cell lung cancer (NSCLC) is surgery. The overall results, however, are very poor with only about 12% of cases surviving 5 years from diagnosis [2]. Only 20% of tumours are suitable for potentially curative resection [3], and many of these ultimately die from secondaries unsuspected at the time of surgery. The principal reason for this is the tendency for these tumours to spread early in their natural history, invariably before diagnosis. Thus surgery cannot realistically be expected to benefit all but a small minority of cases.

For the same reasons, radiotherapy (another local treatment) is unlikely to make much impact in what is essentially a disseminated disease in most cases. Nevertheless, it has been the mainstay of treatment for localized, inoperable NSCLC, despite a dearth of evidence to support it as a curative agent. Historically there have been two randomized trials evaluating radiotherapy and both have been criticized for using orthovoltage equipment and/or suboptimal radiotherapy techniques [4, 5].

One much more recent trial does warrant a second look, since it was intended originally to test the value of modern radiotherapy planning and treatment techniques [6]. Planned in 1981, this Southeastern Cancer Study Group (SECSG) trial was designed to evaluate the role of immediate megavoltage radiotherapy in locally advanced, inoperable NSCLC. Since few investigators were willing at that time to randomly assign patients to a "no treatment" or "placebo" arm, patients in the "no radiotherapy" arm were given single agent vindesine. A third arm of the study combined radiotherapy with vindesine. The SECSG trial used a 60 Gy in 6 weeks schedule which was based on the results of the Radiation Therapy Oncology Group study 73-01 [7]. In the early 1980s, when the SECSG trial was being designed, vindesine was reported to be very active in NSCLC. Since then, much less encouraging results have been reported [8]. A total of 319 patients were randomized between the three arms in the SECSG trial. The response rate in the vindesine arm was only 10%, compared to 30% in the radiotherapy arm and 34% in the combined arm. Crossover from vindesine to radiotherapy and vice versa was permitted. Thirty-six (of 98) vindesine patients "crossed over" and their objective response rate was 22%. The response rate to vindesine in 25 evaluable radiotherapy failures was just 4%. More importantly, overall survival in the three arms was identical. Thus the authors conclude that immediate radiotherapy does not prolong survival in these patients. Furthermore, of the 13 2-year survivors in the vindesine alone arm, six ultimately received thoracic radiation and seven did not. So it is unlikely that *delayed* radiotherapy materially affected the survival of these patients. The fundamental conclusion and the title of this paper [6] is "Thoracic radiotherapy does not prolong survival in patients with locally advanced, unresectable NSCLC". This finding does not necessarily contradict the observation that long-term survival is occasionally seen following radiotherapy alone in NSCLC. It seems most likely that a small proportion of cases where small tumours are treated before widespread dissemination could experience survival extension as a result of radical radiotherapy, and that trials like that of the SECSG are too small to demonstrate this.

Chemotherapy

The only hope of influencing the natural history of the disease for most patients lies with systemic therapy. Unfortunately standard chemotherapeutic agents have, at best, only marginal activity in NSCLC. Until very recently only five drugs (ifosfamide, mitomycin, cisplatin, vinblastine and vindesine), when tested as single agents in large numbers, produced major responses in 15% or more of cases [9]. Newer agents, including navelbine, taxol and gemcitabine, offer some promise, but it is unlikely that even these alone, or in combination, will be effective enough to cure NSCLC.

End-points Other than Cure

There are two other worthwhile objectives in cancer therapy that fall short of permanent eradication of the disease (cure). These are extension of life and improved quality of life. The terms "curative" and "palliative" are self-explanatory, but there is not a widely used adjective to describe those treatments (e.g. chemotherapy in advanced small cell lung cancer) which produce extension of life as well as palliation, but fall short of cure. I have suggested the term "retardative", implying a slowing or temporary reversal in growth of the tumour [10]. Evidence is beginning to emerge suggesting that chemotherapy can have both palliative and retardative effects on NSCLC.

Does Chemotherapy Prolong Life in NSCLC?

Chemotherapy has been tested in randomized trials in several different contexts in NSCLC:

1. Neo-adjuvant chemotherapy prior to surgery in cases of borderline operability.
2. Adjuvant chemotherapy following "curative" surgery.
3. Chemotherapy in inoperable, but still localized disease where standard therapy would be *radical* radiotherapy.
4. Chemotherapy in advanced disease where standard therapy would be supportive/palliative care.

Trials of Neo-adjuvant Chemotherapy Prior to Surgery in Cases of Borderline Operability

Opinions vary on the role of surgery in stage IIIA NSCLC. This category includes patients with locally invasive primary tumours or tumours associated with ipsilateral mediastinal lymph node involvement. In four separate studies totalling 1180 patients who underwent resection, the 5-year survival rates ranged from 14% to 30% [11–14]. Variations in staging investigations and in the definition of complete resection contribute to the difficulty in interpreting uncontrolled data. There is, however, no doubt about the legitimacy of examining neo-adjuvant chemotherapy in this context. Unfortunately there are only two randomized trials [15, 16] and both are far too small to convince many that neo-adjuvant chemotherapy should become standard practice. Nevertheless they are of interest.

In the trial from Barcelona [15] 60 patients with stage IIIA NSCLC were randomly assigned to receive either surgery alone or three courses of chemotherapy (mitomycin $6\,mg\,m^{-2}$, ifosfamide $3\,g\,m^{-2}$ and cisplatin $50\,mg\,m^{-2}$: MIC) followed by surgery. All patients received mediastinal radiotherapy after surgery. Eighteen out of 30 patients (60%) randomized to chemotherapy achieved an objective response. Three patients in the MIC arm did not undergo surgery; two refused and one had progressive disease within the liver detected after chemotherapy had commenced. Four patients in the MIC arm had unresectable tumours compared to three in the surgery alone arm. The median survival was 26 months in the patients treated with chemotherapy prior to surgery, compared with 8 months in those treated with surgery alone ($p < 0.001$). Rosell and colleagues were unable to continue with this trial since some of his surgical collaborators felt it would be unethical to randomize further patients to surgery alone (pers. comm.).

The second trial is from the MD Anderson Cancer Centre in Texas [16]. Sixty patients with "resectable stage III" NSCLC were randomly allocated to three cycles of preoperative chemotherapy (cyclophosphamide, etoposide and cisplatin) followed by surgery or surgery alone. Those patients achieving an objective response to preoperative therapy went on to receive a further three courses after operation. There were no significant differences in distribution of major prognostic factors between the two arms. "Major" objective responses were seen in 35% of patients following chemotherapy and "minor" responses were observed in 31%. The estimated median survival of patients in the perioperative chemotherapy arm was 64 months compared with 11 months in the surgery alone arm ($p < 0.018$). The authors conclude that "patients with resectable stage III NSCLC should no longer be treated with surgery alone".

This view was voiced prominently in discussion at the IASLC World Lung Cancer Congress in Colorado Springs in 1994, citing both these trials and the huge apparent benefit of chemotherapy. The problem is that the effect of chemotherapy seems quite out of proportion to one's intuitive expectation. The failure of surgery alone is largely due to undetected spread of disease. If currently available chemotherapy was this good at influencing the natural history of subclinical metastatic disease in cases of borderline operability treated with surgery, then one would expect that a similar or greater effect might be observed with adjuvant chemotherapy given in clearly operable cases after "curative" surgery.

It is premature to adopt cisplatin-based neo-adjuvant chemotherapy in stage III NSCLC based on the results of two trials with a total of only 120 patients. Confounding effects resulting from maldistribution of as yet unknown prognostic factors cannot be confidently excluded in small trials such as these. Nevertheless, this is the best evidence available at present and both trials do point to some prolongation of life in stage IIIA NSCLC.

Trials of Adjuvant Chemotherapy Following "Curative" Surgery

Many trials have been undertaken to address the question "Does adjuvant chemotherapy following surgery influence survival in NSCLC?" The vast majority have been far too small to detect the sort of differences likely to emerge, given the limited efficacy of chemotherapy. The most reliable way to assess this evidence and to establish the size of any possible treatment effect is to conduct an overview or meta-analysis of updated individual patient data [17]. Overviews will never be a substitute for individual trials that are big enough to detect differences of magnitude thought clinically important, but they do allow something worth while to be salvaged from otherwise often contradictory data.

The UK Medical Research Council, the Institut Gustave Roussy in Paris and the Instituto di Richerche Farmacologiche "Mario Negri" in Milan have recently collaborated in conducting meta-analyses of all available randomized trials of chemotherapy in NSCLC. Some of the results of this exercise have recently been presented to the Seventh World Lung Cancer Conference in Colorado Springs [18]. Data were available from 14 out of 16 trials dealing with surgery $\pm$ adjuvant chemotherapy. These trials included 4357 patients and 2574 deaths. Hazard ratios (HR) were calculated for a number of pre-specified chemotherapy categories. The HR represents the overall risk of dying on treatment as compared to control. A HR of 1 indicates no difference between treatment and control. A HR of less than 1 favours the chemotherapy group; e.g. a HR of 0.8 represents a 20% relative reduction in the hazard, or risk of death, in the chemotherapy group. A HR of greater than 1 favours the control group. Two important categories, identified prospectively, were: (1) trials using long-term (> 1 year) alkylating agents, and (2) those employing cisplatin-based chemotherapy. The pooled HR of 1.16 (95% CI 1.05–1.28), $p = 0.004$) for the long-term alkylating agent based regimens gives an estimated 16% relative detriment of chemotherapy. This is equivalent to an absolute worsening of survival of 6% at 5 years. In contrast, the seven cisplatin-based trials give a pooled HR of 0.87 (95% CI 0.73–1.04, $p = 0.124$), suggesting a relative survival benefit from chemotherapy of 13%. Although not statistically significant by conventional criteria, the authors point out that the result is equivalent to an absolute improvement in survival of 5% from 47% to 52% at 5 years. The 95% CIs suggest the results are compatible with a 10% improvement or a 1% detriment from chemotherapy at 5 years. The survival curves for cisplatin-based trials appear to diverge at around 6 months, with the possible benefit to cisplatin-based chemotherapy maintained over time.

Chemotherapy plus *Radical* Radiotherapy vs. *Radical* Radiotherapy Alone

The modern era of chemotherapy investigation in NSCLC began with the demonstration of the activity of cisplatin as a single agent. All trials commenced since 1984 have incorporated this drug. Consequently this provides a convenient subdivision historically, but possibly also marks a watershed in efficacy.

Trials including Cisplatin

It is clear that in the pre-cisplatin era chemotherapy was nowhere near active enough to be expected to influence the natural history of NSCLC. Response rates to cisplatin in combination with other active agents vary from 30 to 50%, but invariably with complete remissions running at 10% only or less. Even the mitomycin, ifosfamide and cisplatin combination (MIC) [19], which is the only thoroughly tested regimen incorporating three drugs having single agent activity around the 20% mark, induces objective responses in only 52% of cases, with 10% complete remission (CR) [20]. However, three trials have shown a statistically significant benefit for the chemotherapy arm. The trial of Schaake-Koning et al. [21] differed from the others in using cisplatin concurrently with radiotherapy as a radiosensitizer. This was a three-arm trial comparing radiotherapy alone, radiotherapy plus weekly cisplatin, and radiotherapy plus daily cisplatin. Survival with the daily cisplatin arm was significantly better than with radiotherapy alone. There was no effect on distant recurrence rate and the authors concluded that the effect observed was due to improved local control.

The other two trials demonstrating a significant effect of cisplatin combinations are more orthodox chemotherapy trials, with the chemotherapy given before radiotherapy (in the CALGB) trial, and before and after radiotherapy (in the French trial), with the intention of exerting an independent effect.

In the French trial [22], patients randomized to chemotherapy plus radiotherapy received three courses of cisplatin, cyclophosphamide, vindesine and lomustine (VCPC) prior to radiotherapy and a further three courses afterwards. The two arms were not well balanced for the key prognostic factor of performance status, with 84% of the combined modality arm having a Karnofsky index ⩾ 80%, compared with only 76% of those in the radiotherapy arm. It is also worth noting that five patients in the chemotherapy plus radiotherapy arm proceeded to surgery after three courses of VCPC. When first published in 1991 the survival trend was in favour of the combined modality arm but did not reach statistical significance. A more recent update [23], with longer follow-up, showed a 2-month prolongation of median survival resulting from the maximum 6 months of chemotherapy, and a logrank test giving a "p" value <0.02. Local control in both arms of the trial was very poor (16% and 15%) despite a radiotherapy dose of 65 Gy in 6.5 weeks.

The trial from the CALGB [24], testing this question, restricted entry to a subset of cases with good prognostic features, and the randomization was to just two doses of cisplatin 100 $mg\,m^{-2}$ and four doses of vinblastine 5 $mg\,m^{-2}$ over a 4-week period, followed by radiotherapy, or to radiotherapy alone. The trial was closed after 180 cases had been randomized, but 25 patients (14%) were excluded as being ineligible. Hence the results are based on 155 cases. The response to chemotherapy was poor given the tight entry criteria, with only 4% CR, 22% partial remission (PR) and a further 10% with minor responses. Despite this, there was a remarkable impact on survival with a doubling of 3-year survivors (from 11% to 23%). Given the deliberate policy of selecting only those cases with good prognostic features for this trial, it is also surprising that there is an excessive early death rate in the radiotherapy alone arm. The implication may be that there was an imbalance in the two arms for unidentified prognostic features favouring the chemotherapy arm. Many feel it was a mistake to discontinue the trial early on the basis of interim group sequential analysis. Only 155 eligible cases had been randomized, and although the difference between the two arms was statistically significant, the degree of benefit to the combined arm is difficult to quantify with such relatively small numbers, and the risk of unidentified imbalances influencing the result is a real problem. We have argued [25] that, for such an important issue, we have to have a more precise measure of survival advantage before there is widespread adoption of chemotherapy in inoperable NSCLC. Indeed, the CALGB trial is being repeated by an inter-group co-operative trial in the USA and preliminary results were reported at the Colorado Springs meeting in June 1994 [26].

In addition to the two arms compared in the CALGB trial, a third arm of hyperfractionated radiotherapy (with no chemotherapy) was added in the inter-group (RTOG-8808, ECOG-4588) trial. Patients with stage II, IIIA and IIIB unresectable NSCLC were eligible if their Karnofsky performance (KP) score was greater than 60, with weight loss less than 5%. In practice, two-thirds of cases had a KP $>90\%$. Between January 1989 and January 1992, 490 cases had been randomized and 452 were available for analysis with a minimum follow-up of 1 year. Grade IV toxicity (mainly haematological) occurred in 50% of cases in the chemo/radiotherapy arm with 3.5% treatment-related deaths. The results so far are given in Table 15.1.

Table 15.1 Interim results of inter-group trial RTOG-8808, ECOG-4588

Trial arm	Conv. RT	Hyperfr. RT	CT/Conv. RT
12-month survival (%)	46	51	60
24-month survival (%)	19	24	32
Median survival (months)	11.4	12.3	13.8

The combined modality arm was statistically significantly superior to either radiotherapy alone arm ($p = 0.03$). It is interesting also to note that the benefit of chemotherapy was confined to adenocarcinoma patients. There was no significant benefit to patients with squamous tumours. Clearly, the definitive results of this trial will be influential.

Overview of Chemotherapy in Locally Advanced NSCLC

These two fully published trials described above [22, 24], along with nine other completed trials addressing the question of chemotherapy incorporating cisplatin with radiotherapy versus radiotherapy alone in unresectable NSCLC, have also been the subject of a meta-analysis of updated individual patient data initiated by the UK Medical Research Council [27]. In all there were available data from some 1780 randomized patients. In addition, the same group performed a meta-analysis of individual patient data on 11 similar trials, *not* including cisplatin, with 1253 patients. Only two of the individual trials gave conventionally significant results in favour of the combined approach. These have been discussed already. The pooled HR was 0.90 (95% CI 0.83–0.97, $p = 0.006$), corresponding to an absolute benefit from chemotherapy of 3% (CI 1–5%), from 16% to 19% alive at 2 years. The trials using cisplatin-based chemotherapy provide the most information (more than 50%) and the strongest evidence for an effect in favour of chemotherapy. The HR for cisplatin-based trials (0.87, CI 0.79–0.96%, $p = 0.005$) gave an estimated absolute benefit of 4% (CI 1–7%) at 2 years.

Randomized Trials of Chemotherapy in Advanced Disease

Finally, the MRC-initiated overview of trials testing chemotherapy in NSCLC has examined those in advanced disease where the randomization was between chemotherapy plus supportive/palliative care versus supportive/palliative care alone [28]. Updated individual patient data from eight trials conducted in the post-cisplatin era with a total of 778 patients (761 deaths) were analysed. The HR was 0.73 ($p < 0.0001$) or a reduction in the risk of death of 27%, which is equivalent to an absolute improvement in survival of 10% at 1 year (95% CI 5–15), or an increased median survival of 1.5 months (95% CI 1–2.5 months). Thus proportionately this effect of cisplatin-based chemotherapy is greatest (lowest HR) in the most advanced disease. At first sight, this may seem an unexpected result. However, given that this is the only setting where chemotherapy is the sole anti-cancer treatment employed, and indeed the only anti-cancer treatment available, it is perhaps not as surprising as it might seem.

Treatment Effect in Patient Subgroups

In the meta-analysis described here, predefined subgroups of patient having cisplatin-based chemotherapy were investigated to assess whether there was any evidence of a differential size of treatment effect between such categories. Data on age, sex, stage, histology and performance status were available on 92–99% of patients. There was no evidence that this effect of chemotherapy was more or less apparent in any of the subgroups under these headings [18, 27, 28].

The consistency of results in the different settings examined in these overviews lends weight to the conclusion that cisplatin-based regimens improve survival in NSCLC.

Effects of Chemotherapy on Symptoms and Quality of Life

The history of chemotherapy is marked by dramatic effects in rare cancers, resulting in cure for a proportion of patients, and by severe, even life-threatening toxicity. Both of these factors have militated against serious consideration and evaluation of the use of chemotherapy for palliation. This is quite astonishing given the remarkable palliative effects of chemotherapy in chemotherapy-incurable tumours that have been known for many years (e.g. ovarian cancer, low-grade lymphomas, SCLC, etc.). The belief that unless you were striving for and seen to be approaching cure, your efforts were somehow wasted has been an important brake on progress in this area. Consequently, techniques for describing and measuring palliation and quality of life are in their infancy.

Three factors have gradually changed opinion and hence interest in the use and scientific evaluation of non-curative chemotherapy in advanced malignant disease:

1. The subjective toxicity of chemotherapy has reduced substantially in recent years (e.g. carboplatin replacing cisplatin in ovarian cancer; much better antiemetic therapy with high-dose metoclopramide and then the $5HT_3$ antagonists). The result of this is a much more acceptable trade-off between symptom relief and side-effects.
2. Evidence has emerged demonstrating that many patients are prepared to accept significant short-term toxicity for a small chance of life prolongation [29].
3. There has been an acceptance that cure for common advanced cancers is not "just around the corner", and that other worth while objectives warrant consideration.

Describing Palliation in NSCLC

There are very few worthwhile published data on symptom control with chemotherapy (or anything else) in NSCLC, and what there are often suffer from the many pitfalls that beset the scientific approach to quantifying palliation. Consider 20 hypothetical patients with NSCLC. Twelve of them have cough and eight do not. As a result of a palliative treatment such as chemotherapy, six of the 12 have improved at a specified later time-point, three are the same and three have worsened. This may be described as "50% improved". Some reports of chemotherapeutic palliation in NSCLC with chemotherapy do just that [30]. Obviously the eight without cough at the start of the same palliative treatment cannot improve. However, they may develop cough during the same time period, while receiving the same "palliative" therapy. If four did and four remained free from cough the figures would be rather different; namely 6/20 improved (30%),

7/20 stayed the same (35%) and 7/20 deteriorated (35%). So now, with the same 20 patients behaving in the same way, the result appears to have shifted from "50% improvement" to "5% *more* cases deteriorated than improved". This is certainly not a far-fetched example, since advanced lung cancer patients who are not improving are usually deteriorating. Describing the treatment in the second way makes it look distinctly less promising than in the first way. But it is more honest, and if adopted in the only really valid context for palliation testing, namely within a randomized trial, offers a more powerful tool, since a systemic palliative like chemotherapy, if given to all patients in one arm of a trial, may be shown to prevent or delay the development of symptoms, as well as relieve them, when compared to controls.

Another weakness inherent in the simple description given above is that no account is taken of symptom severity. A change from having a severe cough to a mild, occasional cough clearly represents improvement as much as the reverse would represent deterioration. So there does need to be a simple scoring system to allow changes to be quantified.

In any group of patients with advanced NSCLC, some will die during the observation period of any palliation assessment. These will in general be the most ill, most symptomatic patients. A dead patient has no symptoms and so there is likely to be selective removal of the worst cases during any palliative experiment. This clearly biases the result in favour of the palliative modality. Supposing five of the 12 hypothetical cases with cough die before the post-treatment evaluation, and none of the eight without cough does so, then the change from 12/20 (60%) with cough beforehand to 7/15 (47%) with cough at the end appears to show an improvement in the symptom, when clearly none had occurred. Again, restricting symptom control studies to randomized trials goes a long way towards avoiding these hazards, since if attrition is equal the problem is non-existent, and if it is unequal then one is ideally placed to make value judgements between quantity and quality of life. With these thoughts in mind we are undertaking a comparison of symptom control in advanced NSCLC between standard treatment alone and standard treatment plus chemotherapy.

MIC Randomized Trials of Palliation in Advanced NSCLC

This study is part of two major trials of chemotherapy employing mitomycin, ifosfamide and cisplatin (MIC) under way in the UK. The MIC1 trial compares MIC (to a maximum of four courses) followed by radical radiotherapy versus radical radiotherapy alone in limited (stage III), inoperable NSCLC. The MIC2 trial is for patients with more advanced disease where radical radiotherapy is inappropriate. In this trial, ambulatory patients under 75 are randomly allocated to receive MIC (again to a maximum of four courses), plus whatever other palliative treatment may be required versus palliative treatment alone. Currently, over 700 patients have been randomized in the two trials. The symptom control study involves 109 of these patients (as of November 1994), 45 in the MIC1 trial and 64 in the MIC2 trial.

This is a questionnaire-based study, administered by experienced oncology nurses independently of the physician responsible for the patients. An example of part of the questionnaire is given in Table 15.2. These questions are asked immediately prior to commencing therapy and at fixed time points thereafter.

Table 15.2 Part of the MIC questionnaire

	None	A little	Quite a bit	Very much
Do you have a cough?	[ ]	[ ]	[ ]	[ ]
Do you get breathless on mild activity like dressing?	[ ]	[ ]	[ ]	[ ]
Do you get breathless when walking on the flat?	[ ]	[ ]	[ ]	[ ]
Do you get breathless on stairs or walking uphill?	[ ]	[ ]	[ ]	[ ]
Have you coughed blood?	[ ]	[ ]	[ ]	[ ]
How much pain are you getting?	[ ]	[ ]	[ ]	[ ]
Have you noticed any loss of appetite?	[ ]	[ ]	[ ]	[ ]
Have you been worrying?	[ ]	[ ]	[ ]	[ ]
Have you been depressed?	[ ]	[ ]	[ ]	[ ]
Have you been feeling generally ill?	[ ]	[ ]	[ ]	[ ]
Do you feel tired or lethargic?	[ ]	[ ]	[ ]	[ ]

During and after treatment, questions relating to side-effects are included. To allow simple quantitation, and hence comparison of what are intrinsically subjective phenomena, scores are allocated as follows:

None = 0
A little = 1
Quite a bit = 2
Very much = 3

Mean scores for each symptom (in all patients, including those without the symptom at the start) at each time-point, in both arms of the trial, can easily be calculated and compared statistically. The time-points chosen were as follows:

Chemotherapy arm:

1. Pretreatment.
2. Three weeks following first course (week 3).
3. Three weeks following second course (week 6).
4. Three weeks following third course (week 9).
5. Three weeks following fourth course (week 12).

No chemotherapy arm:

1. Pretreatment.
2. Week 3.
3. Week 6 or min. 3 weeks following radiotherapy if given.
4. Week 9 or min. 6 weeks following radiotherapy if given.

Attrition rates were similar in the two arms in both trials during these observation periods.

Figure 15.1 illustrates the mean scores for breathlessness on moderate exertion (walking on the flat) for patients in both arms of the MIC2 trial, over the observation periods given above. The scores are similar at the start, but the trends indicate a greater improvement in the chemotherapy arm than in the palliative care arm. This difference is not statistically significant. Figure 15.2 illustrates the results for cough in the MIC1 trial. In Figure 15.3 (*overleaf*) the format is different. Here, the *change* in mean score between the pretreatment level and the "6" week time-point are charted for all symptoms, for all patients in

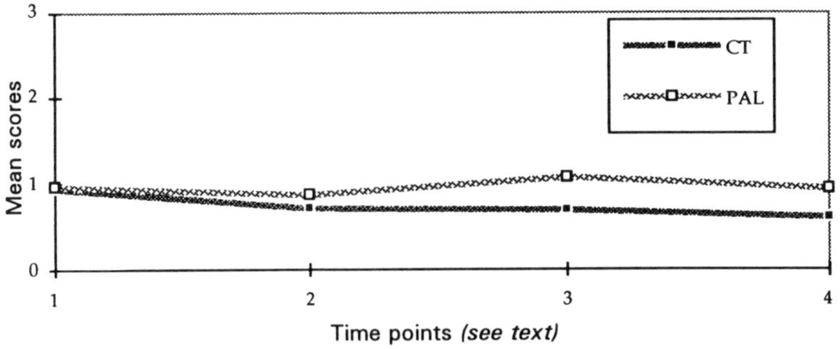

Figure 15.1 Change in mean symptom scores with time reported by patients in chemotherapy (CT) and palliative care (PAL) arms of the MIC2 trial for *breathlessness on moderate exertion* (see text for description of scoring)

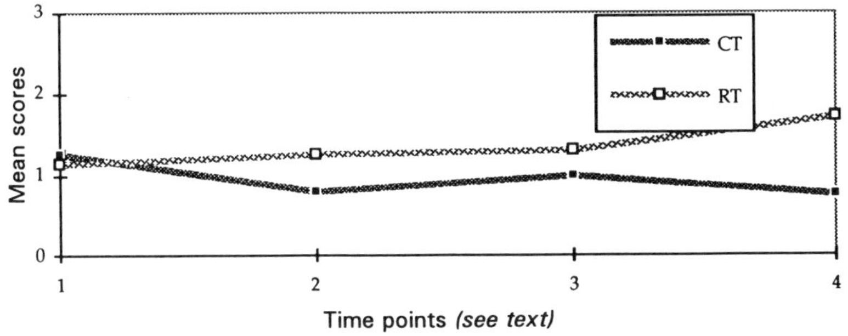

Figure 15.2 Change in mean symptom scores with time reported by patients in chemotherapy (CT) and radiotherapy (RT) arms of the MIC1 trial for *cough* (see text for description of scoring)

the symptom control part of the MIC2 trial. A minus score indicates improvement and a plus score deterioration. It can clearly be seen that there is a consistent trend in all parameters for those patients having chemotherapy to experience either greater improvement or less deterioration than in the palliative care arm. In each case the change, numerically, is small. This is because *all* patients are included. Those without a particular symptom at the start or later on will have the effect of reducing the mean change in score for the whole population. This tends to hide those patients who experience major improvements or deteriorations (as some did).

As for treatment-related side-effects, these were assessed in the same way, although pretreatment data on nausea and vomiting, for instance, were not collected. We have already reported phase II toxicity data for MIC elsewhere [19], but used the opportunity of the present symptom evaluation study to reassess important subjective side-effects including nausea and vomiting. Figure 15.4 (*overleaf*) shows the proportion of patients in the chemotherapy arms reporting nausea and vomiting either during or between courses of MIC in the two ongoing trials. It is clear that very few experienced moderate or severe nausea and vomiting, although some did. This must be weighed against any improvement in tumour-related symptoms.

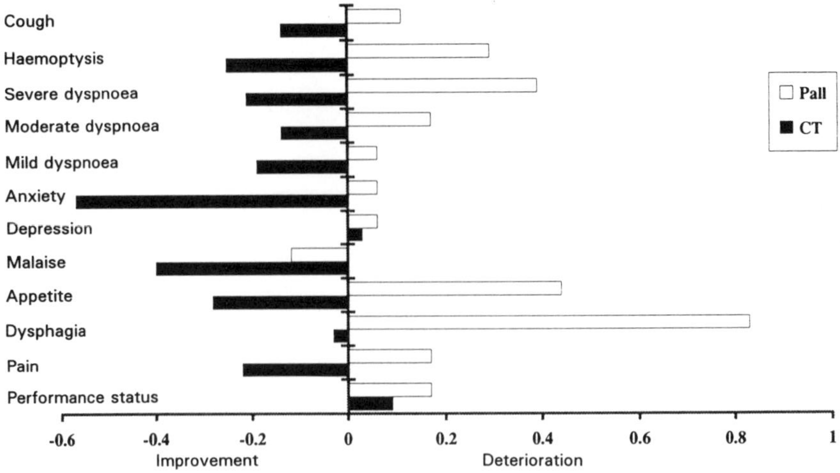

Figure 15.3 MIC2 trial: mean change in symptom score for all symptoms (in all patients in symptom control study) comparing pretreatment level and "6" week time-point

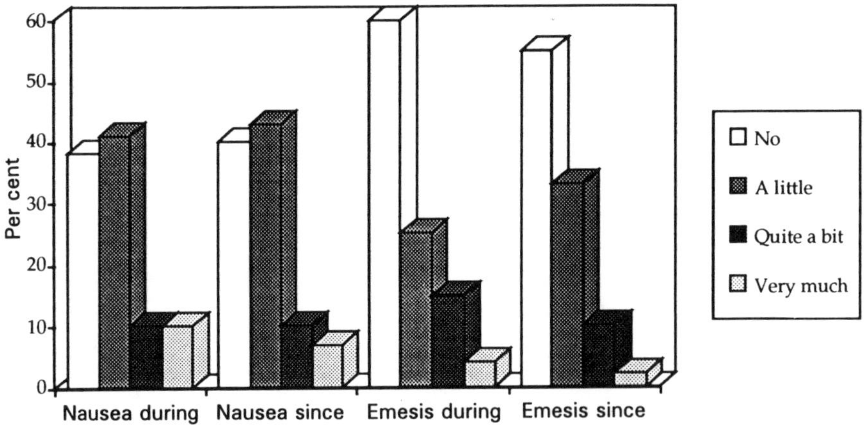

Figure 15.4 The percentage of 58 patients having MIC chemotherapy responding to the following questions:

1. Did you feel sick during your last course of treatment?
2. Have you been feeling sick since your last course of treatment?
3. Did you vomit during your last course of treatment?
4. Have you vomited since your last course of treatment?

Answers: "No", "A little", "Quite a bit", "Very much"

These data must be interpreted with caution since the numbers are small and the study continues. There is, however, a suggestion that chemotherapy is at least as good a palliative as radiotherapy or other conventional measures, and may turn out to be better. Since this chapter was written, the MIC trials have been completed, analysed and reported to the 8th World Lung Cancer Conference, Dublin, 1997. With over 800 patients randomized between chemotherapy and standard treatment, there is a significant survival advantage for MIC chemotherapy. Furthermore, in 176 patients assessed for quality of life during the early weeks of treatment, gains in symptom improvement far outweighed side-effects, and overall there was again a significant advantage for chemotherapy over standard care [32–35].

Conclusions

The role of chemotherapy in inoperable NSCLC is still controversial [31]. All the indications are that combinations including cisplatin confer a small, but real, prolongation of survival. Contrary to what many health economists believe, most patients do want the chance to live longer, even at the expense of some short-term deterioration in their quality of life. The economics of health care worldwide increasingly is demanding high-quality information so that priorities can be determined. Overviews with meta-analysis of patient data from similar randomized trials have become a fashionable, if rather unrefined, tool to help address the question of survival duration. A meta-analysis cannot include statements concerning changes in symptoms, toxicity and performance status. Nor can it help determine which precise chemotherapy treatment one should employ. Therefore large, well-designed and well-executed randomized trials are still needed if more time and money is not going to be wasted in the search for better treatments in lung cancer. The two MIC trials, now with over 700 cases randomized, are attempting to evaluate both quantity and quality of life in inoperable NSCLC, using a regimen which is certainly as effective as any other currently under evaluation. Gradually the weight of evidence is beginning to support the use of chemotherapy in the non-curative setting of NSCLC.

Acknowledgements

I gratefully acknowledge the help and advice of Jane Cook, Cindy Billingham and Charlotte Woodroffe in the symptom control study, and my thanks to Asta Medica for financial support towards this section of our work.

References

1. Parkin DM, Saxo AJ (1993) Lung cancer: worldwide variation in occurrence and proportion attributed to tobacco use. Lung Cancer (suppl) 9:1–16.
2. Squires TS, Tong T (1993) Cancer statistics. CA Cancer J Clin 43:7–26.
3. Rudd R (1991) Chemotherapy in the treatment of non-small cell lung cancer. Resp Dis Prac 7:12–15.
4. Berry RJ, Laing AH, Newman CR, Peto J (1977) The role of radiotherapy in treatment of inoperable lung cancer. Int J Radiat Oncol Biol Phys 2:433–439.
5. Roswit B, Patno ME, Rapp R et al. (1968) The survival of patients with inoperable lung cancer: a large-scale randomized study of radiation therapy versus placebo. Radiology 90:688–697.

6. Johnson DH, Einhorn LH, Bartolucci A et al. (1990) Thoracic radiotherapy does not prolong survival in patients with locally advanced, unresectable non-small cell lung cancer. Ann Intern Med 113:33–38.
7. Perez CA, Pajak TF, Rubin P et al. Long-term observations of the patterns of failure in patients with unresectable non-oat cell carcinoma of the lung treated with definitive radiotherapy. Report by the Radiation Therapy Oncology Group. Cancer 59:1874–1881.
8. Einhorn LH, Loehrer PJ, Williams SD et al. (1986) Random prospective study of vindesine versus vindesin plus high-dose cisplatin versus vindesine plus cisplatin plus mitomycin C in advanced non-small-cell lung cancer. J Clin Oncol 4:1037–1043.
9. Kris M, Cohen E, Gralla R (1985) An analysis of 134 phase II trials in non-small cell lung cancer (NSCLC) (Abstr). Proc of the IV World Conf on Lung Cancer, Toronto, 4:39.
10. Cullen MH (1983) Acceptable damage to normal tissue. In: Stoll B (ed) Cancer treatment: end-point evaluation. Wiley, Chichester, pp139–171.
11. Watanabe Y, Shimizu J, Oda M et al. (1991) Aggressive surgical intervention in N_2 non-small cell cancer of the lung. Ann Thorac Surg 51:253–261.
12. Martini N, Flehinger BJ (1987) The role of surgery in N_2 lung cancer. Surg Clin North Am 67:1037–1049.
13. Mountain CF (1990) Expanded possibilities for surgical treatment of lung cancer: survival in stage IIIA disease. Chest 97:1045–1051.
14. Naruke T, Goya T, Tsuchyia R, Suemasu K (1988) The importance of surgery to non-small cell carcinoma of lung with mediastinal lymph node metastasis. Ann Thorac Surg 46:603–610.
15. Rosell R, Gomez-Codina J, Camps C, Maestre J, Padille J, Canto A, Mate JL, Li S, Roig J, Olazabal A, Canela M, Ariza A, Skacel Z, Morera-Prat J, Abad A (1994) A randomized trial comparing preoperative chemotherapy plus surgery with surgery alone in patients with non-small-cell lung cancer. N Engl J Med 330:153–158.
16. Roth JA, Fosella F, Komaki R, Ryan MB, Putnam JB, Lee JS, Dhingra H, De Caro L, Chasen M, McGavran M, Atkinson EN, Hong WK (1994) A randomized trial comparing perioperative chemotherapy and surgery with surgery alone in resectable stage III non-small cell lung cancer. J Natl Cancer Inst 86:673–680.
17. Peto R (1987) Why do we need systematic overviews of randomised trials? Stat Med 6:233–240.
18. Stewart LA, Pignon JP, Parmar MKB, Arriagada R, Souhami RL on behalf of the NSCLC Collaborative Group (1994) A meta-analysis of adjuvant chemotherapy in non-small cell lung cancer (NSCLC) using updated individual patient data. Lung Cancer II (suppl 2): 49–50.
19. Cullen MH, Joshi R, Chetiyawardana AD, Woodroffe CM (1988) Mitomycin, ifosfamide and cisplatin in non-small cell lung cancer: treatment good enough to compare. Br J Cancer 58:359–361.
20. Cullen MH (1994) Trials of radical radiotherapy versus chemotherapy plus radical radiotherapy in non-small cell lung cancer. Semin Oncol 21(3 suppl 4):34–41.
21. Schaake-Koning C, Van Den Bogaert W, Dalesio O et al. (1992) Effects of concomitant cisplatin and radiotherapy on inoperable non-small cell lung cancer. N Engl J Med 326(8):524–530.
22. Le Chevalier T, Arriagada R, Quoix E et al. (1991) Radiotherapy alone versus combined chemotherapy and radiotherapy in unresectable non-small cell lung carcinoma. J Natl Cancer Inst 83:417–423.
23. Le Chevalier T, Arriagada R, Quoix E et al. (1991) Impact of chemotherapy (CT) on survival of locally advanced non-small-cell lung cancer (NSCLC): results of a randomized study in 353 pts (Abstr). Lung Cancer 7(suppl):159.
24. Dillman RO, Seagren SL, Propert KJ et al. (1990) A randomized trial of induction chemotherapy plus high dose radiation versus radiation alone in stage III non-small cell lung cancer. N Engl J Med 323:940–945.

25. Souhami RL, Spiro SG, Cullen MH (1991) Chemotherapy and radiation therapy as compared with radiation therapy in stage III non-small-cell cancer. N Engl J Med 324:1136.
26. Sause W, Scott C, Taylor S, Johnson D, Livingston R, Komaki R, Emami B, Curran W, Byhardt R, Fisher G, Turrisi A (1994) RTOG 8808 ECOG 4588, preliminary analysis of a phase III trial in regionally advanced unresectable non-small cell lung cancer. Lung Cancer II (suppl 1):179.
27. Arriagada R, Stewart LA, Pignon JP, Souhami RL, LeChevalier T on behalf of the NSCLC Collaborators Group (NSCLCCG) (1994) Combined radio-chemotherapy in the management of locally advanced non-small cell lung cancer (NSCLC). Lung Cancer II (suppl 2):146–147.
28. Souhami RL, Stewart LA, Arriagada R, Parmar MKB, Le Chevalier T, Pignon JP (1994) A data-based meta-analysis of randomised trials of chemotherapy versus best supportive care (BSC) in advanced non-small cell lung cancer (NSCLC). Lung Cancer II (suppl 2):24–25.
29. Slevin, M, Stubbs L, Plant HJ, et al. (1990) Attitudes to chemotherapy; comparing views of patients with cancer with those of doctors, nurses, and general public. Br Med J 300:1458–1460.
30. Hardy JR, Noble T, Smith IE (1989) Symptom relief with moderate dose chemotherapy (mitomycin-C, vinblastine and cisplatin) in advanced non-small cell lung cancer. Br J Cancer 60:764–766.
31. Green MR (1991) Unresectable stage III non-small-cell lung cancer: lessons and directions from clinical trials research. J Natl Cancer Inst 83:382.
32. Cullen MH, Billingham LJ, Dunn J (1997) Abstract 8. Lung Cancer 18 (suppl 1):4.
33. Cullen MH, Billingham LJ, Woodroffe CM, Gower N, Souhami RL, Chetiyawardana AD, Joshi R, Rudd R, Trask C, Spiro S (1997) Abstract 10. Lung Cancer 18 (suppl 1):5.
34. Cullen MH, Woodroffe CM, Billingham LJ, Chetiyawardana AD, Joshi R, Ferry D, Connolly CK, Bessell E (1997) Abstract 11. Lung Cancer 18 (suppl 1):5.
35. Billingham LJ, Cullen MH, Woods BW, Chetiyawardana AD, Joshi R, Cook J, Woodroffe CM (1997) Abstract 26. Lung Cancer 18 (suppl 1):9.

16 – Non-Curative Chemotherapy for Gastric Cancer

G. Middleton and D. Cunningham

Introduction

Although the incidence of gastric cancer is declining, it is still one of the leading causes of cancer deaths worldwide. The incidence of proximal tumours is increasing and these are technically more difficult to resect. Eighty per cent of tumours are too advanced at presentation to be operated upon with curative intent. In the UK in 1990, death from gastric cancer constituted 6% of all cancer deaths, accounting for some 10 000 people. This chapter examines the treatments available for the palliation of advanced gastric cancer.

Systemic Therapies

Any worthwhile treatment for advanced gastric cancer should either prolong life without a decrease in its quality or, in the absence of a survival benefit, lead to maintenance of good quality of life or an improvement in those with poor quality of life at the start of treatment. Most trials assess impact on survival by calculation of median survival. However, response rates for individual chemotherapy regimens in many trials are less than 50%, with complete response rates much less than this. Thus comparisons of these regimens are unlikely to demonstrate any survival differences by analysing median survival [1]. The rationale for the use of median survival as the major end-point in some trials is that response rates are perceived to provide no clinically useful information. Further analyses of outcome in patients responding to chemotherapy versus non-responders is scientifically suspect. These beliefs are based on the following:

1. Patients with better performance status at randomization are likely to live longer but are also more likely to respond to chemotherapy.
2. Patients demonstrating a response will live longer, simply because the technical definition of response includes that it be for at least 1 month.
3. There is a wide variation in response rate in individual trials for any one chemotherapy regimen.
4. Chemotherapy may negatively influence outcome in non-responders. Patients with non-measurable or non-assessable disease (and therefore

patients in whom it is not possible to define a response) represent the majority of patients with advanced gastric cancer.

5. Response rate in some trials is not assessed by accurate methods of bidimensional measurement such as are obtainable by CT.

However, regimens which demonstrate superior activity in comparison trials but do not show a survival benefit may provide potential patient benefit since

1. In colorectal cancer, attainment of complete or partial response or stabilization of disease for > 4 months strongly correlates with symptomatic improvement [2].
2. In colorectal cancer, a response to chemotherapy is associated with a longer survival even after corrections for the guarantee time effect and the distribution of prognostic variables at the time of randomization [3].

Whether these results are applicable to advanced gastric cancer is unknown, but they provide a rationale for incorporating response rates as an end-point in trials and for separately analysing the survival of responders and non-responders, provided that these two groups are balanced for prognostic variables at time of randomization and the guarantee time effect is taken into account.

Many patients with advanced gastric cancer do have measurable disease: only 33 of the 640 gastric cancer patients included in the Royal Marsden Hospital database have non-measurable or non-assessable disease.

Only two of ten trials included in Tables 16.2(a) or 16.2(b) below make any attempt to explore the issues of quality of life and neither of these trials performed a formal quality-of-life analysis. With the growing awareness of the potential importance of quality-of-life analysis in assessing the role of chemotherapy in a non-curative context, some ongoing phase III comparisons of combination regimens have included a quality-of-life component. There is a need for validated add-on modules specific to assessment of quality of life in gastric cancer patients.

In a cost-conscious environment, attention must also focus on the economic impact of palliative chemotherapy to assess whether the cost of provision of chemotherapy, with the ancillary costs of antiemetic requirement for hospitalization and so on, is outweighed by the benefits of reduced requirements for supportive care services. The optimal way to assess whether chemotherapy is better than no specific treatment beyond palliative measures, such as provision of adequate analgesia and so on is by randomized best supportive care comparisons. Positive results in favour of chemotherapy then lead to the question of the most effective regimen.

Best Supportive Care Comparisons

Randomized trials of chemotherapy versus best supportive care are necessary to decide if potentially toxic treatment offers any benefit over no treatment. Median survival in most phase II efficacy or phase III randomized comparisons is usually around 6–8 months. Such figures appear to provide little justification for treatment, especially as quality-of-life issues are often not addressed. Accrual of patients to best supportive care comparisons is difficult, as patients are keen to be given what is perceived as active treatment. They are difficult to justify if previous trials with a best supportive care arm show clear benefit for chemotherapy.

Table 16.1 Studies incorporating best supportive care or initial expectant treatment

Reference	No.	Median survival	Quality-of-life (QOL)assessment	
Murad et al. [4]				
Modified FAMTX (MTX = 1000 mg m^{-2})	30	10/12*	No formal QOL assessment. Only 3% with grade IV toxicity (leucopenia and infection)	
vs.				
BSC	10	3/12		
Pyrhonen et al. [6]				
FEMTX	17	12+/12*	No formal QOL assessment. Significant prolongation of progression-free survival	
vs.				
BSC	19	3+/12		
Glimelius et al. [5]			Quality-of-life adjusted survival	Subjective Response >4/12 duration
ELF 7 or FLV 3	10	10/12+	7/12*	7/10*
vs.				
Expectant treatment (ELF 3 and FLV 1)	8	4/12	2/12*	2/8

* Reaches levels of conventional status significance.
BSC = best supportive care.

Table 16.1 shows the details of randomized trials with a best supportive care arm. A Brazilian study represents the only published report available in which initial accrual included a best supportive care arm without allowing subsequent administration of chemotherapy [4]. This was closed prematurely after ten patients had been randomized to control and 12 to treatment (modified FAMTX with a methotrexate dose of 1000 mg m^{-2}). This demonstrated a median survival of 10 months in the treatment arm, against 3 months in non-treated patients. Responders had a median survival of 16 months. There was no formal quality-of-life analysis. A group from Sweden, who have published extensively on the palliative and survival benefits of chemotherapy in advanced colorectal cancer, randomized patients to receive either initial or delayed chemotherapy using ELF (etoposide, leucovorin, 5-FU) or FLV (5-FU, leucovorin) in advanced gastric cancer [5]. Ten patients were randomized to initial treatment and eight to best supportive care, four of whom subsequently received chemotherapy. Median survival was 10 months in those that received initial treatment, against 4 months in those receiving delayed therapy. Quality of life was assessed by a structured questionnaire with an added psychological component and demonstrated a 5-month improvement in maintenance of high-quality life or improvement in quality of life without hospitalization. This suggests that earlier institution of chemotherapy offers more effective palliation than waiting for symptoms to develop.

A Finnish study, presented in abstract form, showed a significant extension of progression-free time and survival in patients treated with FEMTX (5-FU, epirubicin, methotrexate) compared to patients receiving no chemotherapy [6]. Quality-of-life analyses were not included. The Swedish group conclude that the survival and symptom control benefits demonstrated by these trials need to be confirmed and extended and have initiated a multicentre best supportive care versus chemotherapy randomized trial.

Much work is directed at defining the optimal combination chemotherapy regimen and deciding whether combination regimens offer any advantages over single agent chemotherapy.

Suitable End-points

Single Agent vs. Combination Regimen Trials

Table 16.2(a) shows some randomized comparisons of combination chemotherapy against single agent treatment with an analysis of enrolment criteria (measurable versus non-measurable disease), assessment of response (CT or otherwise), along with survival, quality of life, toxicity and response data where applicable. Included among these is the Eastern Central Oncology Group (ECOG) trial comparing 5-FU/methyl-CCNU, FAMe, Adriamycin and mitomycin C and the Georgetown FAM regimens, since an early Southwestern Oncology Group study demonstrated no benefit for the addition of methyl-CCNU to a bolus 5-FU regimen [7].

Two North Central Collaborative Trials Group trials randomized patients to FA (5-FU, Adriamycin) FAM (5-FU, Adriamycin, mitomycin C), FAC (5-FU, Adriamycin, cisplatin), FAMe (5-FU, Adriamycin, methyl CCN), and FAMe alternating with triazinate as a single agent bolus 5-FU [8, 9]. None of the combination regimens improved time to progression or performance status compared with single agent 5-FU. These trials included fewer than 25 patients with measurable disease and thus these data cannot be used to assess the survival or subjective benefits in those with measurable disease or to calculate response rates.

FAM showed a clear survival advantage for FAM compared to 5-FU/methyl-CCNU, FAMe and Adriamycin/mitomycin C. All patients had measurable disease and FAM demonstrated a 39% overall response rate compared to 14% for 5-FU and methyl-CCNU. Surprisingly, response was greatest in those with performance status scores of 2–3 when FAM was used (44%) and where weight loss was greater than 5%. This translated to an improved median survival for this poor prognostic group. Although this suggests that combination chemotherapy may be most effective in those with advanced (and by implication measurable) disease, such findings of improved outcomes in patients with performance status scores of 3 are unusual and patients with poor performance status such as this often do poorly with chemotherapy.

Recently, a group from Seoul have reported the results of a randomized comparison of 5-FU, Adriamycin and mitomycin C and 5-FU/cisplatin (FP) against 5-FU alone [10]. The FAM regimen was not the Georgetown regimen and involved a much higher 5-FU dose given as 12 h infusions on 5 consecutive days. The 5-FU single agent dose was high, with 5000 mg m^{-2} being given 3-weekly again by split 12 h infusions. There was no survival or response rate difference between the FAM and 5-FU arms in this trial, possibly due to the high cumulative dose used in the 5-FU alone arm offsetting any advantage from the addition of Adriamycin and mitomycin C. The addition of platinum doubled the response rate and led to significant improvement in time to progression (21.8 weeks for FP, 9.1 weeks for 5-FU ($p \leqslant 0.005$), but there was no improvement in overall survival. The groups were well balanced for prognostic factors. The lack of a

Table 16.2(a) Randomized comparisons of combination chemotherapy vs. single agent 5-FU

Regimen	No.	Eligibility	Assessment	Response (CR)	Median survival	QOL	Toxicity	Reference
Bolus 5-FU	9	Measurable	Not by CT	23%	NA	NA	Increased myelotoxicity for combination	Baker et al. [7]
5-FU/me CCNU	29			21%				
Bolus 5-FU	51	Meas. and non-meas. ⩽ 25%	Not by CT	2/11	7+/12	No difference in symptoms, weight or performance status	Greater thrombocytopenia and less diarrhoea and stomatitis with FAM compared with bolus 5-FU	Cullinan et al. [9]
5-FU/adria	49	meas. in each arm		3/11	7+/12			
FAM	51			5/13	7+/12			
Bolus 5-FU	69	Meas. and non-meas. ⩽ 20% meas.	NA	NA	6+/12	No improvement in performance status or weight gain	More grade 3, 4 or 5 (NCI) nausea and vomiting with combination regimens	Cullinan et al. [8]
FAMe	53	in each arm			6+/12			
FAMe + TzT	79				7+/12			
FAP	51				6+/12			
5-FU/Me CCNU	44	Measurable	CT-assessable disease excluded	11% (2%)	13/52	NA	FAM least toxic with low-level myelosuppression, nausea and vomiting	Douglass et al. [27]
FAMe	39			18% (10%)	22/52			
Adria./mito. C	46			22% (7%)	18/52			
FAM	46			35% (4%)	30/52			
5-FU (12 h inf.)	94	Measurable or evaluable	CT included	26%	30.6/52	NA	Low incidence of grade 3 myelosuppression	Kim et al. [10]
FAM (not Georgetown)	28			25%	29.3/52		More nausea and vomiting and neuropathy with FP	
FP	103			51% (4%)	36.9/52			

NA = not assessed.

difference in overall survival may relate to the low complete response (CR) rate attained (4%) or the addition of non-measurable disease (48/103 in the FP arm).

An earlier randomized comparison of FAB (5-FU, Adriamycin, BCNU) vs. Adriamycin alone showed that the combination improved time to progression and overall survival by both the Gehan–Wilcoxon test (sensitive to differences occurring early in time) and the log rank test (sensitive to later differences), but that no difference was seen in either test for patients with non-measurable disease [11]. For the overall group, the time to progression and survival advantage reached significance only by the Gehan–Wilcoxon test, which suggests that the addition of patients with non-measurable disease may dilute any survival benefit accruing from combination regimens and strengthening the hypothesis that combination regimens benefit patients with measurable disease more than those with non-measurable disease, where by implication disease is limited.

In this study, the most favourable influences on therapy were predominant lymph node involvement, two or fewer metastatic sites, weight loss of < 10% and performance status scores of 0–1. The authors concluded that the combination exerts a moderate benefit on survival, but that if the disease is too advanced or the natural history of the disease is still relatively long (non-measurable disease) this effect will be minimized.

Combination chemotherapy would appear to lead to benefits over single agent treatment in those with measurable disease, but increasing dose intensity of the single agent drug may offset this, as shown in the Korean study [10], indicating a role for single agent protracted infusional treatment with 5-FU which can deliver high quantities of the drug with minimal toxicity. Although the addition of platinum did not provide an overall survival benefit in the Korean trial, it did improve time to progression. Improvements in disease-free survival are important as they imply an increase in normal or near normal quality of life.

Randomized Comparisons of Combination Regimens

The results of four randomized studies comparing platinum-containing against non-platinum-containing regimens are included in Table 16.2(b), which summarizes some comparisons of various combination chemotherapies.

The Gastrointestinal Tumour Study Group (GITSG) had originally adopted the FAMe regimen as its standard therapy. In a three-way comparison of FAMe with the platinum-containing regimen FAP and FAT (using the antifol triazinate) randomizing 247 patients [12], FAP resulted in a significant survival advantage over FAMe, with median survival of 31+ weeks vs. 23+ weeks and 1-year survival rates of 32% against 15%. FAP achieved equivalent responses to FAT. This trial accrued patients with and without assessable disease, but the treatment groups were well balanced for prognostic variables and there were equivalent numbers of patients with non-measurable disease in each arm. This trial may have underestimated the impact of the addition of platinum, as only 66% of the prescribed 5-FU dose was delivered in the FAP arm (compared to $\geqslant$ 97% in the other two arms) and only 69% of the FAP courses were accompanied by platinum (87% for triazinate in FAT).

The phase III comparison of PELF (using 300 mg m^{-2} of 5-FU, modulated with 200 mg m^{-2} of folinic acid for 4 days and 3-weekly epirubicin and platinum) with FAM shows a significant improvement in response rate and a trend towards

Table 16.2(b) Randomized comparisons of various combination regimens

Regimen	No.	Eligibility	Assessment	Response (CR)	Median survival	QOL	Toxicity	Reference
FAMe	81	Measurable and non-measurable	NA	15%	23.5/52	NA	Increased toxicity for FAP and FAMe compared to FAT, esp. myelosuppression, but increased dermatitis and mucositis with FAT	GITSG [12]
FAT	81	(33, 30, 38 meas., respectively)		20%	30.3/52			
FAP	85			19%	31.1/52			
FAM	54	Measurable and non-measurable (46 and 76 meas., respectively)	CT included	15% (4%)	5.6/12	NA	Higher non-haematologic toxicity for PELF, but mild	Cocconi et al. [13]
PELF	93			43% (4%)	8.1/12			
FAM	103	Measurable and non-measurable	CT 'strongly recommended'	9%	29/52	NA	Equivalent toxicity	Wils et al. [14]
FAMTX	105	(79 and 81 meas., respectively)		41%	42/52			
FAMTX	30	Measurable or assessable	CT included	33% (10%)	7.3/12	NA	Significantly more myelosuppression, more prolonged hospitalization for sepsis and 4 toxic deaths for EAP vs. FAMTX	Kelsen et al. [15]
EAP	30			20% (0%)	6.1/12			
FEMTX FEMTX-P	123	NA	NA	27%	6–7/12	NA	8 toxic deaths	Wils et al. [17]

improved survival which did not reach levels of conventional significance [13]. These trials both suggest that the addition of platinum in combination regimens may be beneficial.

An EORTC study randomized 160 patients with measurable or assessable disease (and a further 41 patients with non-assessable disease were included for toxicity and survival analysis) to either FAM or FAMTX (5-FU, Adriamycin, methotrexate) and demonstrated a significant survival improvement for FAMTX with a 41% objective response rate compared with 9% for FAM and with equivalent toxicity [14]. The FAM response rate in this trial is low, but the majority of responses were CT evaluated and extramurally reviewed. FAMTX has been the subject of a number of completed or ongoing randomized comparisons with various platinum-containing regimens. A trial planned to recruit 130 patients was halted after an interim toxicity analysis performed after 60 patients had been randomized to either EAP (etoposide, Adriamycin, platinum) or FAMTX had shown significantly lower median leucocyte, haemoglobin and platelet counts in the EAP arm [15]. Although there were equivalent numbers in each group requiring hospitalization, principally for febrile neutropenia, the lengths of hospital stay were longer in the EAP arm due to more prolonged neutropenia and there were four toxic deaths in this arm compared to none for FAMTX. There was no significant difference in response or median survival. One of the principle investigators involved in the development of the EAP regimen has stated that he no longer uses this treatment for advanced gastric cancer.

A Spanish group is accruing patients to a phase III trial comparing FLEP (5-FU, leucovorin, epirubicin and cisplatin) against FAMTX [16]. Toxicity data are available and show significant myelosuppression with both regimens and a total of seven toxic deaths (three in the FAMTX arm) with five deaths being due to neutropenic sepsis after 85 patients have been randomized. FEMTX is an evolution of FAMTX, where epirubicin is substituted for Adriamycin in order to decrease the incidence and severity of mucositis and cardiotoxicity associated with Adriamycin. A Dutch–British collaborative trial has assessed the benefit of adding platinum to FEMTX in a comparison of FEMTX vs. FEMTX-P in 123 patients. The response rates were equivalent (27%), as was median survival (6–7 months), and thus platinum does not appear to improve the results obtainable using FEMTX alone [17]. The group concludes that the severe toxicity seen with either regimen requires less toxic protocols to be developed for the palliative treatment of advanced gastric cancer.

We are performing an ongoing study comparing the ECF regimen (epirubicin, cisplatin and protracted infusional 5-FU) developed at the Royal Marsden Hospital with FAMTX, which on the basis of the EAP and FAM comparison data summarized above, appears to be the most appropriate regimen for comparison. Our recently reported phase II data demonstrate an objective tumour response of 71% in 128 patients with measurable disease with a 12% complete response rate [18]. Overall median survival is 8.2 months and 1-year survival was 30%. Toxicity was acceptable, with grade III or IV emesis occurring in 13%, stomatitis in 7%, diarrhoea in 4%, infection in 6%, leucopenia in 21% and thromboyctopenia in 8% of patients. There was a 4.3% treatment-related death rate. The response rate is double that seen with a regimen containing the same drugs but using an unmodulated bolus 5-FU schedule [19]. Our results have recently been confirmed in a GISCAD study which obtained a 59% response rate with a median response duration of 5+ months and acceptable toxicity [20].

Impact of Chemotherapy on Resectability

The treatment of patients with metastatic disease remains non-curative, but for those with unresectable locally advanced disease chemotherapy may potentially downstage the tumour sufficiently to allow resection to be performed in an attempt for cure. The largest trial enrolling patients on the basis of failed laparotomy (33 patients) used perioperative EAP chemotherapy [21]. Nineteen of these went forward to second-look laparotomy and 15 of these were able to undergo complete resection with pathological CR in five patients. Only three patients relapsed initially at a distant site and two of these presented with CNS disease, a sanctuary site, thus demonstrating the ability of chemotherapy to deal with occult micrometastatic disease. However, at the time of publication 60% of disease-free patients had relapsed, principally locoregionally, in spite of gastrectomy and extended lymphadenectomy. A study with similar inclusion criteria also showed a high locoregional relapse rate after potentially curative resection following chemotherapy to downstage disease [22]. Longer term follow-up of trials such as these are needed to decide whether surgery improves outcome beyond chemotherapy alone. One patient with a stage IV tumour resected is disease free more than 3 years out in the EAP study and two patients (one stage IV and one stage IIIA) are disease free in the other study. It seems unlikely that these patients would have achieved such long-term disease-free survival without resection of residual disease.

Although not primarily a trial of neo-adjuvant therapy, using ECF we have obtained an 80% response rate in locally advanced disease [18]. Even though unresectability was assessed by laparotomy in only half of the patients, 11/20 patients were able to undergo complete resection with four having pathological CR in the resection specimen. Median survival for the resected group was no better than the remainder of the patients with locally advanced or metastatic disease included in the study, due to three early postoperative deaths. Again, longer term follow-up is required to assess the impact of resection.

Locally Directed Therapies

Table 16.3 summarizes data from six non-randomized studies comparing the relative value of gastrectomy, bypass procedures and exploratory operation alone with no further definitive procedure with respect to survival and palliation of advanced gastric cancer. Bypass procedures do not improve survival or give useful palliation. Gastrectomy in this series (subtotal gastrectomy or oesophagogastrectomy for tumours of the oesphagogastric junction) is consistently associated with improved survival rates and this is independent of stage (III or IV) and site(s) of metastatic disease. Definitive procedures lead to useful palliation and are preferable in this regard to more conservative surgical approaches. These results are due to alleviation of obstruction, with improvement in nutritional status, prevention of haemorrhage and control of pain. Although total gastrectomy is often not recommended due to the significant morbidity and mortality of the procedure, it may provide a benefit if anatomical considerations demand such an operation, especially in patients presenting with total obstruction. However, there are no randomized comparisons of gastrectomy against other surgical procedures and none comparing it with chemotherapy. For

Table 16.3 Non-randomized trials comparing survival and palliative effects of palliative resections, bypass procedures and exploration alone

Reference	No.	Post-operative mortality	Median survival index	Palliation
Lawrence and McNair [28]	41(T)	NA	8.2[a]	Prolonged period of postoperative adjustment
	67(s)	NA	9.5[a]	Possibly useful for total obstruction
	86(B)	NA	4.2[a]	56.1% achieved > 3/12 symptom control
	239(L)	NA	4.6[a]	No relief from obstruction or bleeding
Stern et al. [29]	39(T and S)	5.1	19.4 (III)[a] 15.5 (IV)[a]	NA
	73(B and L)	5.6	7 (III)[a] 5.6 (IV)[a]	NA
Ekbom and Gleysteen [30]	15(T)	27 } 18	16% 2 yr, 7% 3 yr	88% lasting average 14.6/12 – statistically different
	40(S)	15 } 18		
	20(B)	25	0% 2 and 3 yr	80% lasting average 5.9/12
Boddie et al. [31]	45(T)	17.8	10.4[b]	85.7% achieved "fair" palliation
	21(L)	23.8	3.1[b]	60% achieved "fair" palliation
Hallissey et al. [32]	884(R)	28.6[c] 20.3[c]	} d	NA
	1051(B)	25.9[c] 26.4[c]	} d	NA
	2329(L)	27.4[c] 35.2[c]	} d	NA
Bozzetti et al. [33]	61(T and S)	11.5	8.0[b]	NA
	80(B)	10.0	3.5[b]	NA
	105(L)	4.7	2.8[b]	NA

[a] = mean survival.
[b] = median survival.
[c] = reason for non-curative resection, too advanced disease and presence of distant metastases, respectively.
[d] = overall survival figures not given; statistically significant improvement in 6-, 12-, 18- and 24-month survival for those having resection compared to all other groups in both locally advanced and metastatic disease.
T = total gastrectomy.
S = subtotal gastrectomy.
B = bypass procedure.
L = laparotomy alone.
NA = not assessed.

locally advanced disease, the optimal approach may be to downstage disease to facilitate resection using chemotherapy prior to surgery. This approach has the added benefit of eradication of micrometastatic disease. The decision as to whether a definitive surgical procedure should be performed in patients with metastatic disease for local symptom control, either up front or in disease not responding to chemotherapy, must be made on an individual basis.

Bleeding and obstruction of the cardia and pylorus are amenable to laser therapy. Good results have been obtained with obstruction of the cardia in contrast to more distal lesions. This may relate to poor gastric mobility even if adequate recanalization can be achieved with the laser. Restenosis requires reintervention, but the rate of this can be decreased by concomitant chemotherapy [23]. Using ECF in laser-treated patients, an improvement in weight gain and median survival over patients treated with laser alone was seen, in addition to a reduction in the reintervention rate.

Laser is effective in achieving haemostasis from bleeding tumours, but large tumours present a large surface area which can be difficult to fully coagulate. Lesions high in the fundus are difficult to treat due to problems in manoeuvring the laser tip when the endoscope is retroverted. Exophytic tumours may also present problems with access to the distal margins.

For tumours not responding to high-power laser treatment, low-power interstitial laser photocoagulation may provide long-term haemostatic control [24]. Laser ablation is only applicable to intraluminal tumour. Patients unsuitable for surgery, or where chemotherapy has failed or is not indicated, who have obstruction from primary disease or anastomotic recurrence following total or subtotal gastrectomy, may be considered for stent placement. Insertion of a rigid prosthesis may provide good palliation for inoperable tumours of the cardia and for oesophagojejunal recurrence following total gastrectomy [25]. Suture attachments to anchor the stent to the anterior abdominal wall are successful in reducing subsequent tube migration. Insertion of a rigid prosthesis in a curved lumen adjacent to an anastomosis line carries a high risk of perforation, and flexible self-expanding metal stents have been used to successfully palliate an extramural recurrence causing complete obstruction of the efferent limb of a Billroth II anastomosis [26].

References

1. Oye K, Shapiro MF (1984) Reporting results from chemotherapy trials. J Am Med Assoc 252:2722–2725.
2. Glimelius B, Hoffmann K, Graf M, Pahlman L, Sjoden PO (1994) Quality of life during chemotherapy in symptomatic patients with advanced colorectal cancer. Cancer 73:556–564.
3. Graf M, Pahlman L, Bergstrom R, Grimelius B (1994) The relationship between an objective response to chemotherapy and survival in advanced colorectal cancer. Br J Cancer 70:559–563.
4. Murad A, Santiago FF, Petroianu A (1993) Modified therapy with 5FU, doxorubicin and methotrexate in advanced gastric cancer. Cancer 72:37–41.
5. Glimelius B, Hoffman K, Haglund U, Nyren O, Sjoden PO (1994) Initial or delayed chemotherapy with best supportive care in advanced gastric cancer. Ann Oncol 5:189–190.
6. Pyrhonen S, Kuitunen T, Kouri M (1992) A randomised phase III trial comparing

fluorouracil, epidoxorubicin and methotrexate (FEMTX) with best supportive care in non-resectable gastric cancer. Ann Oncol S3:47.
7. Baker CH, Talley RW, Matter R et al. (1976) A South West Oncology Group Study: Phase III comparison of the treatment of advanced gastrointestinal cancer with bolus weekly 5FU versus methyl CCNU plus bolus weekly 5FU. Cancer 38:1–7.
8. Cullinan SA, Moertel CG, Wieand HF et al. (1994) Controlled evaluation of three drug combination regimens versus fluorouracil alone for the therapy of advanced gastric cancer. J Clin Oncol 12:412.
9. Cullinan SA, Moertel CG, Fleming TR (1985) A comparison of three chemotherapeutic regimens in the treatment of advanced pancreatic and gastric carcinoma: fluorouracil versus fluorouracil and doxorubicin versus fluorouracil, doxorubicin and mitomycin. J Am Med Assoc 253:2061–2067.
10. Kim NK, Park YS, Heo DS et al. (1993) A phase III randomised study of 5 fluorouracil and cisplatin versus 5 fluorouracil doxorubicin, mitomycin C versus 5 fluorouracil alone in the treatment of advanced gastric cancer. Cancer 71:3813–3818.
11. Levi JA, Fox RM, Tattersall MH, Woods RL, Thomson D, Gill G for the Sydney Oncology Group (1986) Analysis of a prospectively randomised comparison of doxorubicin versus 5 fluorouracil, doxorubicin and BCNU in advanced gastric cancer: implications for future studies. J Clin Oncol 4:1348–1355.
12. The Gastrointestinal Tumour Study Group (1988) Triazinate and platinum efficacy in combination with 5 fluorouracil and doxorubicin. Results of a three arm randomised trial in metastatic gastric cancer. J Natl Cancer Inst 80:1011–1015.
13. Cocconi G, Bella M, Zironi S et al. (1994) Fluorouracil, doxorubicin and mitomycin combination versus PELF chemotherapy in advanced gastric cancer: a prospective randomised trial of the Italian Oncology Group for Clinical Research. J Clin Oncol 12:2687–2693.
14. Wils JA, Klein HO, Wagener DJ et al. for the EORTC (1991) Sequential high dose methotrexate and fluorouracil combined with doxorubicin. A step ahead in the treatment of advanced gastric cancer trial of the European Organisation for Research and Treatment of Cancer, Gastrointestinal Tract Co-operative Group. J Clin Oncol 9:827–831.
15. Kelsen D, Atiq AT, Saltz L et al. (1992) FAMTX versus etoposide, doxorubicin and cisplatin: a random assignment trial in gastric cancer. J Clin Oncol 10:541–548.
16. Massuti B, Cervantes A, Anton A (1994) A phase III multicentre randomised study in advanced gastric cancer of fluorouracil + leucovorin + epirubicin + cisplatin (FLEP) versus fluorouracil + Adriamycin + methotrexate + leucovorin. FAMTX toxicity report. Ann Oncol 5 (suppl 8):76–77.
17. Wils JA, Wagener DJTh, Coombes RC et al. (1994) Phase III trial of fluorouracil, methotrexate and epirubicin (FEMTX versus FEMTX plus cisplatin (FEMTX-P)) in advanced gastric cancer. Ann Oncol 5(S8):79.
18. Findlay M, Cunningham D, Norman A et al. (1994) A phase II study in advanced gastro-oesophageal cancer using epirubicin and cisplatin in combination with continuous infusion 5FU (ECF). Ann Oncol 5:609–616.
19. Delfino C, Caccia G, Fein L et al. (1991) Cisplatin (C) epirubicin (E) and 5FU in patients with advanced gastric cancer. Eur J Cancer (ECCO 6) S2:457.
20. Zaniboni A, Labianca R, Martignoni G et al. (1994) ECF is an active feasibile regimen for advanced gastric cancer. A GISCAD Confirmatory Study. Ann Oncol 5(S8): 79–80.
21. Wilke H, Preusser P, Fink U et al. (1989) Pre-operative chemotherapy in locally advanced and non-resectable gastric cancer: a phase II study with etoposide. doxorubicin and cisplatin. J Clin Oncol 7:1318–1326.
22. Plukker JTH, Mulder NH, Sleijfer DTH et al. (1991) Chemotherapy in surgery for locally advanced cancer of the cardia and fundus: phase II study with methotrexate and 5 fluorouracil. Br J Surg 78:955–958.
23. Harper PG, Highley M, Houston N et al. (1992) Significant palliation in advanced

gastric/oesophageal adenocarcinoma with laser endoscopy and combination chemotherapy. Proc Am Soc Clin Oncol 11:472.
24. Barr H, Krasner N (1989) Interstitial laser photocoagulation for treating bleeding gastric cancer. Br Med J 299:659–660.
25. Turnbull A, Kussin S, Kurtz RC, Bains M (1980) Pallitive prosthetic intubation in gastric cancer. J Surg Oncol 15:37–42.
26. Topazian M, Ring E, Grendell J (1992) Palliation of obstructing gastric cancer with steel mesh self-expanding endoprostheses. Gastrointest Endosc 38:58–60.
27. Douglass Jr HO, Lavin PT, Gondsmit A, Klaassen DG, Paul AR (1984) An Eastern Cooperative Oncology Group evaluation of combinations of methyl CCNU, mitomycin C, Adriamycin and 5 fluouroracil in advanced measurable gastric cancer (BST 2277). J Clin Oncol 2:1372–1381.
28. Lawrence W Jr, McNair G (1958) The effects of surgery in patients with incurable gastric cancer. Cancer 11:28–32.
29. Stern JL, Denman S, Elias EG et al. (1975) The evaluation of palliative resection in advanced carcinoma of the stomach. Surgery 77:291–298.
30. Ekbom GA, Gleysteen JJ (1980) Gastric malignancy: a resection for palliation. Surgery 88:476–481.
31. Boddie AW Jr, McMurtrey MJ, Giacco GG, McBride CM (1983) Palliative total gastrectomy and esophagogastrectomy. Cancer 51:1195–1200.
32. Hallissey MT, Allum WH, Rodinsky C, Fielding JW (1988) Palliative surgery for gastric cancer. Cancer 62:440–444.
33. Bozzetti F, Bonfanti G, Audisio RA (1987) Prognosis of patients after palliative surgical procedures for carcinoma of the stomach. Surg Gynecol Obstet 164:151–154.
34. Cazap E, Bruno M, Levy D et al. (1986) A phase II trial of 4 epidoxorubicin in advanced gastric cancer. Proc Am Soc Clin Oncol 5:356.
35. Comis R (1974) Integration of chemotherapy into combined modality treatment of solid tumours. Cancer Treat Rev 1:22–33.
36. Leichman L, Berry BT (1991) Cisplatin therapy for adenocarcinoma of the stomach. Semin Oncol 18 (suppl 3):25–33.
37. Machover D, Goldschmidt E, Chollet P et al. (1986) Treatment of advanced colorectal and gastric adenocarcinomas with 5 fluorouracil and high dose folinic acid. J Clin Oncol 4:685–696.
38. Moertel CG, Levin PT (1979) A phase II–III chemotherapy study in advanced gastric cancer. Cancer Treat Rep 63:1863–1872.
39. Moynihan T, Hansen R, Anderson T et al. (1988) Continuous 5 fluorouracil infusion in advanced gastric carcinoma. Am J Clin Oncol 11:461–464.

17 – Non-Curative Chemotherapy for Colorectal Cancer

G. Middleton and D. Cunningham

Introduction

Approximately 26 000 new cases of colorectal cancer are diagnosed in the UK each year. Twenty-five per cent have metastatic disease at presentation. Table 17.1 presents 5-year survival data and local recurrence rates for tumours operated on with curative intent. Increasing depth of invasion and involvement of local lymph nodes results in progressive worsening of prognosis. For stage III colonic tumours there is around a 50% 5-year survival and this figure may be lower for stage III rectal cancer. Recurrence of rectal cancer often has a locoregional component [1]. This chapter examines specific anti-tumour measures in the treatment of primary and recurrent metastatic colorectal cancer and inoperable local disease.

Systemic Therapies

Best Supportive Care Comparisons

Randomized comparisons of best supportive care versus chemotherapy are important in deciding whether potentially toxic treatments can lead to prolongation of life while at the same time improving or at least maintaining quality of life. This is particularly the case in patients asymptomatic at presentation, where side-effects may negatively impact on quality of life. A Swedish trial randomized 183 patients with asymptomatic non-curable colorectal cancer to immediate treatment with a methotrexate modulated 5-FU regimen or an initial expectant policy with chemotherapy being administered upon the development of symptoms [2]. A 5-month medial survival improvement in the initial treatment arm was demonstrated. There was a highly significant improvement in median duration of symptom-free survival for patients receiving immediate chemotherapy (10 months vs. 2 months). All patients maintained their performance status on treatment.

Two trials have directly compared chemotherapy to best supportive care using a no chemotherapy arm (Table 17.2). An Austrian study randomized 36 patients, with metastatic or inoperable locally recurrent colorectal cancer, to either folinic

Table 17.1 Five-year survival and rates of local relapse following curative surgery for colorectal cancer according to stage

TNM	AJCC/UICC (1986)	Modified Astler-Coller (1954)	Dukes (1958)	5-year survival					Local recurrence rate	
				Crucitti et al. [44] ($n=361$) Colorectal	Moertel et al. [45] ($n=315$) Colon	Wolmark et al. C-01 [46] ($n=172$B 211C) Colon	Willet [47] ($n=533$) Colon	Fisher et al. R-01 [48] ($n=67$B 117C) Rectum	C-01+ ($n=383$) Colon	R-01+ ($n=184$) Rectum
T_1N_0		A		92%			86%			
	Stage I		A		NA	NA		NA	NA	NA
T_2N_0		B_1		82%			73%			
T_3N_0		B_2		76%			65%			
	Stage II		B		NA			57		1.6% perineal
T_4N_0		B_3		NA			51%			
$T_{1-2}N_{1-3}$		C_1		60%		59%	50%		4% anastomotic	6% anastomotic
T_3N_{1-3}	Stage III	C_2	C	55%	51%		39%	35		16.8% pelvic
T_4N_{1-3}		C_3		NA			29%			
M_1	Stage IV	D	D	25%	NA	NA	NA	NA	NA	NA

T_1 = Tumour invades the submucosa.
T_2 = Tumour invades the muscularis propria.
T_3 = Tumour invades through the muscularis propria into the subserosa or into non-peritonealized pericolic or perirectal tissues.
T_4 = Tumour directly invades other organs or structures and/or perforates the visceral peritoneum.
+ = local recurrence as site of first failure.
N_1 = 1–3 pericolic or resected nodes involved.
N_2 = 4 or more pericolic or perirectal nodes.
N_3 = involvement in any node along the course of a vascular trunk and/or apical node involvement.
NA = not assessed.

Table 17.2 Studies incorporating best supportive care or initial expectant treatment arm

Reference	No.	Median survival	Quality-of-life assessment	
Scheithauer et al. [3]				
FLIC	24	11/12*	No difference overall on FLIC scores. Tendency towards improved quality of life in FLIC group, with abnormal scores pretreatment	
vs.				
BSC	12	5/12		
Allen Mersh et al. [38]			Rotterdam	HAD
HAI FUDR	51	14+/12*	13+/12*	11+/12
vs.				
BSC	49	7+/12	6+/12	7/12
Nordic [2]			Symptom-free survival	Progression-free survival
Initial treatment	92	14/12	10/12*	8/12*
vs.				
Expectant treatment (MFL)	91	9/12	2/12 Maintenance of Karnofsky score during treatment with MFL	3/12

*Reaches levels of statistical significance.
BSC = best supportive care.

acid modulated 5-FU and cisplatin (24 patients) or best supportive care alone (12 patients) [3]. The patients' groups had similar pretreatment characteristics, but there was a slightly longer time from original diagnosis to trial entry for the chemotherapy arm. Median time to progression was 6 months for the chemotherapy arm and 2.3 months for patients receiving best supportive care alone: median survival was 11 and 5 months, respectively. Quality of life was assessed two-monthly, with functional living index of cancer (FLIC) scores. Palliative response was assessed by criteria developed by Presant et al. [4]. Overall there were no differences in quality-of-life indices between the two groups (this implies that the doubling of survival time is not accompanied by a worse quality of life), but there was a trend towards improvement in those with advanced FLIC scores at entry (suggesting actual symptom control with chemotherapy – 7/10 symptomatic at trial entry achieving complete or partial palliative response). Numbers in this trial are small, but with the exception of the hepatic arterial infusion (HAI) study mentioned below, this is the only randomized trial of chemotherapy versus best supportive care in advanced colorectal cancer. Taken with the results of the Nordic trial, chemotherapy appears to provide a benefit when compared to best supportive care alone.

The Nordic group have published data on the correlation between objective and symptomatic responses in the context of a randomized comparison of a methotrexate, and a folinic acid modulated 5-FU regimen using a structured questionnaire with an added psychological component [2]. Physicians' and patients' assessment of subjective response was compared. Approximately one-third of patients had an improvement in their overall quality of life and one-quarter had unchanged quality-of-life indices. Improvements were particularly seen for pain. There was close correlation between the patients' assessment of their symptom control and the physicians' assessment of subjective response. Discrepancies occurred in patients with no symptoms at entry (although these should not have been enrolled), with the physicians tending to overestimate the value of treatment. Similarly, for patients with low scores on the combined variables at randomization it was felt that even in the context of an anti-tumour effect, toxicity negatively influenced quality of life. Although this appears to contradict the conclusions from their previous study of asymptomatic patients, it simply underlines the essential requirements for relatively non-toxic regimens in this setting.

There was a close correlation between objective and subjective response, with 100% of the complete response/partial response (CR/PR) patients gaining subjective response and none of the patients with stable disease deteriorating subjectively (these two groups consisted of half of the entire patient population). The duration of CR/PR and SD was around 8 months. Thus, response appears to correlate with symptomatic improvement. The failure of improved response rate to translate to improved median survival is a common one and is partly due to the low rate of CR attained in many trials. However, The Swedish group have also published an analysis of the correlation between objective response to chemotherapy and survival in advanced colorectal cancer and have shown that a response to chemotherapy is associated with a longer survival, even after correction for the guarantee time effect and the distribution of prognostic variables [5].

Inclusion of stable disease of greater than 4 months as an end-point in trials is important as this would, in the absence of symptomatic deterioration, be of positive benefit when compared to the poor prognosis of untreated patients (around 6 months).

The Optimal Regimen?

Research into the optimal chemotherapy regimen centres around refining dosing schedules and methods of modulation of 5-FU as combination chemotherapy does not add much in terms of worthwhile palliation.

Two recent meta-analyses have compared folinic acid (FA) and methotrexate (MTX) modulated 5-FU to 5-FU alone [6, 7]. FdUMP, a 5-FU metabolite, binds to thymidylate synthase in the presence of 5,10-methylene tetrahydrofolate. Folinic acid increases stabilization of the covalent ternary complex thus formed, by increasing intracellular CH_2FH_4 levels. In the meta-analysis of folinic acid modulation [6], nine trials comprising 1381 patients randomized were reviewed. Objective response was doubled with FA modulation - 23% against 11%. The differences in response rate were highly significant for all studies and all schedules, except where a higher 5-FU dose as control was used and here statistical significance was lost. Median survival was not improved (around 11 months for both treatments). The confidence intervals for the survival odds ratios for all trials individually crossed the unity line. Trials using a higher dose of 5-FU as control showed a non-significant trend favouring the control arm. Why do improved response rates not lead to improved survival? When duration of response is analysed it is usually at least 6 months and this would be expected to translate to a survival benefit. Three-quarters of patients do not respond to the treatment and together with a CR of $<5\%$ this may rduce any trend towards increased survival. This analysis, like many individual trials, makes no mention of impact on symptom control of the various regimens, but data from the Nordic trial showing correlation of response to symptom control suggest that modulation may provide such benefit by increasing the response rate. Modulation appears to provide similar chemotherapeutic efficacy using a lower dose of 5-FU, as a higher dose of 5-FU alone and any decrease in the toxicity of the regimen will have a symptomatic impact. There was almost a doubling of grade 3 or greater non-haematological toxicity in the 5-FU arm, compared to the FA modulated 5-FU arm, in the only published trial included in the meta-analysis to use non-equivalent 5-FU doses [8].

Data from an NCCTG collaborative study compared six different 5-FU based regimens [9]. This trial was not included in the meta-analysis. There was a significant survival advantage for FA modulated 5-FU over 5-FU alone (12 months vs. 7.7 months): subset analyses revealed this to be limited to patients with no measurable disease. This subset represents patients with a low tumour burden and thus these results are to be expected on the basis of the superiority of FA modulated 5-FU in the adjuvant setting, where the focus of attack is occult micrometastatic disease. There was a statistically significant improvement in symptom control for the modulated arm (documented by physicians' assessment of symptoms), with more than 50% deriving benefit. These results were not correlated with response, but modulation led to a quadrupling of responses, with an 8-month median time to progression for responders in all groups. These results are consistent with those of the meta-analysis which suggests that FA modulation is unlikely to provide a median survival benefit in advanced disease and also with the Nordic study which demonstrated subjective improvements in half of the patients treated (greater than in the 5-FU alone arm and possibly related to the improved response rates of moderate duration).

The optimal folinic acid dose for use as modulation was analysed in an NCCTG trial comparing high- and low-dose FA. There was no difference in response rate, median survival or palliative effects, but a statistical increase in leucopenia, stomatitis and diarrhoea, together with increased hospitalization at almost double the cost, for the high-dose FA arm [10].

In addition to its effects on DNA, 5-FU also inhibits RNA synthesis. 5-FU is converted to 5-FUMP in the presence of phosphoribosylpyrophosphate (PRPP) and upon phosphorylation to the triphosphate incorporated into RNA with resultant cytotoxicity. MTX is a purine inhibitor and this directly leads to intracellular accumulation of PRPP. A total of 1178 patients, enrolled in eight trials, were included in the meta-analysis of MTX modulation [7]. The single agent 5-FU response rate was reproducible and again doubled with modulation. There was a similar reduction in the response effect when higher 5-FU doses were used as the control arm. In contrast to the results obtained with folinic acid modulation, there was a statistically significant survival advantage, with a 13% reduction in odds of death from modulated treatment. However, the upper 95% confidence interval approached unity. Thus MTX and FA modulated 5-FU yield equivalent benefits over 5-FU alone. This was the conclusion of the meta-analysis investigative committee on examination of data from trials directly comparing the two regimens. Although NCCTG data indicated the superiority of FA over MTX modulation in terms of a statistically significant improvement in response rate and median survival, these regimens were not comparable as almost twice the amount of 5-FU was used in the FA modulated arm. A trial utilizing equivalent 5-FU doses demonstrated their equivalence in terms of response rate, symptom relief and survival, but FA modulation was found to be easier to administer and had reduced toxicity [11].

A randomized trial of 500 mg m^{-2} of MTX, followed by 600 mg m^{-2} of 5-FU and 200 mg m^{-2} of leucovorin vs. 5-FU/leucovorin in equivalent dose vs. 5-FU 1200 mg m^{-2} bolus given two-weekly, demonstrated equivalent actuarial survival for single and double modulation. Response rates for the different modulated regimens were not statistically different [12].

The short half-life of 5-FU suggests that for an individual bolus dose there will only be a small percentage of cells in S-phase susceptible to the effects of the drug. One way to overcome this limitation is protracted infusional 5-FU (PIF) schedules. The results of a randomized Mid-Atlantic Oncology Programme trial demonstrated superior response rate with PIF compared to a 5-day 500 mg m^{-2} unmodulated bolus schedule, using a dose of 300 mg m^{-2} per 24 h - 30% against 7% [13]. Median survival was the same at around a year. Thus the net result was similar to those seen for modulated bolus 5-FU. No quality-of-life study was performed, but there was a statistically significant reduction in neutropenia and stomatitis at the expense of palmar plantar erythema, a side-effect unique to the PIF schedule.

We have recently reported a similar response rate to PIF, 24%, in the context of a randomized comparison of PIF ± interferon α 2B subcutaneously 3 weekly [14]. The median survival was just under 1 year for 5-FU alone and 328 days for the combination. There were no measurable differences in quality of life between the two groups using the EORTC questionnaire. There was an overall symptomatic response of 68% for the entire group. For PIF, improvements in pain were seen in 65%, weight loss in 85% and anorexia in 78%. Toxicity was significantly greater with the addition of interferon, with increased mucositis, alopecia and neutropenia.

A further randomized phase III trial performed at the Royal Marsden Hospital analysed the value of inclusion of interferon to a bolus 5-FU regimen [15]. The Wadler schedule of 750 mg m^{-2} continuous intravenous infusion for 5 days followed by the same dose weekly, ± 10 Mu interferon three times weekly, were compared in 106 patients eligible for assessment. There was no difference in response rate, progression-free survival or overall survival, but significantly more toxicity in the form of leucopenia, depression and alopecia in the interferon-treated group. Four toxic deaths occurred in patients receiving interferon, compared with none for 5-FU alone.

A group from Indiana have reported results of a trial with very similar design: no statistically significant differences in response or response duration was seen [16]. The same interferon-containing regimen has been compared against 370 mg m^{-2} 5-FU modulated with 200 mg m^{-2} folinic acid for 5 days every 28 days in a large multicentre trial [17]. The regimens were equivalent with respect to response and survival: diarrhoea, nausea and vomiting and stomatitis were more frequently observed with the 5-FU and leucovorin regimen, whereas fatigue, somnolence and fever were more frequently seen in the interferon arm.

Two groups independently assessed the value of the addition of interferon to different folinic acid modulated 5-FU regimens, with the result that neither demonstrated any clinical benefit but significantly more toxicity for the arm receiving interferon in addition [18, 19]. These results are partly to be expected as interferon appears to exert its 5-FU modulation via FdUMP stabilization of thymidine synthetase; folinic acid also acts via thymidine synthetase. Interferon changes the pharmacokinetics of 5-FU, with decreased clearance, increased half-life, increased serum concentration and decreased catabolism, but the addition of folinic acid to interferon and 5-FU decreases the area under the curve to near that of single agent 5-FU.

Cisplatin and 5-FU combinations are widely used in the treatment of oesophageal cancer and head and neck cancers. The Mid Atlantic Oncology Programme evaluated the addition of cisplatin to a PIF regimen using 20 mg m^{-2} of cisplatin per week and found no improvement beyond that obtained with PIF alone [20]. A randomized trial of a 5-FU and cisplatin combination versus NCCTG folinic acid modulated 5-FU demonstrated that the cisplatin-containing regimen, while providing improvements in median time to progression of death, did not improve median survival, response rate or median duration of response and the investigators concluded that the addition of cisplatin did not provide therapeutic benefit [21].

N-phosphono-acetyl-L-aspartate (PALA) is a *de novo* pyrimidine synthesis inhibitor, decreasing uridine pools and thus effectively increasing 5-FU metabolite activity at its molecular targets. This pyrimidine synthesis inhibition also has the spin-off of increased PRPP levels, which favours the formation of 5-FU nucleotides. Early trials of PALA-modulated 5-FU used high PALA doses, as PALA has been shown to have some single agent activity in preclinical trials. Toxicity considerations resulted in reductions of the 5-FU dose to levels which in retrospect, were unlikely to be effective [22]. As a modulator, however, low-dose PALA is effective in inhibiting pyrimidine synthesis, allowing 5-FU dose escalation without undue toxicity. Most trials use 250 mg m^{-2} of PALA, 24 h before 5-FU administration either as a single weekly high-dose infusion or in bolus schedules. The most recent of these phase II studies demonstrates a 35% response rate and a median response duration of 11 months. Median survival was 18 months [23]. These figures compare to those seen using FA-modulated 5-FU and PIF. Fifteen of 16 responders developed hepatic abnormalities, all with increases in bilirubin, and six patients developed ascites apparently not related to progressive disease. This may be due to decreased bilirubin glucuronidation secondary to decreased hepatic uridine and decreased hepatic protein synthesis.

What recommendations can be drawn from these date on 5-FU biomodulation? On the basis of phase III evidence, the addition of cisplatin or alpha interferon does not appear to be of value and double modulation seems to provide no clinical benefit. The NCCTG FA-modulated 5-FU regimen and PIF would appear to be the best choices for comparison. Phase II data on PALA modulation must be confirmed in phase III trials. A direct comparison of PIF and 5-FU/FA has not been published, although the South Western Oncology Group has presented, in abstract form, data which when peer reviewed and mature will be important [24]. This directly compares seven regimens, including NCCTG 5-FU/FA, a high-dose FA modulated regimen, single agent 5-FU, a weekly high-dose infusion regimen, PALA modulation, PIF and FA modulated PIF. Both PIF regimens show response rates of 25% compared to 15% for NCCTG 5-FU/FA and hazard ratios show a trend towards improved survival in the infusional arm compared to unmodulated bolud 5-FU, while survival in the NCCTG arm is no different to the unmodulated arm. There was greater grade 4 toxicity for NCCTG when compared to PIF. The PALA modulated regimen had a response rate of 10%. This trial includes a quality-of-life component. We are conducting a randomized comparison of NCCTG against PIF in the adjuvant setting, together with quality-of-life monitoring. Although not directly applicable to metastatic disease, early data from the safety monitoring committee demonstrates a much more favourable therapeutic profile for PIF, with significantly less grade 3–4 neutropenia, stomatitis and diarrhoea.

A Role for Second-Line Therapy?

There are few data on the value of second-line treatment in refractory disease. PIF and FA modulated 5-FU can salvage some patients refractory to single agent 5-FU. We obtained a 27% PR rate using PIF in patients previously treated with single agent 5-FU [25]. In an overview of six phase II trials using FA/5-FU, an objective response rate of 12% was seen in patients pretreated with unmodulated 5-FU [26]. What, however, is an acceptable strategy for those who have progressed on these regimens? There are a number of reports on the use of CPT-11 as second-line therapy and results are promising [27–29]. These trials do not separately analyse results for those receiving single agent 5-FU, modulated 5-FU or oral fluoropyrimidines as initial therapy.

We obtained 0/6 responses using PIF in patients who had failed folinic acid modulated 5-FU [14], but a small Italian study using a similar protocol achieved an 8% response rate with 50% stabilization, ranging in duration from 3 to 9 months [30]. This group has investigated the mechanisms of resistance of cell lines to various 5-FU schedules. Lines resistant to fluoropyrimidines given by bolus schedules still retain full sensitivity to a 7-day continuous exposure (7-day resistant clones are, however cross-resistant to bolus exposure) [31]. Two mechanisms appear to be responsible – decreased incorporation of 5-FU metabolites into RNA in short-exposure resistant clones and impaired polyglutamation of CH_2 FH_4, leading to rapid recovery from (TS) inhibition on cessation of drug exposure in 7-day resistant clones. Thus disease resistant to bolus 5-FU regimens might respond to PIF, but also if bolus regimens lead to an RNA-directed mechanism of resistance, then RNA-directed modulators such as MTX might be more appropriate than TS-directed modulation using folinic acid, and conversly FA might be an appropriate modulation for PIF if resistance is TS based. This group is currently piloting a hybrid regimen consisting of MTX modulated bolus 5-FU alternating with FA modulated infusional 5-FU and have found it to be twice as active and half as toxic as FA modulated 5-FU as used at their institution, yielding a 42% response rate with a 7+ month median duration of response [32].

Only well-designed randomized trials, preferably with a best supportive care arm, will be able to assess whether any further treatment in refractory disease is better than no treatment at all.

Locally Directed Therapies

Hepatic Arterial Chemotherapy

Systemic therapy aims to deal with both metastatic disease and any locoregional component. For local disease alone, strategies specifically targeted to this are intuitively appealing. Established colorectal hepatic metastases derive their blood supply from the hepatic artery, whereas normal hepatocytes have a dual supply from hepatic artery and portal vein. High first-pass extraction rates allow large increases in hepatic exposure to drugs administered via the hepatic artery when compared to intravenous infusion. Fluorodeoxyuridene (FUDR) is most favourable in this regard, with an extraction ration of 0.95, allowing 100–400 tmes increased hepatic exposure. There have been five randomized trials of HAI FUDR against systemic fluoropyrimidine therapy [33–37], all demonstrate response rates around 50% for HAI accompanied by marked change in natural history, with a definite delay in progression of liver metastases but a much higher death rate from extrahepatic progression. This is not surprising, as HAI will have no effect on occult extrahepatic micrometastatic disease. Side-effects are not trivial, with a 25% rate of sclerosing cholangitis and a 37% gastrointestinal complication rate at 12 months, necessitating stoppage of treatment in more than 50% of patients at 6 months in a large recent study [37].

If the liver metastases are, at the time of institution of treatment, the most obvious disease, a survival advantage might be expected. Trial designs incorporating crossover to HAI after progression on systemic therapy make the interpretation of overall median survival figures difficult. Data from Memorial Sloan Kettering showed median survivals of 9.5 months against 3.4 months for those who crossed over against those who did not [35]. There was a median survival of the initial HAI group of 17 months compared to 8 months in the non-crossed over group.

The design of the recent French multicentre trial makes the only valid comparison between those who received HAI and those who did not [37]. Only 50% in the control arm of systemic therapy (and 30% in the HAI arm) actually received some systemic treatment. A 2-year survival of 23% vs. 13% and median survival of 15 months against 11 months were obtained for the group receiving HAI. These small survival benefits in patients with disease apparently confined to the liver by delay in hepatic progression are accompanied by significant toxicity. Good quality-of-life data become important with such a relatively toxic treatment. HAI requires preliminary hepatic angiography, laparotomy and often prophylactic cholecystectomy.

A group at the Charing Cross and Westminster Medical School have recently published the results of a randomized comparison of HAI FUDR against best supportive care and have shown a prolongation of median survival from 226 days to 405 days for the treated group and a similar prolongation in normal quality life [38]. The HAI-treated group tended to die of extrahepatic disease as to be expected, as FUDR provides no systemic spillover to eradicate micrometastatic disease. The median Karnofsky score of the treated patients was 90%, with a range of 90–100%. Such excellent performance status patients often form a relatively small proportion in trials of systemic therapy. We have separately analysed the results of patients treated with PIF at our institution who have ECOG scores of 0–1; these patients had median survivals of 543 days, a much higher figure than the HAI arm in the above best supportive care comparison. Further, there was a 5% mortality rate due to the catheter placement procedure in the HAI trial. The authors plan to perform a trial assessing the benefit of the addition of HAI to conventional systemic chemotherapy. The MRC are accruing to a randomized trial comparing HAI 5-FU and intravenous folinic acid against folinic acid modulated intravenous 5-FU. The extraction ratio of 5-FU is 0.35 and therefore HAI 5-FU should provide good systemic spillover. HAI 5-FU does not lead to hepatobiliary toxicity. These trials are important in assessing any future role, if any, for hepatic arterial therapy.

Resection of Hepatic Metastases

Although not strictly considered a palliative measure, those with a limited number of colorectal liver metastases without any obvious extrahepatic disease should be considered as candidates for radical excision. A large German retrospective study showed 2% 3-year survival for those with unresectable liver metastases [21]. Patients who were considered resectable but were not treated fared better, but there were no 5-year survivors. Patients who were resected had a 40% 5-year survival, if the 5% postoperative mortality was excluded. Those who had incomplete resections did no better than untreated patients. Those who underwent "curative resection" but eventually relapsed had a shift forward of 1-year in survival, with good palliation in symptomatic patients.

Recurrence of liver metastases after resection can be successfully dealt with by repeat resection. Recent French data show a 35% liver recurrence rate after "curative surgery", but a 3-year survival of 33% with less than 1% surgical mortality for repeat resections [39]. Similarly, a third hepatectomy appeared to offer benefit, with a 12-month survival rate of 81% in this series.

Laser

Patients with inoperable colorectal liver metastases, those unfit for surgery or those who refuse surgery may benefit from interstitial laser photocoagulation (ILP). Grade 1 or 2 necrosis can be achieved for tumours less than 4 cm in diameter, as assessed by dynamic CT scanning, and no regrowth was seen in the area of a grade 1 response in a series of 21 patients [40]. Those who achieve lesser degrees of necrosis inevitably develop progression within 2–3 months. In this series, estimation of impact on survival is difficult in view of concomitant chemotherapy and small numbers, but at least 37% 2-year survival was seen. The same arguments applied to HAI with high extraction rate fluoropyrimidine can be applied to ILP as single modality treatment, and indeed chemotherapy during ILP could be potentially modulated by the thermic effects of the treatment. Laser offers advantages over cryosurgery, in that it can be done under local anaesthetic and is minimally invasive.

Laser also has potential in the palliation of symptoms in inoperable rectal and distal sigmoid cancers [27]. Local symptom control of 88% using a Nd:YAG laser, with 67% complete control of bleeding, 88% relief from obstructive symptoms and 80% control of faecal incontinence, was obtained in one study. Only 3/17 required further laser intervention, which was successful in two patients. Complications are minimal and hospital stay averages 2–3 days. It is easy to perform and controllable, due to direct visualization via the flexible endoscope. By contrast, radiotherapy may result in fistula formation, soft-tissue necrosis and abscess formation, as well as diarrhoea, vaginitis and dermatitis. Radiation therapy is effective in palliation of mass effect, bleeding or discharge in some two-thirds of patients with a recurrence, but such palliation is short lived, and symptoms recur in the majority of patients. In one series, median duration of symptom control was 5 months, with a 12-month median survival – a short duration of palliation with respect to duration of survival [41].

Chemoradiation for Localized Disease

Patients with inoperable rectal cancer may be treated in order to downstage their tumours sufficiently to allow an attempt at resection. Workers at the Memorial Sloan Kettering treated patients with unresectable disease using either radiation together with folinic acid modulated 5-FU or radiation alone [42]. Although small numbers prevented the results reaching statistical significance, there was a higher rate of pathological complete remission, lower incidence of positive nodes and the complete resection rates with negative margins were higher in the patients who received combined modality therapy.

Pelvic Exenteration

Laser has advantages over diathermy and cryotherapy in that the former cannot be used above the peritoneal reflection and requires anaesthesia, while the latter may result in prolonged rectal discharge after treatment. Those who develop intractable symptoms unresponsive to local measures present a difficult problem. In one series of patients undergoing pelvic exenteration for uncontrollable symptoms, over half had developed these after treatment with pelvic irradiation. Twenty patients were treated with palliative intent, specifically for pelvic pain, some patients having obstruction, fistula, bleeding or urinary symptoms [43]. Five patients died in the postoperative period, with a median survival of 10 months; no patient demonstrated local recurrence. Late complications included fistula formulation and obstruction, but good pain control was seen in two-thirds of those who left hospital. Although no form of quality-of-life analysis was included, the authors felt that the procedure had led to substantial improvements in this. The number of patients suitable for such procedures is small: strict patient selection, coupled with the surgeon's experience, will always be major determinants of outcome.

Conclusions

With the judicious use of specific systemic and locally directed therapies, patients with metastatic and inoperable local disease can expect improvements in symptom control, quality of life and survival beyond that provided by best supportive care measures alone. Patient selection is critical; patients with poor performance status generally do badly on chemotherapy and such an option is usually inappropriate. However, for patients in relatively good health chemotherapy can be justified when instituted early in the course of disease, when tolerance of treatment and response will be greatest. Meticulous attention to toxicity and response are essential requirements to its successful use.

References

1. Stipa S, Nocolatti V, Botti C et al. (1991) Local recurrence after curative resection for colorectal cancer: frequency risk factors and treatment. J Surg Oncol S2:155–160.
2. The Nordic Gastro-intestinal Tumour Adjuvant Therapy Group (1992) Expectancy or

primary chemotherapy in patients with advanced asymptomatic colorectal cancer – a randomised trial J Clin Oncol 10:904–911.
3. Scheithauer W, Rosen H, Kornek GV et al. (1993) Randomised comparison of combination chemotherapy plus supportive care with supportive care alone in patients with metastatic colorectal cancer. Br Med J 306:752–755.
4. Presant CA, Wiseman C, Blayney D et al. (1990) Proposed criteria for serial evaluation of quality of life in cancer patients. J Natl Cancer Inst 82:322–323.
5. Glimelius B, Hoffman K, Graf W et al. (1994) Quality of life during chemotherapy in symptomatic patients with advanced colorectal cancer. Cancer 75:556–562.
6. The Advanced Colorectal Cancer Meta-analysis Project (1992) Modulation of fluorouracil by leucovorin in patients with advanced colorectal cancer – evidence in terms of response rate. J Clin Oncol 10:896–903.
7. The Advanced Colorectal Cancer Meta-analysis Project (1994) Meta-analysis of randomised trials testing the biochemical modulation of fluorouracil by methotrexate in metastatic colorectal cancer. J Clin Oncol 12:960–969.
8. Valone FH, Friedman MA, Wittlinger PS et al. (1989) Treatment of patients with advanced colorectal carcinoma with fluorouracil alone, high dose leucovorin plus fluorouracil or sequential methotrexate, fluorouracil and leucovorin: a randomised trial of the Northern California Oncology Group. J Clin Oncol 7:1427–1436.
9. Poon MA, O'Connell MJ, Moertel CG et al. (1980) Biochemical modulation of fluorouracil. Evidence of significant improvement in survival and quality of life in patients with advanced colorectal carcinoma. J Clin Oncol 7:1407–1417.
10. Gerstner J, O'Connell MJ, Wieand HS et al. (1991) A prospectively randomised clinical trial comparing 5FU combined with either high or low dose leucovorin for the treatment of advanced colorectal cancer. Proc Am Soc Clin Oncol 10:134.
11. The Nordic Gastrointestinal Tumour Adjuvant Therapy Group (1993) Biochemical modulation of 5FU. A randomised comparison of sequential methotrexate 5FU and leucovorin versus sequential 5FU and leucovorin in patients with advanced symptomatic colorectal cancer. Ann Oncol 4:235–240.
12. Abad A, Garcia P, Gravalos C et al. (1992) Phase III trial with methotrexate, 5FU and high dose leucovorin versus 5FU leucovorin vs 5FU in advanced and metastatic colorectal cancer. Proc Am Soc Clin Oncol 11:A459.
13. Lokich JJ, Ahlgren JD, Gullo JJ et al. (1989) A prospective randomised comparison of continuous infusion fluorouracil with a conventional bolus schedule in metastatic colorectal carcinoma; a Mid Atlantic Oncology Programme Study. J Clin Oncol 7:425–432.
14. Hill ME, Cunningham D, Findlay M et al. (1994) A randomised phase III trial of infusional 5FU +/− interferon α 2B in colorectal cancer and a parallel study measuring tumour FDG uptake of positron emission tomography. Ann Oncol 5:(S8)238.
15. Hill ME, Norman AR, Cunningham D et al. (1995) The Royal Marsden Phase III trial of 5FU with or without interferon α in advanced colorectal cancer. J Clin Oncol (in press)
16. York M, Grecco FA, Figlin RA et al. (1993) A randomised phase III trial comparing 5FU with or without interferon α 2A for advanced colorectal cancer. Proc Am Soc Clin Oncol 12:590.
17. The Corfu – A Collaborative Group (1993) 5FU plus interferon α 2A versus 5FU plus leucovorin in metastatic colorectal cancer. Results of a multicentre multinational phase III study. Proc Am Soc Clin Oncol 12:562.
18. Kosmidis P, Tsavaris N, Skarlos D et al. (1993) Fluorouracil 5FU and folinic acid with or without alpha 2B interferon in advanced colorectal cancer. A prospective randomised trial. Proc Am Soc Clin Oncol 12:A635.
19. Seymour MT, Slevin M, Cunningham D et al. (1994) A randomised trial to assess the addition of interferon α 2A to 5FU and leucovorin in advanced colorectal cancer. Ann Oncol 5(S8):237.

20. Lokich JJ, Ahlgren JD, Cantrell J et al. (1991) A prospective randomised comparison of protracted infusion 5FU with or without weekly bolus cisplatin in metastatic colorectal carcinoma. A Mid Atlantic Oncology Programme Study. Cancer 67:4–19.
21. Scheele J, Stangl R, Altendorf-Hoffman A et al. (1990) Hepatic metastases from colorectal cancer. Impact of surgical resection on a natural history. Br J Surg 77:1241–1246.
22. Martin DS, Kemeny NE (1992) Modulation of fluorouracil by *N* (phosphonacetyl) L asparate: a review. Semin Oncol 19(S2):49–55.
23. Kemeny N, Ponty JA, Selter K et al. (1992) Biochemical modulation of bolus fluorouracil by PALA in patients with advanced colorectal cancer. J Clin Oncol 10:747–752.
24. Leichman CG, Fleming TR, Muggia FM et al. (1993) Fluorouracil 5FU schedules and modulation in advanced colorectal cancer. A Southwest Oncology Group (SWOG) screening trial. Proc Am Soc Clin Oncol 12:A583.
25. Findlay M, Hill A, Cunningham D (1994) Protracted venous infusion 5FU and interferon α in advanced refractory colorectal cancer. Ann Oncol 5:239–243.
26. Arbuck SG (1987) 5FU/leucovorin: biochemical modulation that works? Oncology 1:61–71.
27. Bugat R, Suc E, Rougie Y et al. (1994) CPT11 (irinotecan) as second line therapy in advanced colorectal cancer (CRC). Preliminary results of a multicentric phase II study. Proc Am Soc Clin Oncol 13:586.
28. Rothenburg ML, Eckardt JR, Burris HA et al. (1994) Irinotecan (CPT11). A second line therapy for patients with 5FU refractory colorectal cancer. Proc Am Soc Clin Oncol 13:578.
29. Shimada Y, Yoshno M, Watia A et al. (1993) A phase II study of CPT 11 a new camptothecin derivative, in metastatic colorectal cancer. J Clin Oncol 11:909–913.
30. Mori A, Bertogli S, Guglielmi A et al. (1993) Activity of continuous infusional 5FU in patients with advanced colorectal cancer clinically resistant to bolus 5FU. Cancer Chemother Pharmacol 33:1791–1780.
31. Aschele C, Sobrero A, Fadaran NA et al. (1992) Novel mechanisms of resistance to 5FU in human colorectal cancer (HCT-A) sublines following exposure to two different clinically relevant dose schedules. Cancer Res 52:1855–1864.
32. Sobreor A, Aschele C, Guglielmi A et al. (1994) High activity and low toxicity of alternating bolus in continuous infusion 5FU with schedule orientated biochemical modulation in advanced colon cancer patients. Proc Am Soc Clin Oncol 13:588.
33. Chang AE, Schneider PD, Sugarbaker PH, Simpson C, Culane M, Steinberg NM (1987) A prospective randomised trial of regional versus systemic continuous 5 fluordexoyuridine chemotherapy in the treatment of colorectal liver metastases. Ann Surg 206:688–693.
34. Hohn DC, Stagg RJ, Freidman MA et al. (1989) A randomised trial of continuous intravenous versus hepatic intraarterial floxuridine in patients with colorectal cancer, metastatic to the liver. J Clin Oncol 7:1646–1654.
35. Kemeny N, Daley J, Reichman B, Guillet N, Bothet J, Oderman P (1987) Intrahepatic or systemic infusion of fluordexoyuridine in patients with liver metastases from colorectal carcinoma. A randomised trial. Ann Intern Med 107:459–465.
36. Martin JK, O'Connell MJ, Wieand HS et al. (1990) Intra-arterial floxuridine versus systemic fluorouracil for hepatic metastases from colorectal cancer. Arch Surg 125:1022–1027.
37. Rougier P, Leplanche A, Huguier M (1992) Hepatic arterial infusion of floxuridine in patients with liver metastases from colorectal carcinoma. Long term results of a prospective randomised trial. J Clin Oncol 10:1112–1118.
38. Allen Mersh TG, Earlam S, Ford DC et al. (1994) Quality of life and survival with continuous hepatic artery floxuridine infusion for colorectal liver metastases. Lancet 344:1255–1260.

39. Nordlinger B, Vaillant DJC, Guiguet N et al. (1994) Survival benefit of repeated liver resections for current colorectal metastases: 143 cases. J Clin Oncol 12:1491–1496.
40. Amin Z, Donald JJ, Masters A et al. (1993) Hepatic metastases: interstitial laser photocoagulation with real time US monitoring and dynamic CT evaluation of treatment. Radiology 187(2):339–347.
41. Rostock RA, Zajac AJ, Gallagher J. Radiation therapy in treatment of colorectal cancer. In: Ahlgren JD, Macdonald JS (eds) Gastrointestinal oncology, pp366–367.
42. Minsky BD, Cohen MA, Vemeny N et al. (1992) Enhancement of radiation induced downstaging of rectal cancer by fluorouracil and high dose leucovorin chemotherapy. J Clin Oncol 10:79–84.
43. Yeung RS, Moffat FL, Falk RE et al. (1993) Pelvic exenteration for recurrent and locally advanced primary colorectal adenocarcinoma. Cancer 72:1853–1858.
44. Crucitti F, Soffel L, Batista D et al. (1991) Prognostic factors in colorectal cancer, current status and new trends. J Surg Oncol (suppl. 2):76–82.
45. Moertel C, Flemming T, McDonald J (1992) The Inter Group Study of fluorouracil plus levamisole, levamisole alone as adjuvant therapy for stage C colon cancer – a final report. Proc Am Soc Clin Oncol 11:161.
46. Wolmark N, Fisher B, Rockette H et al. (1988) Postoperative adjuvant chemotherapy or BCG for colon cancer: results from NSABP protocol C-01. J Natl Cancer Inst 80:30–36.
47. Willett C, Tepper JE, Cohen A et al. (1984) Local failure following curative resection of colonic adenocarcinoma. Int J Radiat Oncol Biol Phys 10:645–651.
48. Fisher B, Wolmark N, Rockette H et al. (1988) Postoperative adjuvant chemotherapy or radiation therapy for rectal cancer. Results from NSABP Protocol R-01. J Natl Cancer Inst 80:21–29.
49. Brown SG, Barr M, Matthewson K et al. (1986) Endoscopic treatment of inoperable colorectal cancers with the YAG laser. Br J Surg 73:949–952.
50. Graf W, Pahlman L, Bergstrom R et al. (1994) The relationship between objective response to chemotherapy and survival in advanced colorectal cancer. Br J Cancer 70:559–563.
51. Paul MA, O'Connell MJ, Weiand HS et al. (1991) Biochemical modulation of fluorouracil with leucovorin. Confirmatory evidence improved therapeutic efficacy in advanced colorectal cancer. J Clin Oncol 9:1967–1972.
52. Scheithauer W, Depischi D, Kornek G et al. (1994) Randomised comparison of fluorouracil and leucovorin therapy versus fluorouracil, leucovorin and cisplatin therapy in patients with advanced colorectal cancer. Cancer 73(6):1562–1568.

18 – Non-Curative Chemotherapy for Gynaecological Cancer

J.A. Prendiville and M.E. Gore

Epithelial Ovarian Cancer

Introduction

Epithelial ovarian cancer (EOC) accounts for 90% of malignant ovarian tumours, is the fourth commonest cause of cancer death among women in the Western world and the leading cause of gynaecological cancer mortality. Cytotoxic treatment has evolved from single agent therapy, primarily with the alkylating agent melphalan, to aggressive platinum-based combination chemotherapy. Platinum-based treatment produces complete remission rates of 20–60% in patients with advanced disease (i.e. FIGO stages III or IV), depending on the extent of residual disease [1–4]. However, only 20% of patients with advanced disease will survive for 5 years despite chemotherapy, and these are largely patients who had initial radical debulking of the tumour [2, 5]. The majority of women (70–80%) present with advanced disease and therefore most women with advanced EOC receive chemotherapy which is non-curative. Even among those women who receive chemotherapy for FIGO stages Ic or II disease, many will relapse and require further chemotherapy which will also be non-curative.

There are several factors which predict for poor prognosis and define a group of patients who receive non-curative chemotherapy, i.e. patients refractory to first-line chemotherapy and those who relapse after first-line treatment. Poor prognostic factors at presentation include: a high volume of post-surgical residual disease, less differentiated histology, more advanced stage, clinically measurable disease, the presence of ascites and older age. Stage and the volume of residual disease are the most important of these [5, 6–10].

Histological grade (i.e. degree of cellular differentiation) is probably the third most important prognostic factor, particularly in patients with early stage disease, and the observation appears to be independent of which grading classification has been used [7, 11–13]. While histological grade (degree of cellular differentiation) is an important independent prognostic factor, histological type appears to have limited prognostic significance that is independent of histological grade, clinical stage or extent of disease, although conflicting data have been published [9, 14–18]. However, a relationship between prognosis and histological type has been identified with serous, endometrial and clear cell tumours, although significantly less so. There are therefore patients with apparently favourable pathological types (serous well-differentiated, mucinous and endometrioid of all grades) and unfavourable pathological types (serous poorly differentiated, unclassified and clear cell of all grades [7]). Age also has an influence on prognosis, survival decreasing for every 5-year increase in age past the age of 40 [7].

Failure of elevated CA125 values to fall during the early cycles of chemotherapy predicts for a high probability of residual tumour at second-look surgery and therefore is a further poor prognostic factor for survival [19]. Most patients with advanced EOC have residual tumour at second look [20] and their 3-year survival is 23–27% compared with 83% for patients with no evidence of disease [21]. In patients who have a negative second laparotomy (i.e. pathological complete remission; pCR), a higher histological grade in the original tumour predicts for an increased recurrence rate (grade 1, 22%; grade 2, 39% and grade 3, 56% [22]). As many as 50–60% of patients with advanced stage EOC who experience a pCR will ultimately relapse [22, 23].

The definition of non-curative chemotherapy for EOC is a relative one. First-line treatment for EOC is usually given with curative intent, but as has been shown, the 5-year survival for patients with advanced disease is still disappointingly low. It is therefore important to consider the basic principles of first-line chemotherapy for advanced disease and the chemotherapy regimens received by patients. Most women presenting with EOC will require second- or third-line chemotherapy and as these chemotherapy regimens are invariably non-curative, we will focus on such treatments in this review.

First-Line Chemotherapy for Advanced Disease

There is now a consensus that cytoreductive surgery followed by platinum-based combination chemotherapy should be standard first-line treatment for patients with advanced stage EOC. However, a quantitative statistical overview (meta-analysis) of 8139 patients from 45 different randomized trials has produced no firm conclusions on what drugs, doses or schedules have the greatest impact on survival [24]. Nevertheless, this meta-analysis by the Advanced Ovarian Cancer Trialists Group (AOCTG) has observed that (1) for survival up to 6 years, immediately delivered platinum-based regimens were marginally better than single agent or combination non-platinum treatments, and that (2) for survival between 2 and 8 years, platinum combinations are marginally better than single agent platinum regimens at the same dose. With respect to this latter observation, there remains uncertainty as to whether the difference seen with platinum-based combinations is due to the addition of other drugs or to the higher doses of cisplatin administration compared to those used in earlier single agent cisplatin trials. In addition, combination therapy results in increased toxicity and this is an important consideration if survival advantages are small. The AOCTG also noted (3) that there was no apparent difference in survival between treatment with cisplatin and carboplatin, although there was no follow-up beyond 4 years. The role of Adriamycin in platinum-based combinations remains uncertain, although as a single agent it yields a response of 30% in untreated patients [25]. A meta-analysis of 1200 patients treated in four randomized trials comparing CAP (cyclophosphamide, Adriamycin and cisplatin) with CP (cyclophosphamide and platinum) demonstrated a statistical benefit for CAP, with a 7% increase in the pCR rate and an additional 6% increase in 6-year survival [26]. The analysis could not clarify whether the benefit observed with CAP was due to a greater dose intensity or to the presence of Adriamycin. However, a recent larger meta-analysis of 31 randomized trials in advanced EOC concluded that Adriamycin did have a statistically significant impact on survival and that this was at least equal in magnitude to platinum [27].

Against this background most patients with advanced stage EOC now receive treatment with single agent carboplatin or a platinum analogue in combination with cyclophosphamide, with or without Adriamycin. Although platinum-based chemotherapy has undoubtedly improved response rates, complete remission rates and median survival, the most optimistic 5-year survival rates in patients with advanced disease remain 20–25% [28]. It must be emphasized, however, that in the pre-platinum era the largest series of advanced stage patients treated with single agent melphalan demonstrated that approximately 20% of patients who responded and only 9% of the entire group were alive at 5 years.

The issues of cumulative dose and dose intensity (dose expressed as a function of time) in first-line treatment for EOC remain controversial. A prospective randomized comparison of six cycles of CAP (normal cumulative or total dose) with 12 cycles of CAP (twice the normal cumulative dose but at normal dose intensity) in advanced EOC did not show a statistically significant correlation between mean cumulative dose and either pCR or survival [29]. With respect to dose intensity, a retrospective analysis of randomized studies of first-line chemotherapy published between 1975 and 1989 demonstrated an improvement in objective response rates of between 12% and 16% and an improvement in median survival of between 2 and 4 months when the total dose intensity of cisplatin, doxorubicin or cyclophosphamide was increased by 1 unit (defined in terms of mg m^{-2} per week for each drug; [30]). However, there was no difference in objective response rates or median survival in a prospective randomized trial comparing low and high dose in a CP combination where the high-dose arm delivered nearly twice the dose intensity of the low-dose arm, though both received the same cumulative dose.

Paclitaxel has been shown to be active in recurrent disease (see below) and a number of studies, either ongoing or recently closed, are evaluating its place as part of the first-line treatment of EOC. The Gynaecological Oncology Group (GOG) have recently reported a randomized study in poor prognosis patients (suboptimally debulked) of cisplatin-paclitaxel vs. CP and shown a highly significant survival advantage for the former [31]. This regimen has become the gold standard treatment in the USA. However, many feel that this result needs to be confirmed.

Chemotherapy for Recurrent Disease

Epithelial ovarian cancer at presentation is a rewardingly chemosensitive neoplasm in most patients, but frustrating because of its propensity to relapse and its poor response to further chemotherapy. Chemotherapy options for those patients who relapse or for those with disease refractory to first-line treatment are invariably non-curative and include:

1. Retreatment with platinum analogues, single agent or in combination.
2. Retreatment with non-platinum drugs only.

3. Endocrine therapy.
4. Intraperitoneal treatment.

While there are many factors predicting for those patients who may require further chemotherapy, as discussed in the introduction to this section, there are unfortunately only a few factors that predict for response to chemotherapy in this setting. Patients requiring further treatment will include those who did not respond well to first-line chemotherapy or may even have progressed (primary drug resistance) and those who responded to first-line chemotherapy but relapsed after a disease-free interval (no proven drug resistance). Blackledge and colleagues showed that response in phase II trials was related to the interval between the end of initial treatment and the start of therapy for relapse [32]. The choice of second-line chemotherapy for EOC is influenced by these factors, i.e. the distinction between those patients whose neoplasm may still be platinum sensitive (i.e. initial response to platinum-based therapy and relapse more than 12 months after cessation of treatment) and those with platinum-resistant disease (i.e. progression during or within 12 months of first-line platinum-based chemotherapy).

Platinum Regimens

Seltzer and colleagues were probably the first to clearly document the value of retreating patients with cisplatin who had previously responded to this agent as first-line treatment; in a small study of 11 women the overall response to a rechallenge with cisplatin-based regimens was 72% (36% CR; [33]). However, Seltzer's group could not fully assess the role of cisplatin rechallenge, in that the drug was used in combination with other agents, nor did they address the issue of the relationship between the treatment-free interval and response.

Gore et al., in a 1990 study of 54 patients, examined the effect of rechallenging with cisplatin or carboplatin patients who previously responded to one or other platinum analogue: 43 patients were treated with a different analogue, 11 patients with the same analogue [34]. There was a non-statistically significant difference in response between patients (35%) who crossed over to the other platinum drug and those who were treated with the same analogue (9%) and there was no difference in survival between the two groups. However, survival was significantly improved for all responders compared to non-responders ($p = 0.001$). Crucially, they noted that a powerful prognostic factor for predicting response to further platinum rechallenge was the duration of the treatment-free interval, with response rates as follows: treatment-free interval < 1 year, 17%; 1–2 years, 27%; and > 2 years 57% (Table 18.1). The treatment-free interval also predicted for survival in the patients who responded.

Table 18.1 Relationship between response and treatment-free interval from the end of previous therapy and the initiation of platinum rechallenge in ovarian cancer (Combined data from Gore et al. [34] and Markman et al. [35])

Treatment-free interval	*n*	Response rate
< 12 months	64	22%
12–24 months	26	31%
> 24 months	36	69%

These data were later confirmed in an analysis of 72 patients for the Memorial Sloan Kettering (Table 18.1; [35]). The patients for analysis were selected on the basis of having been treated with two or more cisplatin/carboplatin-based chemotherapy regimens (though all with cisplatin initially), and having a treatment-free interval of 4 or more months between treatments; only three patients had demonstrated progressive disease with initial chemotherapy, while the other 69 patients demonstrated an initial response. The response rates in this study were: treatment interval < 1 year 27% (5% pCR); 1–2 years, 33% (11% pCR); and more than 2 years 59% (22% pCR). Seven patients achieved a pCR with both initial cisplatin treatment and again when rechallenged with cisplatin treatment, but this was shorter at rechallenge (median 14 months) than with initial treatment (median 35 months). The overall median survival of patients who responded to second-line cisplatin-based therapy was approximately 2 years from the initiation of second-line cisplatin: interestingly, the treatment-free interval was not shown to influence the subsequent survival. A smaller prospective study of 19 patients by Gershenson and colleagues demonstrated 100% response (50% CR) in patients rechallenged with cisplatin who had demonstrated an initial response to cisplatin and lends further weight to the strategy of rechallenge with platinum analogues at relapse [36]. One great advantage of platinum rechallenge is that if single agent carboplatin is used toxicity may be minimal.

Other single agent platinum analogues have also been tested in relapsed disease, including iproplatin and zeniplatin. Iproplatin was tested in 97 patients who had recurrences after prior cisplatin or carboplatin administration. A response rate of 12% was observed in 78 patients with platinum-resistant disease, with an overall response rate of 26% among 19 patients whose disease was still to be considered platinum sensitive [37]. Zeniplatin appeared to show definite but modest activity in early phase II studies examining its effect in the treatment of relapsed EOC, but further development of the drug was curtailed because of its severe renal toxicity [38, 39].

While rechallenge with single agent platinum analogues in platinum-sensitive recurrent disease produces encouraging response rates, these may be improved when platinum-based combination chemotherapy is used. Weekly cisplatin in combination with epirubicin or etoposide in 40 patients with recurrent platinum-sensitive EOC produced a 60% (25% CR) response rate, a median duration of response of 7 months and a median survival of 13.5 months. As previously observed, the longer the disease-free interval, the greater the likelihood of response to the salvage treatment [40]. Carboplatin in combination with cyclophosphamide produced a response rate of 46% in 13 patients with platinum-sensitive disease, but only 20% in 15 patients with platinum-resistant disease [41]. This latter study produced a higher than expected response rate in platinum-resistant disease, although its definition included patients with treatment-free intervals of up to 12 months.

Recent phase II studies at the Royal Marsden Hospital have demonstrated that continuous infusional 5-FU, together with bolus cisplatin and epirubicin (ECF) at 3-weekly intervals, is a very active chemotherapy regimen in both primary breast cancer and advanced gastric cancer [42, 43]. We are currently examining its efficacy in recurrent EOC and have treated 30 patients, 16 with primary platinum-resistant EOC (relapsed less than 4 months from last treatment) and 14 with possible platinum-sensitive EOC (relapsed between 4 and 12 months from last treatment). The overall response rate was 43%, with a median duration of response of 7+ months (range 2+ to 13+ months). The response rate in the platinum-resistant group was surprisingly high, 25%. ECF is generally well tolerated but side-effects from infusional 5-FU, including palmar plantar erythema, stomatitis and enteritis, can be encountered [42, 43].

Non-platinum regimens

Unfortunately, the greater number of patients requiring salvage chemotherapy will have platinum-resistant disease, often following more than one previous treatment. Several chemotherapy agents have been identified which are useful in this setting, including taxol, hexamethylmelamine, anthracyclines, alkylating agents and etoposide. Other agents currently being studied and therefore with less established efficiency include gemcitabine, topotecan and the oral platinum agent JN 218.

Taxanes

The taxanes, taxol (paclitaxel) and taxotere (docetaxel), exert their anti-tumour effect by promoting tubulin polymerization, stabilizing microtubules. The formation of stable microtubules inhibits the normal dynamic reorganization of the microtubule network that is essential for cell division [44]. Taxol is extracted from the bark of the Pacific yew tree (*Taxos brevifolia*); taxotere is a semisynthetic analogue of taxol, prepared from extracts of needles of the European yew tree (*Taxos baccata*).

The novel mechanism of action of taxol no doubt contributes to the encouraging response rates seen in patients with EOC whose disease is or has become refractory to cytotoxics with different mechanisms of action, in particular platinum drugs. Phase II studies of single agent taxol have demonstrated a response rate of 18.5–37% in platinum-refractory EOC (Table 18.2; [45–50]). However, the duration of response is disappointingly low, usually 3–6 months. Patients who still have potentially platinum-sensitive EOC achieve higher response rates of 40–44% [46, 49] to single agent taxol. These data suggest that, from a practical point of view, in the palliative treatment of patients with platinum-sensitive recurrent EOC, taxol is not clearly superior to rechallenge with further platinum-based chemotherapy, particularly for those patients relapsing after 2 years in whom a 59% response rate to more platinum treatment might be expected.

Taxol was initially perceived as an unusually dangerous drug because of two potentially dangerous toxicities, i.e. major hypersensitivity reactions and disturbances of cardiac rhythm. However, as investigators have become increasingly familiar and confident with the agent, methods of controlling its toxicities have been devised [51, 52]. The former side-effect is abrogated by steroid premedication and the latter is no more frequently encountered than with some other chemotherapeutic agents in clinical use. The predominant adverse effects are leucopenia, anaemia and neuropathy (reviewed by Spencer and Faulds [52]). Leucopenia, predominantly neutropenia, is the principal dose-limiting toxicity, but it is usually of short duration (3–10 days) and rarely delays the next cycle of treatment or results in febrile episodes. Neutropenia does not appear to be

Table 18.2 Phase II single agent studies of taxol in ovarian cancer

Study authors	Patients evaluable for response	No. of prior chemotherapies	Planned 3-weekly dose of taxol ($mg\,m^{-2}$)	Platinum-sensitive (%)	Platinum-persistent (%)	All patients (%)
Thigpen et al. [49]	43	1	170	44	33	37
Trimble et al. [50]	652	⩾ 3	135	–*	22	22
Einzsig et al. [45]	29	1	250	–	–	21
McGuire et al. [46]	40	⩾ 1	200–250	40	24	30
Seewaldt et al. [47]	100	⩾ 3	135†	–*	25	25
ten Bokkel Huinink et al. [48]	286	⩾ 1	135–175	–*	18.5	18.5

*No platinum-sensitive disease patients entered.
†G-CSF support.

cumulative and may be less severe with a 3 h infusion than 24 h infusion at the same dose. Anaemia and thrombocytopenia are rarely troublesome. Essentially, neuropathy is the most common neurotoxic effect of taxol and is frequent as the dose approaches 250 mg m^{-2}. It is dose related, cumulative and exacerbated by concomitant use of platinum analogues. Motor and sensory neuropathies, myopathy effects and CNS effects are less commonly described. A significant side-effect of taxol, particularly as it relates to its use in relapsed, therefore non-curative, disease is alopecia which is invariable.

Hexamethylmelamine

Hexamethylmelamine (HMM) has been investigated since 1964 as an anti-tumour agent for EOC. The mechanism of HMM cytotoxicity is unknown, but its molecular structure is similar to that of alkylating agents. The drug's role in primary combination chemotherapy and in salvage therapy is unclear. Response rates of 30–40% have been demonstrated in untreated patients [53, 54]. Moore and colleagues treated 44 evaluable patients with 100–300 mg day^{1} of HMM for 14 days on a 4-week cycle, the largest reported series of patients with persistent or recurrent EOC treated with single agent HMM [55]. The overall response rate was 20% (six CR, three PR) and there was a significant survival advantage among responding patients in whom the progression-free survival was 55% (overall survival was 88% at 3 years). All patients had received at least one previous chemotherapy regimen and 97% of patients had received a platinum analogue. However, another study in 52 patients with advanced EOC who were treated with single agent HMM at 260 mg m^{-2} orally per day for 14 days followed by 14 days off the drug found no objective responders and 42% of patients progressed while on treatment [56].

Vergote and colleagues examines hexamethylmelamine at a dose of 260 mg m^{-2} per day p.o. for 14 days each month in 50 patients with platinum-resistant disease [57]. In 39 patients with primary platinum-resistant disease, the response rate was only 8%, but of seven patients who relapsed within 6 months of receiving cisplatin, four (57%) responded to hexamethylmelamine. Hexamethylmelamine may therefore be of value in the treatment of patients with EOC who relapse early after platinum treatment.

Etoposide

Etoposide (VP-16-213) is a semi-synthetic podophyllotoxin which has clinically established chemotherapeutic activity in lymphoma, small cell lung cancer (SCLC) and non-seminomatous germ-cell tumours of the testis. In very recent years the drug has been reinvestigated as a useful palliative treatment for primary or secondary platinum-resistant EOC, particularly when administered orally. Etoposide inhibits the function of the DNA enzyme topoisomerase II and demonstrates most activity during the late S and early G2 phases of the cell cycle when topoisomerase II is functional. Consequent to this cell cycle phase specificity, it is not surprising that it is schedule dependent in vitro [58]. Marked clinical schedule dependency has also been demonstrated in patients with SCLC in whom the response to one i.v. dose was 10%, compared with 90% when the same total i.v. dose administered was divided into five daily fractions [59]. There is also some evidence that an even longer 8-day schedule is less myelotoxic than a 5-day schedule [60].

Etoposide has established clinical activity in the treatment of relapse and primary-resistant EOC. Seymour and colleagues have analysed five reported studies in such patients conducted between 1985 and 1990, in which 240 patients were treated with an overall response rate of 21% [61]. The studies all employed 3- or 4-day intravenous or oral schedules [62–66]. More recently, and against the background of the reported schedule dependency in SCLC, there have been two further reported studies of etoposide in the second-line treatment of EOC, employing 14-day oral schedules repeated at 3-weekly intervals [61, 67]. Seymour and colleagues demonstrated a 24% overall response rate in 47 patients with etoposide 50 mg p.o. b.d. which was similar to the previously reported 3- or 4-day schedule. In addition, toxicity for most patients was mild, and sporadic severe myelotoxicity was encountered, with two treatment-related deaths. They were forced to modify their schedule (originally 50 mg p.o. b.d. for 14 days) to 7 days treatment escalating to 10 then 14 days if well tolerated. Hoskins and Swenerton conducted a similar study in a cohort of 31 patients, demonstrating an overall response rate of 26%. The original study design allowed for etoposide to be delivered orally at 100 mg m^{-2} per day, but this proved to be too toxic in the first seven patients and the subsequent 24 patients received the drug at 100 mg p.o. stat [67]. Interestingly, this group did not dose modify further as the previous study did, although the later group may have encountered more toxicity by allowing the entry of ECOG 3 patients and more heavily pretreated patients into the study.

Etoposide is a useful but perhaps more importantly convenient, second- or third-line treatment for EOC. The outpatient nature of the treatment has to be balanced against the almost definite development of alopecia which may be too high a price for some women to pay for what is essentially palliative therapy. Also, there are reports of severe sudden neutropenia and deaths have been seen. Phase II studies have not suggested the same schedule dependency as seen with SCLC, but randomized trials have not been conducted. In the absence of these, the protracted oral schedule of 100 mg p.o. daily (single or divided dose) for 14 days every 3 weeks still seems a reasonable chance. However, the more cautious schedule of starting with 7 days treatment, and escalating to 10 then 14 days if well tolerated, seems a pragmatic approach in the palliative setting, particularly when risk factors for severe toxicity apply, e.g. performance status ECOG 3, hepatic and renal impairment and previous myelosuppressive treatment.

Endocrine Therapy

Endocrine manipulations are of proven therapeutic efficacy in many tumours arising from tissues under hormonal control, e.g. breast, prostatic and endometrial cancer. Levels of oestrogen receptors and progesterone receptors have some predictive value for response to endocrine treatment in breast and endometrial cancer, as do levels of androgen receptors in prostatic cancer, though the relationship is not a simple one. The endocrine gland origin of EOC and the presence of oestrogen and progesterone receptors in approximately 50% of EOC tumours does suggest that a similar role for endocrine manipulation

Table 18.3 Published trials of progestational agents in recurrent or refractory ovarian carcinoma (After Ahlgren et al. [72])

Study	Agent	Dose	Pt no.	Response (%)	Duration (months)
Jolles [73]	HP	250 mg kg^{-1}	10	10	4+
Varga and Henriksen [74]	HP	1250–7000 mg week^{-2}	8	12	3
Malkasian et al. [75]	DHPM	100–800 mg day^{-1}	9	22	30, 40
Kauffman [76]	MPA	2000–3000 mg day^{-1}	11	9	18+
Malkasian et al. [77]	MPA	100–400 mg day^{-1}	19	5	44
Slayton et al. [78]	MPA	1000 mg week^{-1}	19	0	-
Mangioni et al. [79]	MPA	500–800 mg day^{-1}	33	15	5–8+
Aabo et al. [80]	MPA	600 mg m^{-2} per day	27	4	5
Trope et al. [81]	MPA	500 mg day^{-1}–500 mg week^{-1}	25	4	3+
Hamerlynck et al. (EORTC) [82]	MPA	500 mg day^{-1}–1000 mg week^{-1}	41	2	5
Malfetano et al. (EORTC) [83]	MPA	150 mg day^{-1}	24	43	-
Geisler [71]	MA	800–400 mg day^{-1}	23	43	4–65+
Sikic et al. (NCOG) [84]	MA	800–400 mg day^{-1}	47	8	4–18
Ahlgren et al. (HAOP) [72]	MA	800–400 mg day^{-1}	35	0	-

might exist for the treatment of patients with EOC. While the results of clinical trials of endocrine therapy for recurrent or refractory EOC have been variable and mostly disappointing, the non-toxic nature of such therapy and the observed clear benefits for those individual patients that do respond ensure its continuing use in the palliative setting.

Oestrogen and androgen therapy have both been attempted in patients with EOC. A phase II study demonstrated a 28% partial response rate in 14 patients with advanced disease who received 15–30 mg diethystilboestrol daily, some patients having previously received radiotherapy or chemotherapy or both [68]. High-dose androgens in the form of fluoxymesterone 10 mg p.o. twice daily have also been tested in a phase II study of 16 patients with advanced refractory EOC, but no responses were seen [69]. No other trials have been reported of single agent oestrogen or androgen stimulation and these agents are not now used in clinical practice.

Medroxyprogesterone acetate (MPA) and megestrone acetate (MA) are synthetic progestational agents, MPA being 20–35 times as potent as progesterone and with a duration of activity of 20–30 days. The mechanism of action of progestational agents is unknown, but it may be partly due to a direct inhibition of RNA/DNA synthesis in the EOC cell [70]. Of 14 phase II studies exploring the efficacy of progestational agents in recurrent or refractory EOC, response rates vary from 0% to 43% and the duration of response ranges from 3 to 65+ months (Table 18.3). It is interesting to note that while most studies have been conducted with MPA, the response rates are almost invariably lower than those produced with other progestational agents. The highest response in any trial of a progestational agent was 43% to megestrone acetate, reported by Geisler in 23 patients with advanced EOC [71]. Two further larger trials conducted by the NCOG and the

MAOP failed to confirm this apparently superior activity of MA [72, 84]. Geisler's study may have produced unexpectedly good results because it included previously untreated patients and patients who had received initial suboptimal chemotherapy; in addition, only those with papillary serous histology were treated. There is no evidence from 14 phase II studies of progestational agents that higher doses are associated with better results, although there are suggestions that it is possible to use too low a dose. MPA at 400 mg day^{-1} is a good compromise dose and this is the practice of our institution.

Intraperitoneal Chemotherapy

In the last 16 years intraperitoneal chemotherapy has evolved from a pharmacological model into an established treatment option for a subset of patients with EOC. This form of regional drug delivery has mainly been used as a salvage treatment for patients with EOC, although recently encouraging results have been obtained utilizing this technique as part of initial therapy for EOC. Numerous phase I and II studies have been performed with virtually all the drugs with established activity against EOC. However, these studies have usually contained less than 40 patients, are non-randomized and therefore little better than feasibility studies. The basic pharmacological principle underlying intraperitoneal chemotherapy is that if the concentration of drug within the tumour can be increased, then response rates and survival may also improve. The peritoneal cavity can be exposed to 10–1000-fold higher concentrations of certain drugs than would be measured in the systemic circulation.

Cisplatin is the most frequently administered intraperitoneal chemotherapy in relapsed EOC and, as with systemic chemotherapy for relapsed disease, a history of previous response to intravenous treatment, a greater than 6-month progression-free survival and very small volume disease all predict for a further response when intraperitoneal treatment is initiated [35]. A retrospective analysis by Markman and colleagues of two phase II trials of intraperitoneal cisplatin therapy in 89 patients with persistent/recurrent ovarian carcinoma showed an overall response rate of 56% and 33% CR rate in the 52 patients who previously demonstrated a response to systemic cisplatin treatment, compared with 11% and 3% respectively in the 37 patients who were not prior responders to systemic treatment [35]. However, the most important factor defining the patients who may respond to intraperitoneal therapy is the size of the tumour nodules being treated. In the same retrospective analysis described above, 41 patients with microscopic disease or very small volume macroscopic disease (largest tumour nodule $\leqslant 0.5$ cm) was 34%, in contrast to 5% for 39 patients whose largest tumour mass was >1 cm in maximum diameter [35]. Markman also reported a study of 41 patients with relapsed small volume disease (largest tumour nodule < 1 cm) and demonstrated a pCR rate of 43% in 30 patients who had previously experienced a response to intravenous platinum-based treatment, compared with a pCR rate of only 9% in 11 patients who had failed to respond to systemic treatment [85]. A further study by Markman of intraperitoneal cisplatin and etoposide showed a 40% response rate in 25 patients with favourable pretreatment characteristics [86].

Intraperitoneal chemotherapy is still experimental and is a relative complex treatment requiring considerable commitment from the patient and therefore is not a particularly obvious choice for a palliative treatment. Furthermore, since only patients with small volume disease are likely to benefit and these patients tend to be asymptomatic, such an approach cannot be decided as palliative. Most workers in this field regard intraperitoneal chemotherapy as a treatment with curative rather than non-curative intent.

Conclusions

The majority of patients with advanced EOC, and virtually all patients with relapsed EOC, present the clinical dilemma of non-curable disease. Most centres now treat bad prognosis advanced disease and good prognosis (stage IC and II) disease with platinum-based combination chemotherapy. Response rates nearing 80% are used to justify this intensive though well-tolerated approach. However, most patients with advanced disease that are treated will eventually relapse and die of their disease. Stage IV disease has a particularly bad prognosis, and some centres such as our own offer these patients entry into phase II studies of new treatments. For example, cisplatin, epirubicin and infusional 5-FU is currently being investigated in this context by the London Gynaecological Oncology Group.

Similarly, patients with refractory and relapsed EOC can legitimately be treated by phase II drugs and novel therapies, considering the poor prognosis of these patients when treated with conventional treatment. However, when planning these approaches it is important to consider the toxicity of the new treatment compared to standard chemotherapy, e.g. rechallenge with carboplatin, HMM, etoposide, etc. Objective tumour responses in EOC are often followed by good palliation of symptoms which may be difficult to control otherwise, e.g. intestinal obstruction, intermittent abdominal pain. As with all non-curative treatments, the severity of symptoms, the ability to control them by methods other than chemotherapy, the chances of obtaining a response and the toxicity of treatment all need to be considered by doctor and patient together before chemotherapy is either started or withheld.

Cervical Cancer

Carcinoma of the uterine cervix is the fourth most common malignancy in Western women and the second leading cause of death from gynaecological malignancy. The widespread use of cytological screening has brought an increase in early detection and subsequent cure of precancerous and early lesions. In the past there was a situation similar to that which exists now in non-Western countries, i.e. cervical cancer being the most frequent tumour in the female population and the leading cause of death from malignancy in women.

Cervical cancer is best treated with either radiation therapy or radical surgery or both. Standard therapy varies according to the stage of disease and consists of total abdominal hysterectomy ± lymph node dissection ± radiation therapy with external beam radiation ± brachytherapy ± chemotherapy [87]. Attempts have been made to combine surgery, radiation and chemotherapy in aggressive primary treatment regimens, but at present this approach has not proved to be superior to standard therapy which does not include chemotherapy [87]. The improvements in overall survival for women with cervical cancer in the last two decades reflected a trend towards early diagnosis rather than improvement in treatment, since stage-specific 5-year survival rates remain unchanged. These are approximately 80% for early stage disease (Ia to IIa), 60–70% for stage IIb, and 40–50% for stage III [87]. Very occasional patients with stage IV disease may be cured by aggressive radiation treatment with pelvic exenteration [88]. For those patients who fail this approach or who are considered ineligible for it or who develop recurrent disease, systemic chemotherapy may be employed, but it is nearly always non-curative. Considering all stages, the recurrence rate for cervical carcinoma is approximately 35% [89]. The majority of patients with recurrent disease are not suitable for further curative surgery.

The vast majority of patients with carcinoma of the cervix have squamous cell histology and the role of chemotherapy has been best defined in this setting. Although a moderately chemosensitive tumour, chemotherapy for patients with recurrent and/or advanced squamous cell carcinoma (SCC) of the cervix has been characterized by short duration of response and little or no survival advantage [87, 90]. An additional challenging factor for chemotherapy in SCC of the cervix is the treatment of recurrent disease within a prior radiation field, as responses to chemotherapy tend not to occur in these areas [91–93].

Single Agent Platinum

Cisplatin is the most active single agent and is generally associated with a 30–40% overall response rate (reviewed in [87]) and the median duration of response to single agent cisplatin is 4–5 months, with the median duration of survival 6–7 months. The GOG have performed studies to determine the optimum dose schedule of cisplatin in SCC of the cervix [94]. A total of 444 evaluable patients with recurrent or refractory disease were randomized to receive first-line chemotherapy with one of three different cisplatin dosing regimens: 50 mg m^{-2} stat, 100 mg m^{-2} stat or 20 mg m^{-2} per day for 5 days; each treatment was cycled every 3 weeks. Cisplatin scheduling had no effect on median survival (less than 7 months), although overall response rates to the three arms were 21%, 31% and 25%, respectively, with a non-statistically significant trend towards improved efficacy for 100 mg m^{-2} of cisplatin as compared with the 50 mg m^{-2} regimen. A further study looking at cisplatin scheduling compared 50 mg m^{-2} stat with 50 mg m^{-2} as a 24 h infusion, both every 3 weeks, showed no difference in overall response rate which was 17% and 18%, respectively, and median length of survival which was 6–7 months [95]. Median duration of response in the five regimens examined in these two studies ranged between 4.1 and 5.5 months.

Carboplatin has been evaluated in a small number of patients. A phase II study of carboplatin 260 mg m^{-2} on day 1 and cisplatin 50 mg m^{-2} on day 2, every 4 weeks, in 42 women with advanced recurrent SCC of the cervix produced an overall response rate of 28.6% (one CR and 11 PRs [97]). For all patients and for responders, median progression-free interval was 4.4 and 9.5 months, respectively, and the median survival was 8.9 months and 9.5 months, respectively. Platinum analogues such as carboplatin and iproplatin appear less active than cisplatin in cervical cancer. In a GOG randomized study comparing carboplatin 400 mg m^{-2} with iproplatin 270 mg m^{-2}, each cycled every 4 weeks, response rates of 15% (175 patients) and 11% (177 patients), respectively, were observed, with median survivals of 6.2 and 5.5 months, respectively [96]. None of the differences was statistically significant. Other smaller non-randomized phase II studies of carboplatin or iproplatin in the treatment of SCC of the cervix have demonstrated response rates in the order of 25%, with no apparent improvement in survival [97–99].

Platinum-based Combination Regimens

Platinum-based combination chemotherapy regimens produce more promising overall response rates than are produced with single agent treatment. A review of 16 non-randomized phase II studies of cisplatin-based combination chemotherapy in the treatment of recurrent/refractory SCC of the cervix has concluded that the improvement in objective response rates is largely due to the increased number of partial responses and such regimens appear to have no effect on CR rates or median survival, as compared with single agent cisplatin therapy [87]. Some of these studies do, however, have strikingly improved overall response rates. A combination of cisplatin, vinblastine and bleomycin, alternating with 5-FU, doxorubicin, vincristine and cyclophosphamide, produced a 62% response rate among 43 patients [93]. This combination of drugs has not been tested in other studies. However, cisplatin, vinblastine and bleomycin in combination but in a non-alternating regimen produced a response rate of 66% in 33 patients, with a median response duration greater than 6 months for complete responders and 4.5 months for partial responders, and a median survival duration of 10 months for complete responders and 11 months for partial responders [100]. A combination of cisplatin, bleomycin and ifosfamide has produced overall response rates of 69% (34 patients) and 67% (14 patients) in two studies [101, 102], while the same combination in a third study of 20 patients produced an overall response rate of only 15% [103]. Another study examining the combination of cisplatin with 5-FU observed an overall response rate of 67% in 48 patients [104], although a further three studies examining the same regimen observed response rates of only 22–50% [105–107].

There are three reported randomized trials of combination cisplatin chemotherapy in the treatment of recurrent or refractory cervical carcinoma, but in only one of these is there a comparison between treatment with single agent cisplatin and combination cisplatin therapy [108]. This was a three-arm study, but poor patient accrual resulted in closure of the cisplatin only arm after only nine patients were entered, although in these an overall response rate of 33% was observed with a median response duration of 7.3 months and a median survival duration of 17.0 months. Results from the other two arms were disappointing, with an overall response rate of 25% for cisplatin plus mitomycin C, a median response duration of 7.2 months and a median survival duration of 7.0 months. The overall response rate of the third arm (cisplatin, mitomycin C, vincristine, bleomycin) was 22%, median response duration 5.4 months and median survival duration 6.9 months. Results are awaited from two further randomized studies comparing single agent cisplatin-based with combination cisplatin-based treatment from the EORTC and the GOG. The combination therapies being tested by these two groups are cisplatin, mitomycin C, vindesine and bleomycin (EORTC) and cisplatin, dibromodulcitol and ifosfamide (GOG).

Non-Platinum Drugs

Other standard non-platinum chemotherapeutic agents which have significant single activity in the treatment of advanced or recurrent cervical carcinoma include doxorubicin, ifosfamide, mitolactol and vincristine [109–116]. However, the response rates associated with these drugs are in the order of 20% and they are therefore only rarely used as single agent treatment in the setting of first-line treatment for SCC of the cervix. Recently, a phase II trial of ifosfamide, 5-FU and leucovorin was completed in 30 patients with recurrent SCC of the cervix and a relatively high response rate of 53% (33% CR) was obtained, considering that the regimen did not contain platinum [117]. Response rates outside and within the irradiated area were 68% and 27%, respectively, the median progression-free interval was 7 months and the median overall survival was 12 months.

Endometrial Cancer

Patients with advanced endometrial cancer (stage II, tumour outside the corpus but not outside the true pelvis; stage III, disease involvement of the bladder, rectum or extension outside the pelvis; stage IV metastatic disease) have a very poor prognosis, with 27% and 9% of patients, respectively, alive at 5 years [118]. The mainstay of treatment is hormonal therapy with progestogens, such as hydroxyprogesterone, medroxyprogesterone or megestrol acetate, all of which give similar results.

Endocrine Treatment

Patients with well-differentiated tumours tend to have the highest progesterone receptor positivity and this correlates with response; 63% and 58% of endometrial adenocarcinomas are rich in progesterone or oestrogen receptors, respectively [119]. These authors considered tumours were rich in a particular receptor if more than 40% of the epithelial cells were positive for the receptor in a immunohistochemical assay. They also showed that nearly 40% of tumours contain both oestrogen and progesterone receptors, but that 30% of patients expressed these receptors poorly – only 5% of the 111 tumours investigated were completely devoid of any oestrogen or progesterone receptor. It has been suggested that response to hormone therapy depends on a number of factors, but that the tumour hormone receptor status is particularly important. It has been reported that 89% of patients with progesterone-positive tumours respond to hormone manipulation compared to 64% of patients with oestrogen receptor positive tumours, whereas only 10–20% of patients with negative tumours respond [104, 120]. Other factors that predict for response to hormone therapy include the histological grade of the tumour, disease-free survival and site of metastases, with responses being commonest in pulmonary and lymph node disease and less common in pelvic recurrences, particularly in sites of previous irradiation.

Lentz has recently reviewed the literature on hormone therapy for advanced and recurrent endometrial cancer and showed the GOG data which demonstrates that the overall response rate for medroxyprogesterone acetate 50 mg orally three times a day is 14% [121]. The response rate to a slightly higher daily dosage

(200 mg) increased the response rate to 26% in a subsequent GOG study, but increasing the dose further to 1 g per day had no further effect and only 18% of patients responded to this high-dose regimen [120, 122]. Similar response rates have been found for other progestational agents, namely, megestrol acetate (320 mg daily orally) 11% and hydroxyprogesterone caproate (1 g per week i.m.) 14% [123, 124]. Response rates to tamoxifen 20–40 mg daily orally are approximately 20% [125]. Attempts have been made to increase the concentration of progesterone receptors in tumours by giving tamoxifen and medroxyprogesterone acetate sequentially and although response rates can be increased to 35%, there are no randomized data to support this approach [126]. Gonadatrophin-releasing hormone analogues have also been assessed and in one trial of 17 patients an overall response rate of 35% was seen [127]. Response rates to hormonal agents vary widely, but in one large review of over 1000 patients it was suggested that the average duration of response was 16–28 months [104]. The major advantage of hormone therapy for advanced endometrial cancer is that generally it is well tolerated with few side-effects, so that the therapeutic ratio is high. Patients occasionally complain of fluid retention with a feeling of bloating and sometimes indigestion, but generally speaking the main side-effect, particularly of progestogens, is one of wellbeing and increased appetite.

Chemotherapy

Muss reviewed the data on chemotherapy and showed that the most active agents in this condition are the platinum drugs, anthracyclines and 5-FU, giving response rates of 20–30%; however, response durations are short, 3–6 months [128]. Other agents that give response rates of 10–20% include hexamethylmelamine, mitozantrone, vincristine, cyclophosphamide and ifosfamide. Combination chemotherapy can give higher response rates, with Adriamycin, cyclophosphamide and cisplatin-containing regimens being the most commonly used. In four trials containing a total of 75 patients, the response rate to cisplatin plus Adriamycin was 61%; when cyclophosphamide was added to this combination in five trials of 157 patients the response rate was 46%; but when platinum was left out of this combination in four trials of 154 patients the response rate fell to 34%. Combination chemotherapy, particularly when platinum- and Adriamycin-based, is associated with increased toxicity, but response durations appear not to be increased. Randomized data in 223 patients, however, suggest that single agent Adriamycin is inferior to a cisplatin–Adriamycin combination, with response rates being 35% and 66%, respectively, and the progression-free interval increasing from 3.9 to 6.2 months; this was statistically significant ($p < 0.05$). However, there were no overall survival differences between the two arms of this trial [129].

A number of phase II studies have examined the role of combination chemoendocrine therapy and one randomized study suggests a survival benefit for the addition of megestrol acetate and tamoxifen to a cyclophosphamide, Adriamycin, 5-FU combination [130]. In this study, response rates were increased from 15% to 43% in favour of the combination therapy and this was statistically significant. However, there were no survival differences between the two arms of the study and the number of patients (43) in the trial was very small. Chemotherapy needs to be reserved for fit patients and consideration should be given to entering these patients into randomized prospective studies.

Vulvar Cancer

Carcinoma of the vulva is a rare malignancy, accounting for 3–4% of all gynaecological malignancies. Despite the accessibility of the lesion, patients often delay seeking medical help and up to 50% of patients have FIGO stage III or IV disease at time of initial diagnosis [131]. Surgery, plus or minus radiotherapy, is usually the treatment of choice. Chemotherapy has long been thought to be ineffective in this disease, although very limited data exist.

Duxorubicin and bleomycin have both shown limited single agent activity in inoperable SCC of the vulva [132, 133]. Cisplatin has little single agent activity. Combination chemotherapy consisting of bleomycin, vincristine, mitomycin C and cisplatin (BOMP) produced a response rate of 27% in 22 patients [134]. A care report of one women treated with the same regimen showed her to be disease free 20 months after treatment to CR with the same regimen [135]. Infusional 5-FU with or without mitomycin C, but in combination with radiotherapy, produced a response in seven of 15 patients with inoperable disease, all of whom are alive and disease free 5–45 months after treatment [136].

References

1. Conte PF, Bruzzone M, Chiara S et al. (1986) A randomized trial comparing cisplatin plus cyclophosphamide versus cisplatin, doxorubicin and cyclophosphamide in advanced ovarian cancer. J Clin Oncol 4:965–971.
2. Louie KG, Ozols RF, Myers CE et al. (1986) Long term results of a cisplatin-containing combination chemotherapy regimen for the treatment of advanced ovarian carcinoma. J Clin Oncol 4:1519–1585.
3. Nejit J, ten Bokkel Huinink W, van der Burg M et al. (1987) Randomised trial comparing two combination chemotherapy regimens (CHAP-5 vs CP) in advanced ovarian carcinoma. J Clin Oncol 5:1157–1168.
4. Omura GA, Bundy BN, Berek JS et al. (1989) Randomized trial of cyclophosphamide plus cisplatin with or without doxorubicin in ovarian carcinoma: a gynecologic Oncology Group study. J Clin Oncol 7:457–465.
5. Griffiths CT, Fuller AF (1978) Intensive surgical and chemotherapeutic management of advanced ovarian cancer. Surg Clin North Am 58:131–142.
6. Declos L, Quinlan EJ (1969) Malignant tumor of the ovary managed with post-operative megavoltage irradiation. Radiology 93:659–663.
7. Dembo AJ, Bush RS (1982) Current concepts in cancer of the ovary treatment of stages III and IV. Choice of post-operative therapy based on prognostic factors. Int J Radiat Oncol Biol Phys 8:893–897.
8. Griffiths CT (1975) Surgical resection of bulk tumor in the primary treatment of ovarian carcinoma. Symposium on ovarian cancer. Natl Cancer Inst Monogr 42:101–104.
9. Omura GA, Brady MF, Homesley HD, Yordan E, Major FJ, Buchsbaum HJ, Park RC (1991) Long-term follow-up and prognostic factor analysis in advanced ovarian carcinoma: the Gynecologic Oncology Group Experience. J Clin Oncol 9:1138–1150.
10. Smith JP, Day TG (1979) Review of ovarian cancer at the University of Texas Systems Cancer Center, MD Anderson Hospital and Tumor Institute. Am J Obstet Gynecol, 135:984–993.
11. Day TG, Gallager HS, Rutledge FN (1975) Epithelial carcinoma of the ovary: prognostic importance of histologic grade. Natl Cancer Inst Monogr 42:15–21.
12. Decker DG, Mussey E, Williams TJ (1972) Grading of gynecologic malignancy:

epithelial ovarian cancer. In: Proceedings of the 7th National Cancer Congress. J.B. Lippincott, Philadelphia, pp223–231.
13. Ozols RF, Garvin AJ, Costa J et al. (1980) Advanced ovarian cancer: correlation of histologic grade with response to therapy and survival. Cancer 45:572–581.
14. Aure JC, Hoeg K, Kolstad P (1971) Clinical and histologic studies of ovarian carcinoma. Long-term follow up of 900 cases. Obstet Gynecol 37:1–9.
15. Kottmeir HL (1971) Ovarian cancer with special regard to radiotherapy. J Roentgenol Rad Ther Nucl Med 111:417–421.
16. Perez CA, Walz BJ, Jacobson PL (1975) Radiation therapy in the management of carcinoma of the ovary. Natl Cancer Inst Monogr 42:119–125.
17. Smith JP, Rutledge F, Wharton JT (1972) Chemotherapy of ovarian cancer: new approaches to treatment. Cancer 30:1565–1571.
18. Young RC, Hubbard SP, DeVita VT (1974) The chemotherapy of ovarian carcinoma. Cancer Treat Rev 1:99–110.
19. Mogensen O, Mogensen B, Jakobsen A (1990) Predictive value of CA125 during early chemotherapy of advanced ovarian cancer. Gynecol Oncol 37:44–46.
20. Bertelsen K, Jacobsen A, Andersen JE et al. (1987) A randomized study of cyclophosphamide and cisplatin with or without doxorubicin in advanced ovarian cancer. Gynecol Oncol 28:161–169.
21. Bertelsen K (1990) Tumour reduction surgery and long term survival in advanced ovarian cancer. A DACOVA study. Gynecol Oncol 38:203–209.
22. Rubin SC, Hoskins WJ, Hakes TB et al. (1988) Recurrence after negative second-look laparatomy for ovarian cancer: analysis of risk factors. Am J Obstet Gynecol 159:1094–1098.
23. Copeland LJ, Gershenson DM (1986) Ovarian cancer recurrences in patients with no macroscopic tumor at second-look laparotomy. Obstet Gynecol 68:873–874.
24. Advanced Ovarian Cancer Trialists Group (1991) Chemotherapy in advanced ovarian cancer: an overview of randomised clinical trials. Br Med J 303:884–893.
25. Ozols RF, Young RC (1984) Chemotherapy of ovarian cancer. Semin Oncol 11:251–263.
26. Conte PF, Alama A, Rubagooti A et al. (1989) Cell kinetics in ovarian cancer. Relationship to clinicopathologic features, responsiveness to chemotherapy and survival. Cancer 64:1188–1191.
27. A'hern RP, Gore ME (1995) Impact of doxorubicin on survival in advanced ovarian cancer. J Clin Oncol 13:726–732.
28. Ozols RF (1992) Chemotherapy for advanced epithelial ovarian cancer. Hematol Oncol Clin North Am 6:879–894.
29. Bertelsen K, Jakobsen A, Stroyer I et al. (1993) A prospective randomized comparison of 6 and 12 cycles of cyclophosphamide, Adriamycin and cisplatin in advanced epithelial ovarian cancer: a Danish Ovarian Study Group trial (DACOVA). Gynecol Oncol 49:30–36.
30. Torri V, Korn EL, Simon R (1993) Dose intensity analysis in advanced ovarian cancer patients. Br J Cancer 67:190–197.
31. McGuire WP, Hoskins WJ, Brady MF et al. (1995) Taxol and cisplatin (TP) improves outcome in advanced ovarian cancer (AOC) as compared to cytoxan and cisplatin (CP). Proc Am Soc Clin Oncol 14:771.
32. Blackledge G, Lawton F, Redman C et al. (1989) Response of patients in phase II studies of chemotherapy in ovarian cancer: implications for patient treatment and the design of phase II trials. Br J Cancer 59:650–653.
33. Seltzer V, Vogl S, Kaplan B (1988) Recurrent ovarian carcinoma: treatment utilizing combination chemotherapy including cis-diaminedichloroplatinum in patients previously responding to this agent. Gynecol Oncol 21:167–176.
34. Gore ME, Fryatt I, Wiltshaw E et al. (1990) Treatment of relapsed carcinoma of the ovary with cisplatin or carboplatin following initial treatment with these compounds. Gynecol Oncol 36:207–211.

35. Markman M, Reichman B, Hakes T et al. (1991) Responses to second-line cisplatin-based intraperitoneal therapy in ovarian cancer: influence of a prior response to intravenous cisplatin. J Clin Oncol 9:1801–1805.
36. Gershenson DM, Kavanagh JJ, Copeland LJ et al. (1989) Re-treatment of patients with recurrent epithelial ovarian cancer with cisplatin-based chemotherapy. Obstet Gynecol 73:798–802.
37. Weiss G, Green S, Alberts DS et al. (1991) Second-line treatment of advanced measurable ovarian cancer with iproplatin: a Southwest Oncology Group study. Eur J Cancer 27:135–138.
38. Markman M, DeMarco LC, Birkhofer M et al. (1993) Phase II trial of zeniplatin (CL 286 558), a new platinum compound, in patients with advanced ovarian cancer previously treated with organoplatinum-based therapy. J Cancer Res Clin Oncol 119:234–236.
39. Willemse PH, Gietema JA, Mulder NH et al. (1993) Zeniplatin in patients with advanced ovarian cancer, a phase II study with a third generation platinum complex. Eur J Cancer 29A:359–362.
40. Zanaboni F, Scarfone G, Presti M et al. (1991) Salvage chemotherapy for ovarian cancer recurrence: weekly cisplatin in combination with epirubicin or etoposide. Gynecol Oncol 43:24–28.
41. van der Burg ME, Hoff AM, van Lent M et al. (1991) Carboplatin and cyclophosphamide salvage therapy for ovarian cancer patients relapsing after cisplatin combination chemotherapy. Eur J Cancer 27:248–250.
42. Findlay M, Cunningham D, Nomran A et al. (1994) A phase II study in advanced gastro-oesophageal cancer using epirubicin and cisplatin in combination with continuous infusional 5-fluorouracil (ECF). Ann Oncol 5:609–616.
43. Smith IE, Walsh G, Jones A et al. (1995) High complete remission rates with primary neoadjuvant infusional chemotherapy for large early breast cancer. J Clin Oncol 13:424–429.
44. Thigpen JT, Blessing JA, Ball H et al. (1994) Phase II trial of paclitaxel in patients with progressive ovarian carcinoma after platinum-based chemotherapy: a Gynecologic Oncology Group study. J Clin Oncol 12:1748–1753.
45. Einzig AI, Wiernik PH, Sasloff J et al. (1990) Phase II study of Taxol in patients with advanced ovarian cancer. Proc Am Assoc Cancer Res 31:187.
46. McGuire WP, Rowinsky EK, Rosenshein NB et al. (1989) Taxol: a unique antineoplastic agent with significant activity in advanced ovarian epithelial neoplasms. Ann Intern Med 111:273–279.
47. Seewaldt VL, Greer BE, Cain JM et al. (1994) Paclitaxel (Taxol) treatment for refractory ovarian cancer: phase II clinical trial. J Clin Oncol 13:799.
48. ten Bokkel Huinink WW, Eisenhauer E, Swenerton K (1993) Preliminary evaluation of a multicenter randomized comparative study of TAXOL (paclitaxel) dose and infusion length in platinum treated ovarian cancer. Cancer Treat Rev 19:79–86.
49. Thigpen T, Blessing J, Ball H et al. (1990) Phase II trial of Taxol as second-line therapy for ovarian carcinoma: a Gynecologic Oncology Group study. Proc Am Soc Clin Oncol 9:156 (A604).
50. Trimble EL, Adams JD, Vena D et al. (1993) Paclitaxel for platinum-refractory ovarian cancer: results from the first 1000 patients registered to National Cancer Institute Treatment Referral Center 9103. J Clin Oncol 11:2405–2410.
51. Rowinsky EK, Eisenhauer EA, Chaudhry V et al. (1993) Clinical toxicities encountered with paclitaxel (TAXOL). Semin Oncol 20:1–15.
52. Spencer CM, Faulds D (1994) Paclitaxel – a review of its pharmacodynamic and pharmacokinetic properties and therapeutic potential in the treatment of cancer. Drugs 48:794–847.
53. Wharton JT, Rutledge F, Smith JP et al. (1979) Hexamethylmelamine: an evaluation of its role in the treatment of ovarian cancer. Am J Obstet Gynecol 133:833–844.

54. Young RC (1991) Hexamethylmelamine (Altretamine): Early National Cancer Institute trials. Cancer Treat Rev 18:31–35.
55. Moore DH, Valea F, Crumpler LS et al. (1993) Hexamethylmelamine/altretamine as second-line therapy for epithelial ovarian cancer. Gynecol Oncol 51:109–112.
56. Manetta A, MacNeill C, Lyter JA et al. (1990) Hexamethylmelamine as a single second-line agent in ovarian cancer. Gynecol Oncol 36:95–96.
57. Vergote I, Himmelmann A, Franbendal B et al. (1992) Hexamethylmelamine as a second line therapy in platin-resistant ovarian cancer. Gynaecol Oncol 47:282–286.
58. Hill BT, Whelan RDH, Rupniak HT et al. (1981) A comparative assessment of the in vitro effects of drugs on cells by means of colony assays or flow microfluorimetry. Cancer Chemother Pharmacol 7:21–26.
59. Slevin ML, Clark PI, Joel SP et al. (1989) A randomised trial to evaluate the effect of schedule on the activity of etoposide in small-cell lung cancer. J Clin Oncol 7:1333–1340.
60. Slevin ML, Clark PI, Joel SP et al. (1989) A randomised trial to examine the effect of more extended scheduling of etoposide administration in small cell lung cancer (meeting abstract). Proc Am Soc Clin Oncol 8:236 (abstract 921).
61. Seymour MT, Mansi JL, Gallagher CJ et al. (1994) Protracted oral etoposide in epithelial ovarian cancer: a phase II study in patients with relapsed or platinum-resistant disease. Br J Cancer 69:191–195.
62. Eckhardt S, Hernadi Z, Thruzo L et al. (1990) Phase II clinical evaluations of etoposide (VP-16-213, Vepesid registered) as a second line treatment in ovarian cancer. Oncology 47:289–295.
63. Hansen F, Malthe I, Krog H (1990) Phase II clinical trial of VP-16-213 (etoposide) administered orally in advanced ovarian carcinoma. Gynecol Oncol 36:369–370.
64. Hillcoat BL, Campbell JJ, Pepperell R et al. (1985) Phase II trial of VP-16-213 in advanced ovarian carcinoma. Gynecol Oncol 22:162–166.
65. Kavanagh JJ, Moris M, Smalldowe L et al. (1989) A randomised trial of carboplatin versus variably timed continuous infusion etoposide (VP 16) in refractory epithelial ovarian cancer (meeting extract). Proc Am Soc Clin Oncol 8:A637.
66. Kuhnle H, Meerpohl HG, Lenaz et al. (1988) Etoposide in cisplatin-refractory ovarian cancer (meeting abstract). Proc Am Soc Clin Oncol 7:137 (A527).
67. Hoskin PJ, Swenerton KD (1994) Oral etoposide is active against platinum-resistant epithelial ovarian cancer. J Clin Oncol 12:60–63.
68. Long RTL, Evans AM (1963) Diethystilboestrol as a chemotherapeutic agent for ovarian cancer. Mo Med 60:1125–1127.
69. Kavanagh JJ, Wharton JT, Roberts WS (1987) Androgen therapy in the treatment of refractory epithelial ovarian cancer. Cancer Treat Rep 71:537–538.
70. Darwish DH (1978) The effects of sex steroid hormones on the in vitro synthesis of DNA by malignant ovarian tumours. Br J Obstet Gynecol 85:627–633.
71. Geisler HE (1983) Megestrol acetate for the palliation of advanced ovarian carcinoma. Obstet Gynecol 61:95–98.
72. Ahlgren JD, Ellison NM, Gottlieb RJ et al. (1993) Hormonal palliation of chemoresistant ovarian cancer: three consecutive phase II trials of the Mid-Atlantic Oncology Program. J Clin Oncol 11:1957–1968.
73. Jolles B (1962) Progesterone in the treatment of advanced malignant tumours of breast, ovary and uterus. Br J Cancer 16:209–221.
74. Varga A, Henriksen E (1964) Effect of 17-alpha-hydroxyprogesterone 17-*n*-carproate on various pelvic malignancies. Obstet Gynecol 23:51–62.
75. Malkasian GD Jr, Decker DG, Jorgensen EO et al. (1973) 6-dehydro-6, 17-dimethylprogesterone (NSC-123018) for the treatment of metastatic and recurrent ovarian carcinoma. Cancer Chemother Rep 57:241–242.
76. Kauffman RJ (1966) Management of advanced ovarian carcinoma. Med Clin North Am 50:845–856.

77. Malkasian GD Jr, Decker DG, Jorgensen EO et al. (1977) Medroxyprogesterone acetate for the treatment of metastatic and recurrent ovarian cancer. Cancer Treat Rep 61:913–914.
78. Slayton RE, Pagano M, Creech RH (1981) Progestin therapy for advanced ovarian cancer: a phase II Eastern Cooperative Oncology Group trial. Cancer Treat Rep 65:895–896.
79. Mangioni C, Franceschi S, La Vecchia C et al. (1981) High-dose medroxyprogesterone acetate (MPA) in advanced epithelial ovarian cancer resistant to first- or second-line chemotherapy. Gynecol Oncol 12:314–318.
80. Aabo K, Pedersen AG, Hald I et al. (1982) High-dose medroxyprogesterone acetate (MPA) in advanced chemotherapy-resistant ovarian carcinoma: a phase II study. Cancer Treat Rep 66:407–408.
81. Trope C, Johnsson JE, Sigurdsson K et al. (1982) High-dose medroxyprogesterone acetate for the treatment of ovarian carcinoma. Cancer Treat Rep 66:1441–1443.
82. Hamerlynck JVThH, Maskens AP, Mangioni C et al. (1985) Phase II trial of medroxyprogesterone acetate in advanced ovarian cancer. An EORTC Gynecologic Cancer Cooperative Group study. Gynecol Oncol 22:313–316.
83. Malfetano J, Beecham JB, Bundy BN et al. (1993) A phase II trial of medroxyprogesterone acetate in epithelial ovarian cancers. J Clin Oncol 16:149–151.
84. Sikic BI, Scudder SA, Ballon SC et al. (1986) High-dose megestrol acetate therapy of ovarian carcinoma: a phase II study by the Northern California Oncology Group. Semin Oncol 4(suppl 4):26–32.
85. Markman M, Rothman R, Hakes T et al. (1991) Second-line platinum therapy in patients with ovarian cancer previously treated with cisplatin. J Clin Oncol 9:389–393.
86. Markman M, Blessing JA, Major F et al. (1993) Salvage intraperitoneal therapy of ovarian cancer employing cisplatin and etoposide: a Gynecological Oncology Group study. Gynecol Oncol 50:191–195.
87. Alberts DS, Garcia DJ (1994) Salvage chemotherapy in recurrent or refractory squamous cell cancer of the uterine cervix. Semin Oncol 21:37–46.
88. Young RC (1991) Carcinoma of the uterine cervix. In: Wittes RE (ed) Manual of oncologic therapeutics: 1991/1992. Lippincott, Philadelphia, pp200–204.
89. DiSaia PJ (1989) Conservative treatment of the patient with gynaecologic cancer. CA Cancer J Clin 39:135–154.
90. Omura GA (1992) Current status of chemotherapy for cancer of the cervix. Oncology 6:27–32.
91. Hoskin PJ, Blake PR (1991) Cisplatin, methotrexate and bleomycin (PMB) for carcinoma of the cervix: the influence of presentation and previous treatment upon response. Int J Gynecol Cancer 1:75–80.
92. Potter ME, Hatch KD, Potter MY et al. (1989) Factors affecting the response of recurrent squamous cell carcinoma of the cervix to cisplatin. Cancer 63:1283–1286.
93. Sorbe B, Frankendal BO (1984) Bleomycin–Adriamycin–cisplatin combination chemotherapy in the treatment of primary advanced and recurrent cervical carcinoma. Obstet Gynecol 63:167–170.
94. Bonomi P, Blessing JA, Stehman FB et al. (1985) Randomized trial of three cisplatin dose schedules in squamous cell carcinoma of the cervix. A Gynecologic Oncology Group study. J Clin Oncol 3:1079–1085.
95. Thigpen JT, Blessing JA, DiSaia PJ et al. (1989) A randomised comparison of a rapid versus prolonged (24 hr) infusion of cisplatin in therapy of squamous cell carcinoma of the uterine cervix. A Gynecologic Oncology Group study. Gynecol Oncol 32:198–202.
96. McGuire WP, Arseneau J, Blessing JA et al. (1989) A randomised comparative trial of carboplatin and iproplatin in advanced squamous carcinoma of the uterine cervix. A Gynecologic Oncology Group study. J Clin Oncol 7:1462–1468.
97. Arseneau J, Blessing JA, Stehman FB et al. (1986) A phase II study of carboplatin in

advanced squamous cell carcinoma of the cervix (a Gynecologic Oncology Group study). Invest New Drugs 4:187–191.
98. Lira-Puerto B, Silva A, Morris M et al. (1991) Phase II trial of carboplatin or iproplatin in cervical cancer. Cancer Chemother Pharmacol 28:391–396.
99. Weiss GR, Green S, Hannigan EV et al. (1990) A phase II trial of carboplatin for recurrent or metastatic squamous carcinoma of the uterine cervix: a Southwest Oncology Group study. Gynecol Oncol 39:332–336.
100. Wheeler HR, Levi JA, Tatersall MH et al. (1989) Dual non-cross-resistant combination chemotherapy for advanced squamous cervical carcinoma (CACX) Proc Am Soc Clin Oncol 8:165 (A645).
101. Kumar L, Bhargava VL (1991) Chemotherapy in recurrent and advanced cervical cancer. Gynecol Oncol 40:107–111.
102. Ramm E, Vergote IB, Kaern J et al. (1992) Bleomycin-ifosfamide-cisplatin (BIP) in pelvic recurrence of previously irradiated cervical carcinoma. A second look. Gynecol Oncol 46:203–207.
103. Carlson JA, Day TG, Allfgra JC et al. (1994) Methyl-CCNU, doxorubicin and cis-diammine-dichloro-platinum II in the management of recurrent and metastatic squamous carcinoma of the cervix. Cancer 54:211–214.
104. Kauppila A (1984) Progestin therapy of endometrial, breast and ovarian carcinoma. Acta Obstet Gynecol Scand 63:441–450.
105. Bonomi P, Blessing J, Ball H et al. (1989) A phase II evaluation of cisplatin and 5-fluorouracil in patients with advanced squamous cell carcinoma of the cervix: a Gynecologic Oncology Group study. Gynecol Oncol 34:357–359.
106. Coleman RE, Clark JM, Slevin ML et al. (1990) A phase II study of ifosfamide and cisplatin chemotherapy for metastatic or relapsed carcinoma of the cervix. Cancer Chemother Pharmacol 27:52–54.
107. Kim NK, Bang YJ, Kany YK (1989) A phase II trial of 5-fluorouracil (5-FU) infusion and cisplatin (FP) for advanced squamous cell carcinoma of the uterine cervix (SCCUC). Proc Am Soc Clin Oncol 8:166 (A647).
108. Alberts DS, Aristizabal S, Surwit EA et al. (1987) Primary chemotherapy for high risk recurrence cervix cancer. In: Surwit EA, Alberts DS (eds) Cervix cancer. Martinus Nijhoff, Boston, pp161–183.
109. Hannigan EV, Dinh TV, Dillard EA et al. (1989) Ifosfamide in cervical cancer: early phase II results in patients with advanced or recurrent disease. Proc Am Soc Clin Oncol 8:158 (A617).
110. Lira-Puerto V, Morales-Canfield F, Werna J et al. (1984) Activity of mitolactol in cancer of the uterine cervix. Cancer Treat Rep 68:669–670.
111. Malkasian GD,Decker DF, Green SJ et al. (1981) Treatment of recurrent and metastatic carcinoma of the cervix: comparison of doxorubicin with combination of vincristine and 5-fluorouracil. Gynecol Oncol 11:235–239.
112. Stehman FB, Blessing JA, McGehee R et al. (1989) A phase II evaluation of mitolactol in patients with advanced squamous cell carcinoma of the cervix. A Gynecologic Oncology Group study. J Clin Oncol 17:1892–1895.
113. Sutton GP, Blessing J, Homesley HD et al. (1989) Phase II trial of ifosfamide and mesna in advanced ovarian carcinoma: a Gynecologic Oncology Group study. J Clin Oncol 7:1672–1676.
114. Thigpen JT (1987) Single agent chemotherapy in carcinoma of the cervix. In: Surwit E, Alberts D (eds) Cervix cancer. Martinus Nijhoff, Boston, pp119–136.
115. Wallace HJ Jr, Hreschvshvn MM, Wilbanks GD et al. (1978) Comparison of the therapeutic effects of Adriamycin alone versus Adriamycin plus vincristine versus Adriamycin plus cyclophosphamide in the treatment of advanced carcinoma of the cervix. Cancer Treat Rep 62:1435–1441.
116. Wasserman TH, Carter SK (1977) The integration of chemotherapy into combined modality treatment of solid tumors: VII. Cervical cancer. Cancer Treat Rev 4:25–46.

117. Stornes I, Mejlholm I, Jakobsen A (1994) A phase II trial of ifosfamide, 5-fluorouracil and leucovorin in recurrent uterine cervical cancer. Gynecol Oncol 55:123–125.
118. Creasman WT, Weed JC Jr (1985) Carcinoma of the endometrium (FIGO stages I and II): clinical features and management. In: Coppleson M (ed) Gynecologic oncology: fundamental principles and clinical practice. Churchill Livingstone, New York, pp562–574.
119. Sivridis E, Buckley CH, Fox H (1993) Type I and type II estrogen and progesterone binding sites in endometrial carcinomas: their value in predicting survival. Int J Gynecol Cancer 3:80–88.
120. Thigpen JT, Blessing JA, DiSaia P et al. (1986) Oral medroxyprogesterone acetate in advanced or recurrent endometrial carcinoma: results of therapy and correlation with oestrogen and progesterone receptor levels. The Gynecologic Oncology Group experience. In: Baulier EE, Iacobelli S, McGuire WW (eds) Endocrinology and malignancy. Parthenon Publishers, Pearl River, NY, pp446–454.
121. Lentz SS (1994) Advanced and recurrent endometrial carcinoma: hormonal therapy. Semin Oncol 21:100–106.
122. Thigpen JT, Blessing J, Hatch K et al. (1991) A randomised trial of medroxyprogesterone acetate (MPA) 200 mg versus 1000 mg daily in advanced or recurrent endometrial carcinoma: a Gynecologic Oncology Group (GOG) study. Proc Am Soc Clin Oncol 10:A604.
123. Piver MS, Barlow JJ, Lurain JR et al. (1980) Medroxyprogesterone acetate (Depo-Provera) vs. hydroxyprogesterone caproate (Delalutin) in women with metastatic endometrial adenocarcinoma. Cancer 45:268–272.
124. Podratz KC, O'Brien PC, Malkasian GD et al. (1985) Effects of progestational agents in treatment of endometrial carcinoma. Obstet Gynecol 66:106–110.
125. Moore TD, Philips PH, Nerenstone SR et al. (1991) Systemic treatment of advanced and recurrent endometrial carcinoma: current status and future directions. J Clin Oncol 9:1071–1088.
126. Rendina GM, Donadio C, Fabri M et al. (1984) Tamoxifen and medroxyprogesterone therapy for advanced endometrial carcinoma. Eur J Obstet Gynecol Reprod Biol 17:285–291.
127. Gallagher CJ, Oliver RT, Oram DH et al. (1992) Gonadotropin-releasing hormone analog treatment for recurrent progestogen-resistant endometrial cancer. Proc Am Soc Clin Oncol 11:A704.
128. Muss HB (1994) Chemotherapy of metastatic endometrial cancer. Semin Oncol 21:107–113.
129. Thigpen T, Blessing J, Homesley H et al. (1993) Phase III trial of doxorubicin +/− cisplatin in advanced or recurrent endometrial carcinoma: a Gynecologic Oncology Group (GOG) study. Proc Am Soc Clin Oncol 12:A830.
130. Ayoub J, Audet-Lapointe P, Methot Y et al. (1988) Efficacy of sequential cyclical hormonal therapy in endometrial cancer and its correlation with steroid hormone receptor status. Gynecol Oncol 31:327–337.
131. Kucera H, Weghaupt K (1988) The electrosurgical operation of vulvar carcinoma with postoperative irradiation of inguinal lymph nodes. Gynecol Oncol 29:158–167.
132. Deppe G, Buruckner HW, Cohen CJ (1977) Adriamycin treatment of advanced vulval carcinoma. 50:13–14.
133. Trope C, Johnsson JE, Larsson G et al. (1980) Bleomycin alone or combined with mitomycin C in treatment of advanced or recurrent squamous cell carcinoma of the vulva. Cancer Treat Rep 64:639–642.
134. Belinson JL, Stewart JA, Richards A et al. (1990) Bleomycin, vincristine, mitomycin-C and cisplatin in the management of gynecologic squamous cell cancer. Gynecol Oncol 120:387–393.
135. Shimizu Y, Hasumi K, Masubuchi K (1990) Effective chemotherapy consisting of bleomycin, vincristine, mitomycin C and cisplatin (BOMP) for a patient with inoperable vulval cancer. Gynecol Oncol 36:423–427.

136. Thomas G, Dembo A, DePetrillo A et al. (1989) Concurrent radiation and chemotherapy in vulvar carcinoma. Gynecol Oncol 34:263–267.
137. Ahmed F, King DM, Nicol B et al. (1995) Preliminary results of infusional chemotherapy (cisplatin, epirubicin and 5-fluorouracil: ECF) for refractory and relapsed epithelial ovarian cancer. Pers comm.
138. Alberts DS, Garcia D, Mason-Liddil N (1991) Cisplatin in advanced cancer of the cervix: an update. Semin Oncol 18:11–24.
139. Bagley CM Jr, Young RC, Canellos GP et al. (1972) Treatment of ovarian carcinoma: possibilities for progress. N Engl J Med 287:856–862.
140. Belinson JL, Pretorius RG, McClure M et al. (1986) Hexamethylmelamine, methotrexate, 5-fluorouracil as second-line chemotherapy after platinum for epithelial ovarian malignancies. Gynecol Oncol 23:304–309.
141. Benedetti-Panici P, Greggi S, Scambia G et al. (1993) Cisplatin (P), bleomycin (B) and methotrexate (M) preoperative chemotherapy in locally advanced vulvar carcinoma. Gynecol Oncol 50:49–53.
142. Benedeti-Panici P, Scambia G, Greggi S et al. (1990) Doxorubicin and cyclophosphamide alternated with bleomycin and mitomycin C as a second-line regimen in advanced ovarian cancer resistant to cisplatin-based chemotherapy. Oncology 47:296–298.
143. Caldas, C, McGuire P (1993) Paclitaxel (Taxol) therapy in ovarian carcinoma. Semin Oncol 20:50–55.
144. Cannistra SA (1994) Paclitaxel in ovarian cancer: how can we make it better? J Clin Oncol 12:1743–1744.
145. Chambers SK, Lamb L, Kohorn EI et al. (1994) Chemotherapy of recurrent/advanced cervical cancer: results of the Yale University PBM-PFU Protocol. Gynecol Oncol 53:161–169.
146. Coleman R, Clark J, Gore M et al. (1989) A phase II study of mitozantrone in advanced carcinoma of the ovary. Cancer Chemother Pharmacol 24:200–202.
147. Coleman R, Towlson K, Wiltshaw E et al. (1990) Epirubicin for pretreated ovarian cancer (letter). Eur J Cancer 26:850–851.
148. Conte PF (1993) Role of anthracyclines in first line combination chemotherapy of ovarian carcinoma. Bull Cancer 80:152–155.
149. Dembo AJ, Bush RS, Beale FA (1979) Ovarian carcinoma: improved survival following abdominopelvic irradiation in patients with a completed pelvic operation. Am J Obstet Gynecol 134:793–800.
150. Ehrlich CE, Young PC, Cleary RE (1981) Cytoplasmic progesterone and estradiol receptors in normal, hyperplastic, and carcinomatous endometria: therapeutic implications. Am J Obstet Gynecol 141:539–546.
151. Kaern J, Trope C, Abeler V et al. (1990) A phase II study of 5-fluorouracil/cisplatinum in recurrent cervical cancer. Acta Oncol 29:25–28.
152. Kavanagh JJ, Roberts W, Townsend P et al. (1989) Leuprolide acetate in the treatment of refractory or persistent epithelial ovarian cancer. J Clin Oncol 7:115–118.
153. Laatikainen T, Neiminen U, Adlercreutz H (1979) Plasma medroxyprogesterone acetate levels following intramuscular or oral administration in patients with endometrial adenocarcinoma. Acta Obstet Gynaecol Scand 58:95–99.
154. Levi JA, Wheeler HR, Friedlander M et al. (1992) Dual sequential non-cross resistant chemotherapy for advanced stage squamous cell carcinoma of cervix. Gynecol Oncol 45:329–333.
155. McGuire WP 1995 Experimental chemotherapy. Hematol Oncol Clin North Am 6:927–940.
156. Markman M (1991) Intraperitoneal chemotherapy. Semin Oncol 18:248–254.
157. Morris M, Gershenson DM, Burke TW et al. (1994) A phase II study of carboplatin and cisplatin in advanced or recurrent squamous carcinoma of the uterine cervix. Gynecol Oncol 53:234–238.

158. Muggia FM, Muderspach L (1994) Platinum compounds in cervical and endometrial cancers: focus on carboplatin. Semin Oncol 21:35–41.
159. Omura G, Blessing J, Ehrlich C et al. (1986) A randomised trial of cyclophosphamide and doxorubicin with or without cisplatin in advanced ovarian carcinoma. Cancer 57:1725–1730.
160. Ozols RF, Garvin AJ, Costa J et al. (1979) Histologic grade in advanced ovarian cancer. Cancer Treat Rep 63:255–263.
161. Rutledge FN, Mitchell MG, Munsell MF et al. (1991) Prognostic indicators for invasive carcinoma of the vulva. Gynecol Oncol 42:239–244.
162. Slevin ML, Harvey VJ, Osborne RJ et al. (1985) A phase II study of tamoxifen in ovarian cancer. Eur J Cancer Clin Oncol 22:309–312.
163. Stewart LA, Parmar MK (1993) The results of a quantitative overview of chemotherapy in advanced ovarian cancer: What can we learn? Bull Cancer Paris 80:146–151.
164. Sutton GP, Blessing JA, Adcock L et al. (1989) Phase II study of ifosfamide and mesna in patients with previously treated carcinoma of the cervix. A Gynecologic Oncology Group study. Invest New Drugs 7:341–343.
165. Thigpen JT, Vance RB, Khansur T (1993) Second-line chemotherapy for recurrent carcinoma of the ovary. Cancer 71:1559–1564.
166. Tobias JS, Griffiths CT (1976) Management of ovarian carcinoma: current concepts and future prospects. N Engl J Med 294:818–822.

19 – Non-Curative Chemotherapy for Patients with Unknown Primary Cancers

F. Anthony Greco and John D. Hainsworth

Introduction

Cancer of unknown primary site is common, accounting for about 5% of cancer patients. Relatively little attention has been given to this group of patients, and treatment directed against these tumours has been slow to develop. Pessimism concerning the therapy and prognosis of these patients has been one major reason for the lack of effort. The patient with carcinoma of unknown primary is commonly visualized as elderly and debilitated with metastases at multiple sites. Early chemotherapy trials did not seem to provide much palliation and had negligible effect on survival. The heterogeneity of tumours represented in these patients has also made the design of therapeutic studies difficult. Many cancers with different biologies are represented. Effective palliative chemotherapy is now available for many types of advanced cancers, often providing substantial relief of symptoms and extending the length and quality of life. It follows that some patients with carcinoma of unknown primary site have sensitive or treatable tumours. A small minority of these patients have curable metastatic carcinoma (i.e. germ-cell tumours), and these relatively rare examples will not be discussed in detail. However, it must be stressed that precise identification of the lineage and biology of these tumours is often not possible, and a therapeutic plan is desired in an attempt to provide broad coverage for patients with "treatable" cancers. When one reviews the outcome of chemotherapy it is obvious that the major benefit for the majority of the "treatable" patients is palliative in nature (i.e. improvement of quality of life and/or duration of survival).

Recognition of some "treatable" patients within the heterogeneous population has been made possible by the identification of several clinical syndromes that predict chemotherapy responsiveness, and also by specialized pathological techniques which can aid in tumour characterization. Management of patients with cancer of unknown primary sites now requires appropriate clinical and pathological evaluation to identify "treatable" subgroups.

Most patients with cancer of unknown primary site are diagnosed with metastatic cancer after developing symptoms at a metastatic site. History, physical examination, chest radiograph and other appropriate diagnostic studies fail to identify the primary site. A diagnostic biopsy is often the first attempt to characterize the process. The initial light microscopic diagnosis almost always shows one of four histologies, which is used as a guideline for further evaluation of these patients. These four light microscopic pathological diagnoses are poorly differentiated neoplasm, adenocarcinoma, squamous carcinoma and poorly differentiated carcinoma.

Poorly Differentiated Neoplasm

This diagnosis means that the pathologist cannot distinguish carcinoma from other cancers, i.e. lymphoma, melanoma or sarcoma. Establishing the lineage of the tumour is important in this group of patients, since treatable cancers are common. The most frequent tumour for which specific, highly effective therapy is available is non-Hodgkin's lymphoma, representing about 50% of the tumours eventually identified by specialized pathological study [1–4]. Poorly differentiated carcinoma accounts for most of the remaining tumours with melanoma and sarcoma accounting for less than 15% of all patients. The evaluation of the poorly differentiated neoplasm requires specialized pathological studies. Immunoperoxidase staining, electron microscopy and chromosomal analysis are of proven value in the differential diagnosis of these tumours [5–17]. However, it is important to remember that the most common cause of a non-specific light microscopic diagnosis is an inadequate biopsy specimen. Fine-needle aspiration biopsy often provides inadequate amounts of tissue for definitive diagnosis of poorly differentiated tumours, since histology is poorly preserved and the ability to perform special studies is limited by the small biopsy size. A specific diagnosis can often be made simply by obtaining a larger biopsy. Close communication with the surgeon and pathologist is important if repeat biopsy is performed, since some pathological studies require special tissue processing. Some neoplasms remain unclassifiable by light microscopy, and require special pathological study.

Other than non-Hodgkin's lymphoma, most patients will be diagnosed with tumours where only palliative chemotherapy is possible. Treatment is obviously based on the specific diagnosis. In those with *poorly differentiated* carcinoma of unknown primary site, the treatment will be considered in the discussion which follows.

Adenocarcinoma of Unknown Primary Site

Clinical Characteristics

Adenocarcinoma is the most frequent light microscopic diagnosis in patients with neoplasms of unknown primary site, and accounts for approximately 60% of cases. The typical patient with this diagnosis is elderly, and has metastatic tumour at multiple sites. The sites of tumour involvement determine the clinical presentation; common metastatic sites include liver, lungs and bones.

The clinical course is usually dominated by symptoms related to the sites of metastases. During the clinical course, the primary site becomes obvious in only 15–20% of patients [18]. Even at autopsy, 20–30% of patients have no primary site detected. The most common primary sites identified at autopsy are the lung and pancreas [19] (approximately 40% of all cases). Other gastrointestinal sites (stomach, colon, liver) are also frequent, although adenocarcinomas from a wide variety of other primary sites are also occasionally encountered. Adenocarcinomas of the breast and prostate are relatively infrequent in this group of patients, in spite of being common cancer types.

In general, the prognosis for patients with adenocarcinoma of unknown primary site is poor, with a median survival of only 3–4 months. Many patients in this group have widespread metastases and poor performance status at the time of diagnosis. However, several subsets of patients with a much more favourable outlook are a part of this large group and initial evaluation can often identify these more treatable patients.

Pathology

The diagnosis of adenocarcinoma is usually made without difficulty on the basis of light microscopic features, and is based on the formation of glandular structures by neoplastic cells. Since these histological features are shared by all adenocarcinomas, the site of the primary cannot usually be determined by histological examination. Certain histological features are typically associated with a particular tumour type ("papillary features" with ovarian cancer, "signet ring cells" with gastric cancer); however, even these are not specific enough to be used as definitive evidence of the primary site. Immunoperoxidase stains are also of limited utility in identifying the site of origin of most adenocarcinomas. One exception is the stain for prostate-specific antigen, which is quite specific for prostate cancer and should be used in males with suggestive clinical findings. Positive immunoperoxidase staining for oestrogen receptor suggests metastatic breast cancer in women with metastatic adenocarcinoma.

The diagnosis of "*poorly differentiated* adenocarcinoma" does not appear to be the same as "*well-differentiated* adenocarcinoma", since these patients may be distinctive in both tumour biology and responsiveness to systemic therapy. The diagnosis of poorly differentiated adenocarcinoma is usually made when only minimal glandular formation is seen on histological examination. However, this diagnosis is sometimes made in tumours that exhibit positive staining for mucin, but have no glandular features on histological examination. It is clear that adenocarcinoma, poorly differentiated adenocarcinoma and poorly differentiated carcinoma are diagnoses which represent parts of a spectrum of tumour differentiation rather than specific, sharply demarcated entities. Different pathologists may use slightly different criteria for making each of these three diagnoses. It is therefore appropriate to perform additional pathological study with immunoperoxidase staining or electron microscopy in all "poorly differentiated adenocarcinomas". At present, evaluation and treatment of patients with poorly differentiated adenocarcinoma should follow the guidelines outlined for poorly differentiated carcinoma (see section on poorly differentiated carcinoma of unknown primary site, below).

Diagnostic Evaluation

The detection of a primary site is unusual in a patient presenting with adenocarcinoma of unknown primary site. The initial staging evaluation should therefore be performed to evaluate any clinical signs or symptoms and to determine the extent of metastatic disease. Routine initial evaluation should include a thorough history and physical examination (including pelvic examination in females), standard laboratory screening tests (full blood count, biochemistry, urinalysis), and chest radiography. All males should have a serum prostate specific antigen determination, and women with clinical presentation compatible with metastatic breast cancer should undergo mammography, since palliative therapy is available for patients with advanced prostate or breast cancer. Computed tomography of the abdomen can identify a primary site in 10–35% of patients; in addition, it is frequently useful in identifying additional sites of metastatic disease [20, 21]. Additional signs or symptoms should be evaluated with appropriate radiological studies. Extensive radiological evaluation of asymptomatic areas is rarely useful in identifying a primary site, and often results in confusing or false-positive information. Endoscopy of the stomach and colon is also of low yield in asymptomatic patients, although small, occult primary sites are occasionally identified.

Treatment

The group of patients with adenocarcinoma of unknown primary site contains several clinically defined subgroups, for which specific therapy is available. Effective therapy does not exist for most patients who do not fall into one of these subgroups, although some do benefit from empirical chemotherapy.

Women with Peritoneal Carcinomatosis

In women, adenocarcinoma causing diffuse peritoneal involvement usually originates in the ovary, although carcinomas arising in the gastrointestinal tract or breast can occasionally produce this syndrome. Several authors have described women with diffuse peritoneal carcinomatosis who have no primary site found in the ovaries or elsewhere in the abdomen at the time of laparotomy [22–27]. Some have arisen in high-risk families after prophylactic oophorectomy [28]. Many of these patients have histological features typical of ovarian carcinoma, such as papillary configuration or psammoma bodies. When histological features suggest ovarian carcinoma, this syndrome has been termed "multifocal extra-ovarian serous carcinoma" or "peritoneal papillary serous carcinoma". In the early 1980s, several ancedotal reports documented excellent responses to cisplatin-based chemotherapy in women with this syndrome [22, 23, 25, 26]. Several series of such patients treated with cisplatin-based chemotherapy have now been reported [24, 27, 29]. A group of 18 women with abdominal carcinomatosis and no primary site documented at laparotomy were reported from Vanderbilt University [27]. The clinical characteristics in this patient group were similar to those seen in patients with advanced ovarian carcinoma. Metastases in sites other than the peritoneal surfaces were unusual. Histological features frequently seen in carcinoma of the ovary were found in many of these patients; however, only seven of 18 patients had serous adenocarcinoma. Patients were treated according to standard guidelines for the management of advanced ovarian cancer, using initial surgical cytoreduction followed by cisplatin-based combination chemotherapy. Seven of 18 patients had complete clinical response to chemotherapy, and three have remained continuously disease free for more than 4 years after completing treatment. The median survival for the entire group was 23 months.

A similar group of 33 patients was treated with surgical cytoreduction and cisplatin-based chemotherapy at the Mayo Clinic [29]. All of these patients had papillary adenocarcinoma. Median survival of this group was 17 months; three patients were alive 7 years following treatment. In a third group of 31 patients, some of whom received single agent cisplatin or chlorambucil, median survival was 11 months, and two patients were long-term survivors [24].

In summary, some women with metastatic adenocarcinoma involving the peritoneal surface have tumours that are distinct in biology and are often responsive to chemotherapy. The site of origin of these carcinomas is speculative, but some may arise from the peritoneal surface. Optimal management of these patients includes aggressive surgical cytoreduction followed by postoperative chemotherapy. Most of these patients received cisplatin-based combination chemotherapy in the past, but the use of paclitaxel with cisplatin or carboplatin would also be reasonable. Some patients in this group can be expected to have complete response to therapy, but only a small percentage will have prolonged disease-free survival. The majority do obtain substantial palliation, but the therapy is not curative.

Women with Axillary Lymph Node Metastases

Metastatic breast cancer should be suspected in women who have axillary lymph node involvement with adenocarcinoma. Initial lymph node biopsy should include measurement of oestrogen and progesterone receptors; elevated levels provide strong evidence for the diagnosis of breast cancer [30]. If no other metastases are identified with routine staging evaluation, these women may have stage II breast cancer. Modified radical mastectomy has been recommended in such patients, even when physical examination and mammography are normal. In such cases, an occult breast primary is identified in a majority of patients, although the reported rate of identification has ranged from 44% to 82% [31–33]. Primary tumours are usually less than 2 cm in diameter; in occasional patients, only "non-invasive" tumour is identified in the breast [34]. Prognosis following primary therapy is similar to that of other patients with stage II breast cancer [31, 33, 34]. Small numbers of patients have received radiation therapy to the breast following axillary lymph node dissection, with similar results to those achieved with mastectomy [32, 35]. Axillary dissection alone is not recommended, since primary breast tumours will subsequently become manifest in approximately 50% of patients [19, 35]. The benefit of adjuvant systemic therapy following primary therapy is unknown, but it seems reasonable to follow guidelines established for adjuvant therapy of stage II breast cancer.

Women with metastatic sites in addition to axillary lymph nodes may also have metastatic breast cancer. These women should receive a trial of systemic therapy using guidelines for the treatment of metastatic breast cancer. Determination of oestrogen receptor status is of particular importance in these patients, since those with positive oestrogen receptors may derive major palliative benefit from hormonal therapy.

Men with Skeletal Metastases

Metastatic prostate carcinoma should be suspected in men with adenocarcinoma involving predominantly bone, particularly if the metastases are blastic. Elevated serum levels of prostate-specific antigen, or tumour staining with prostate-specific antigen, provides confirmatory evidence of prostate cancer in this clinical setting. Hormonal therapy may provide effective palliation.

Occasional patients have been reported with clinical presentations atypical for prostate cancer, in whom the diagnosis was suggested only by tumour staining for prostate-specific antigen [36, 37]. In general, these patients presented with metastases to the lung, mediastinal lymph nodes or upper abdominal lymph nodes, with no concomitant involvement of bone or pelvic lymph nodes. Some of these patients responded to hormonal therapy.

Other sources of metastatic adenocarcinoma to bone as the first manifestation of disease are bronchus, kidney, thyroid and colon. Therapeutic implications are characteristic of the primary tumour.

Empirical Chemotherapy for Adenocarcinoma of Unknown Primary Site

Most patients with adenocarcinoma of unknown primary site do not fit into any of the specific clinical subgroups outlined above. Systemic therapy has been ineffective in most of these patients, producing low response rates and few complete responses. Patients with poorly differentiated carcinomas as well as those with adenocarcinoma of unknown primary site were included in several of these series. The only drug that has been adequately studied as a single agent is 5-fluorouracil (5-FU); response rates ranged from 0% to 16% [18, 38, 39]. The FAM regimen (5-FU, Adriamycin, mitomycin C) and various modifications have also been used frequently, based on the demonstrated activity of these regimens against gastrointestinal cancers [40–47]. Response rates varied from 7% to 39%. However, median survival remained in the 4–11 month range, and long-term disease-free survivors were not reported.

Cisplatin has been included in several combination regimens reported recently [40, 44, 48–52]. Unlike its important role in the treatment of poorly differentiated carcinoma and poorly differentiated adenocarcinoma, cisplatin has no well-defined role in the treatment of well-differentiated adenocarcinoma of unknown primary site. In general, response rates have been somewhat higher with cisplatin-based regimens, but median survival has not changed and no long-term disease-free survivors have been reported. Toxicity is increased with cisplatin-based regimens, and therefore their routine use is not recommended.

At present, it seems reasonable to consider patients with good performance status for a trial of chemotherapy; regimens containing Adriamycin and mitomycin C have usually produced responses in 20–40% of patients. At present, no compelling evidence exists to include cisplatin in these regimens; however, cisplatin-containing regimens have been incompletely studied, as has the combination of 5-FU and high-dose leucovorin. In patients with widespread metastases and poor performance status, systemic chemotherapy is unlikely to be of benefit, and management may include supportive measures only.

Squamous Carcinoma of Unknown Primary Site

Squamous carcinoma at a metastatic site represents about 5% of cancers of unknown primary site. Treatment is more effective for patients who fit certain clinical syndromes; therefore appropriate evaluation is essential. However, even in the most favourable circumstances the majority of these patients are not cured, but do obtain important palliation and prolongation of survival.

Squamous Carcinoma Involving Cervical Lymph Nodes

The cervical lymph nodes are the most common metastatic site for squamous carcinoma of unknown primary. Patients are usually middle-aged or elderly, and many have a history of substantial tobacco and alcohol use. When the upper or mid-cervical lymph nodes are involved, a primary tumour in the head and neck region should be suspected. Optimal evaluation includes a thorough examination of the oropharynx, hypopharynx, nasopharynx, larynx and upper oesophagus by direct vision and fibrescopy, with biopsy of any suspicious areas. When the lower cervical or supraclavicular lymph nodes are involved, a primary lung cancer should be suspected. Fibreoptic bronchoscopy is indicated if the chest radiograph and head and neck examination are unrevealing. This diagnostic evaluation identified a primary site in 231 of 267 patients (87%) who had metastatic squamous carcinoma in cervical lymph nodes as the first manifestation of malignancy [53].

When no primary site is identified, treatment should be given to the involved neck. All reported series involve retrospective, single institution experiences, often using a variety of treatment modalities [54–68]. It is clear from these results, however, that a substantial percentage of patients can achieve long-term disease-free survival following local treatment modalities. Nevertheless, the majority of patients are destined to relapse. Similar results have been obtained using radical neck dissection, high-dose radiation therapy or a combination of these modalities. Not surprisingly, the bulk of disease in the involved neck influences outcome, with N_1 or N_2 disease having a significantly higher cure rate than N_3 or massive neck involvement. When surgical therapy alone is used as the primary treatment modality, a primary tumour in the head and neck subsequently becomes obvious in 20–40% of patients. The detection of a primary site is less common when radiation therapy is used, presumably due to the eradication of occult head and neck primary sites within the radiation field. Radiation therapy dosages and techniques should be similar to those used in patients with primary head and neck cancer [56]. Most authors recommend that the nasopharynx, oropharynx and hypopharynx be included in the radiation portal.

Patients with low cervical or supraclavicular lymph nodes are more likely to have a primary lung cancer, and treatment results are inferior in this group of patients. Nevertheless, patients with no detectable disease below the clavicle should be treated with the same approach as are patients with higher cervical nodes, since occasional patients will have long-term disease-free survival.

The role of chemotherapy in the treatment of patients with metastatic squamous carcinoma in cervical lymph nodes is undefined. One small non-randomized comparison of patients treated with either local modalities alone or local modalities combined with chemotherapy (cisplatin and 5-FU) showed a higher complete response rate (81% vs. 60%) and longer median survival time (37 months vs. 24 months) in patients receiving chemotherapy [58]. Larger, randomized studies are necessary to verify the role of chemotherapy. The role of neo-adjuvant chemotherapy in locally advanced head and neck carcinoma remains unproven; it is therefore unlikely that its role in this more unusual patient group will be defined in the near future.

Squamous Carcinoma Involving Inguinal Lymph Nodes

Most patients with squamous carcinoma involving inguinal lymph nodes have a detectable primary site in the genital or anorectal areas. In females, careful examination of vulva, vagina and cervix is important, with biopsy of any suspicious areas. Males should have careful inspection of the penis. Digital examination and anoscopy should be performed in both sexes, to exclude lesions in the anorectal area. Identification of a primary site in these patients is important, since curative therapy is available for carcinomas of the vulva, vagina, cervix and anus, even after spread to regional lymph nodes. For the occasional patient in whom no primary site is identified, surgical resection with or without radiation therapy to the inguinal area sometimes results in long-term survival [69].

Squamous Carcinoma Metastatic to Other Sites

Metastatic squamous carcinoma in areas other than the cervical or inguinal lymph nodes usually represents metastasis from a primary lung cancer. Computed tomography of the chest and fibreoptic bronchoscopy should be considered if other clinical features suggest the possibility of lung cancer. Chemotherapy with regimens employed in the treatment of non-small cell lung cancer may be considered in patients with good performance status.

Patients with the diagnosis of "poorly differentiated squamous carcinoma" should be evaluated carefully, particularly if other clinical features are unusual for lung cancer (i.e. young patient, non-smoker, unusual metastatic sites). As with the diagnosis of "poorly differentiated adenocarcinoma", this histological diagnosis is sometimes based on scant histological criteria. Additional pathological evaluation with immunoperoxidase stains or electron microscopy should be considered. When the diagnosis remains unclear, such patients should be considered for a trial of therapy for poorly differentiated carcinoma.

Poorly Differentiated Carcinoma of Unknown Primary Site

Patients with poorly differentiated carcinoma have recently been identified as a distinctive subgroup with specific therapeutic implications. These patients account for approximately 20% of all patients with carcinoma of unknown primary site; an additional 10% of patients have *poorly differentiated* adenocarcinoma. Many early empirical chemotherapy trials included these patients along with the more common patients with adenocarcinoma of unknown primary, since these patients were assumed to have the same poor response to treatment and short survival. It is now clear that some of them have extremely responsive neoplasms, and some are curable with combination chemotherapy. Most of these patients do benefit, at least in a palliative sense, from appropriately administered chemotherapy. Clinical and pathological evaluation is therefore critical in patients with poorly differentiated carcinoma, so that optimal therapy can be administered.

Clinical Characteristics

Clinical characteristics in this diverse group of patients appear to differ substantially from those with well-differentiated adenocarcinoma [70]. The median age of this patient group is younger, although both groups have a wide age range. Patients with poorly differentiated carcinoma often give a history of rapid progression of symptoms and have objective evidence of rapid tumour growth. Most importantly, the location of metastases differs, with lymph nodes, mediastinum and retroperitoneum among the predominant sites of involvement much more frequently in patients with poorly differentiated carcinoma.

Pathological Evaluation

Examination of poorly differentiated carcinoma using light microscopy alone is inadequate to assess these tumours optimally. No light microscopic features have been identified which can distinguish chemotherapy-responsive from non-responsive tumours [71]. Moreover, it is clear that even with careful retrospective review of these cases, some responsive tumours of well-defined types (e.g. germ-cell tumour, lymphoma) cannot be identified [71].

Patients with the light microscopic diagnosis of poorly differentiated carcinoma should therefore undergo additional pathological studies with immunoperoxidase staining and electron microscopy. Because the initial diagnosis of poorly differentiated carcinoma is more specific than "poorly differentiated neoplasm", the frequency of identifying unsuspected tumours of other types (particularly lymphoma) is much lower in this group. However, unsuspected diagnoses may still be suggested; in a series of 87 patients with poorly differentiated carcinoma in whom a large battery of immunoperoxidase stains was performed, other diagnoses were suggested in 16 patients (18%) [72]. These diagnoses were melanoma (eight patients), lymphoma (four patients), neuroendocrine tumour (three patients) and prostate carcinoma (one patient). The diagnosis of poorly differentiated carcinoma was confirmed in 55 patients; in 15 patients, the staining pattern was inconclusive. All four patients with immunoperoxidase features of lymphoma (two of whom had been previously diagnosed as poorly differentiated carcinoma by electron microscopy) had clinical features compatible with lymphoma, and all are long-term survivors following cisplatin-based therapy. Therefore, it appears that immunoperoxidase staining can reliably identify unsuspected lymphomas in this group, and neoplasms thus identified are highly responsive to combination chemotherapy. The eight patients in whom the diagnosis of melanoma was suggested by immunoperoxidase staining are unusual, since three of the eight are long-term survivors following chemotherapy for metastatic disease.

In summary, immunoperoxidase tests are useful in the evaluation of poorly differentiated carcinoma, since they suggest other diagnoses in a minority of patients, some of which have specific therapeutic implications. At present, specific immunoperoxidase staining patterns predictive of tumour responsiveness in this group of patients have not been identified.

Diagnostic Evaluation

The initial diagnostic evaluation of these patients is similar to that described for patients with well-differentiated adenocarcinoma of unknown primary site. A thorough history, physical examination, routine laboratory testing and chest radiograph should be obtained in all patients. Computed tomography of the chest and abdomen should be performed in all patients in this group, due to the frequency of mediastinal and retroperitoneal involvement. Serum levels of human chorionic gonadotropin and alpha-fetoprotein should be obtained in all patients, since significant elevations of these markers suggest the diagnosis of germ-cell tumour. The correlation of other serum tumour markers, such as carcinoembryonic antigen, CA125, CA19-9, and CA15-3 with tumour response to chemotherapy has not yet been evaluated.

Treatment

When specialized pathological studies identify a treatable neoplasm (e.g. lymphoma, Ewing's tumour), specific therapy should be administered. In addition, patients with elevated serum levels of HCG or alpha-fetoprotein and clinical features suggestive of extragonadal germ-cell tumour (e.g. mediastinal or retroperitoneal mass) should be treated with chemotherapy effective for germ-cell tumours, even when histological examination does not lead to a specific diagnosis.

Even after complete clinical and pathological evaluation, the majority of patients will have only the non-specific diagnoses of "poorly differentiated carcinoma" or "poorly differentiated adenocarcinoma". The first suggestion that some of these patients have highly responsive tumours was reported approximately 10 years ago, when small groups of selected patients were reported from two centres [73–76]. Most of these patients were young males with tumour location typical of extragonadal germ-cell tumours; serum levels of HCG or alpha-fetoprotein were frequently elevated. These patients were initially thought to have histologically atypical extragonadal germ-cell tumours, explaining their excellent response to cisplatin-based chemotherapy.

Since these early anecdotal reports, we have further investigated the role of intensive cisplatin-based chemotherapy in patients with poorly differentiated carcinoma or poorly differentiated adenocarcinoma of unknown primary site. In a series of reports, we have documented complete responses and long-term disease-free survival in a small minority of patients with this syndrome [70, 74, 77]. We reported on a group of 220 patients treated between 1978 and 1989 [77]. Most patients in this group did not have clinical characteristics strongly suggestive of extragonadal germ-cell tumour. However, involvement of the mediastinum, retroperitoneum and peripheral lymph nodes was relatively common. Patients received two courses of chemotherapy and were re-evaluated; responding patients received a total of four courses. A total of 116 patients received cisplatin, vinblastine and bleomycin (PVB), and 104 patients received cisplatin and etoposide with or without bleomycin. Of 220 patients, 138 (62%) had major (complete or partial) responses to chemotherapy, with 58 complete responses (26%). Thirty-six patients (16% of the entire group) remained free of tumour after a median follow-up of 61 months (range 11–142).

The achievement of complete responses and long-term survival in a minority of patients in this group has been confirmed by other investigators [52, 78, 79]. Van der Gaast and colleagues treated 40 patients who had poorly differentiated carcinoma or poorly differentiated adenocarcinoma with combination chemotherapy using bleomycin, etoposide and cisplatin. Eighteen of 34 patients (53%) responded to therapy, with four (12%) complete responses and two long-term disease-free survivors [79].

The achievement of complete remissions in a sizeable minority of these patients is therefore reproducible, as is a small cohort (10–20%) of long-term disease-free survivors. At present, combination chemotherapy should include cisplatin and etoposide, since results for this combination are at least as good as previous results using cisplatin, vinblastine and bleomycin, and are achieved with less toxicity. Patients should receive two courses of therapy and be re-evaluated for response; responders should complete a total of four treatment courses. No evidence exists that more prolonged treatment will improve results, and most long-term survivors in reported series received only four treatment courses.

Although these results represent marked improvement, the majority of the patients attain only a useful palliative effect (i.e. amelioration of symptoms and prolongation of survival by several months). This group of patients is heterogeneous, and contains many patients with relatively unresponsive tumours. Recently, several responsive subsets have been identified using clinical and pathological features.

Clinical Characteristics Predictive of Treatment Responsiveness

In our group of 220 patients treated with cisplatin-based regimens, several clinical features were evaluated as potential predictors of response to therapy and survival [77]. These factors included age, sex, smoking history, serum tumour marker status, number of metastatic sites, predominant site of tumour involvement (retroperitoneum/peripheral nodes vs. all others), and light microscopic histology (poorly differentiated carcinoma vs. poorly differentiated adenocarcinoma). Using a Cox multivariate regression analysis, tumour location (retroperitoneum or peripheral lymph nodes) was the most important favourable prognostic feature. Additional independent favourable prognostic features included younger age, no smoking history and metastatic sites.

The importance of some of these clinical features was confirmed in a large group of patients with unknown primary carcinomas reported by Abbruzzese et al. [80]. Although this group of 657 patients was heterogeneous, containing patients with all histological subtypes, the relatively poor outcome in patients with adenocarcinoma (as compared to poorly differentiated carcinoma, squamous carcinoma or neuroendocrine carcinoma) was confirmed. Other favourable clinical features included: limited number of organ sites involved, tumour location in lymph nodes other than supraclavicular, and female sex. Since the patients received a variety of treatment regimens, the effect of therapy could not be addressed.

Neuroendocrine Carcinoma of Unknown Primary Site

Recognition of a broad spectrum of neuroendocrine neoplasia has occurred recently, primarily because of improved pathological methods for making the diagnosis. Most well-described adult neuroendocrine tumours have indolent biology and typical histological features (e.g. carcinoid tumours, islet cell tumours, paragangliomas, pheochromocytoma). A second group of neuroendocrine tumours, typified by small cell lung cancer, have high-grade tumour biology and a typical "small cell" anaplastic appearance by light microscopy. A third group of neuroendocrine tumours, recently recognized, have high-grade biology and no distinctive neuroendocrine features by light microscopy. In this group, the initial diagnosis is usually poorly differentiated carcinoma or poorly differentiated adenocarcinoma; neuroendocrine features are only recognized when immunoperoxidase staining or electron microscopy is performed. Neuroendocrine tumours of unknown primary site occur in each of these three categories, and are considered separately.

Low-Grade Neuroendocrine Carcinoma

Metastatic carcinoid or islet cell tumours are occasionally found at metastatic sites without an obvious primary site. In this situation, the metastatic tumour almost always involves the liver, and is sometimes associated with clinical syndromes from the production of bioactive substances. In some patients, primary sites are subsequently found in the intestine or pancreas.

Carcinoid or islet cell tumours of unknown primary site usually exhibit an indolent biology, and management should follow guidelines established for metastatic tumours of these types with known primary sites. Depending on the clinical situation, appropriate management may include local therapy (resection of isolated metastatis, hepatic artery ligation/embolization), treatment of associated syndromes with somatostatin analogues, 5-FU-based systemic therapy or symptomatic management. Intensive cisplatin-based chemotherapy has not been useful in these patients.

Small Cell Carcinoma

Patients with small cell anaplastic carcinoma at a metastatic site usually have a bronchogenic primary. Computed tomography of the chest and fibreoptic bronchoscopy should be performed, which often identify the primary site. A large number of extrapulmonary primary sites have also been described (e.g.

salivary gland, oesophagus, bladder, prostate, ovary, cervix), and patients with localizing symptoms should have appropriate diagnostic studies performed.

Most patients in this group have widespread tumour of aggressive biology, and should receive combination chemotherapy as recommended for small cell lung cancer.

Poorly Differentiated Neuroendocrine Carcinoma

In 10–15% of poorly differentiated carcinomas, electron microscopy identifies neurosecretory granules; these tumours are called "poorly differentiated neuroendocrine tumours" or "primitive neuroectodermal tumours" on this basis. Neuroendocrine features are observed by light microscopic examination in some of these tumours, while in others the light microscopic diagnosis is "poorly differentiated carcinoma". We previously reported a group of 29 patients with poorly differentiated neuroendocrine tumours [81]. Most patients had clinical evidence of a high-grade tumour, and most had metastases in multiple sites. The retroperitoneum, lymph nodes and mediastinum were frequently involved. We have recently updated our series of these patients. Of 43 evaluable patients, 33 responded to chemotherapy with either a cisplatin-based combination or a combination regimen used in the treatment of small cell lung cancer. Thirteen patients had complete responses and eight remain continuously disease free more than 2 years after completion of therapy. Five patients with involvement at only one site received local modalities only (surgical excision, three; radiation therapy, two), and four have had long-term disease-free survival.

The nature of these tumours in most patients remains unclear. In four patients, specific diagnoses were made either subsequently in their clinical course or at autopsy. Two patients were found to have carcinoid tumours with "undifferentiated" growth pattern (both presented with abdominal carcinomatosis); one had small cell lung cancer, and one had an extragonadal germ-cell tumour with predominant neuroendocrine differentiation. A few similar patients, some with long-term survival following chemotherapy, have been classified as "extrapulmonary small cell carcinoma of unknown primary site'.

The origin of these poorly differentiated neuroendocrine tumours remains unclear, but it is likely that the group is heterogeneous. Some patients may have small cell lung cancer with an "occult" primary site. However, half of the patients had no smoking history, and the absence of pulmonary involvement makes this diagnosis unlikely in most patients. As previously discussed, the clinical behaviour and histological appearance of these poorly differentiated tumours is also atypical of most of the other recognized adult neuroendocrine tumours, which are well-defined clinical entities with indolent biology. However, some of these tumours probably are undifferentiated variants of well-recognized neuroendocrine tumours (e.g. carcinoid tumour), albeit without a recognizable primary site. In the undifferentiated form, the clinical as well as the pathological characteristics no longer resemble the characteristics of the more differentiated counterpart. Metastatic anaplastic carcinoid tumours of gastrointestinal origin have also demonstrated sensitivity to cisplatin-based chemotherapy. It is also possible that some of these neoplasms may represent a previously unrecognized type of neuroendocrine tumour.

Although the nature of these tumours remains undefined, the presence of

Table 19.1 Summary of recommended evaluation and therapy of treatable patient subsets

	Additional clinical evaluation	Special pathologic studies	Special subsets	Treatment	Prognosis
Adenocarcinoma (well differentiated or moderately differentiated)	Abdominal CT scan Men: serum PSA Women: mammogram Serum CA125 Additional studies to evaluate symptoms, signs	Men: PSA stain Women: ER, PR	1. Women: axillary node involvement	Treat as primary breast cancer	Poor for entire group (median survival: 4 months) Better for subgroups (see text)
			2. Women: peritoneal carcinomatosis	Surgical cytoreduction + chemotherapy effective in ovarian cancer	
			3. Men: blastic bone metastases, high serum PSA, or PSA tumour staining	Hormonal therapy for prostate cancer	
			4. Single peripheral nodal site of involvement	Lymph node dissection ± radiotherapy	
Squamous carcinoma	Cervical node presentation: panendoscopy	None	Cervical adenopathy	Radiation therapy ± neck dissection	25–50% 5-year survival
	Inguinal presentation: pelvic, rectal exams; anoscopy		Inguinal adenopathy	Inguinal node dissection ± radiation therapy	Potential long-term survival
Poorly differentiated carcinoma, poorly differentiated adenocarcinoma	Chest, abdominal CT scans; serum HCG, AFP; additional studies to evaluate symptoms, signs	Immunoperoxidase staining Electron microscopy Chromosomal analysis	1. Atypical germ-cell tumours (identified by chromosomal abnormalities only)	Treatment for germ-cell tumour	Treatments results similar to those for extragonadal germ-cell tumour
			2. Neuroendocrine tumours	Cisplatin-based therapy	10–20% cured with therapy; high overall response rate
			3. Predominant tumour location in retroperitoneum, peripheral, otherwise not specific	Cisplatin/etoposide/bleomycin	

neurosecretory granules in patients with poorly differentiated carcinoma identifies a highly treatable subgroup. All of these patients should be considered for a trial of therapy with either a cisplatin-based regimen or a combination proved effective against small cell lung cancer. A few patients with a single tumour site may be curable with local treatment modalities; however, a course of adjuvant chemotherapy should be considered in these patients if clinically feasible.

Conclusions

The recognition of more treatable subsets within the large heterogeneous population of patients with carcinoma of unknown primary site represents a definite advance in the management and treatment of these patients. Treatable subsets can be defined with appropriate clinical and pathological evaluation; Table 19.1 provides a summary of the subsets and outlines the evaluation necessary for their identification. Treatment data remain limited; specific therapy should be considered for each of the recognized subsets, however. Unfortunately, a large group of patients with relatively insensitive tumours remains. Improved therapy for these patients will probably await advances in the treatment of non-small cell lung cancer, pancreatic cancer and the other gastrointestinal cancers, since the majority of insensitive adenocarcinomas arise from these occult primary sites.

References

1. Azar HA, Espinoza CG, Richman AV, Saba SR, Wang T (1982) "Undifferentiated" large cell malignancies: an ultrastructural and immunocytochemical study. Hum Pathol 13:323–333.
2. Gatter KC, Alcock C, Heryet A, Mason DY (1985) Clinical importance of analyzing malignant tumours of uncertain origin with immunohistochemical techniques. Lancet 1:1302–1305.
3. Hales SA, Gatter KC, Heryet A, Mason DY (1989) The value of immunocytochemistry in differentiating high-grade lymphoma from other anaplastic tumours. A study of anaplastic tumours from 1940 to 1960. Leuk Lymphoma 1:59.
4. Horning SJ, Carrier EK, Rouse RV, Warnke RA, Michie SA (1989) Lymphomas presenting as histologically unclassified neoplasms: characteristics and response to treatment. J Clin Oncol 7:1281–1287.
5. Battifora H, Trowbridge IS (1983) A monoclonal antibody useful for the differential diagnosis between malignant lymphoma and nonhematopoietic neoplasms. Cancer 51(5):816–821.
6. Bosl GJ, Ilson DH, Rodriguez E, Motzer RJ, Reuter VE, Chaganti RSK (1994) Clinical relevance of the i(12p) marker chromosome in germ cell tumors. J Natl Cancer Inst 86:349–355.
7. Bosman FT, Giard RWM, Nieuwenhuijen-Kruseman AC, Knijnenburg G, Spaander PJ (1980) Human chorionic gonadotrophin and alpha-fetoprotein in testicular germ cell tumors: a retrospective immunohistochemical study. Histopathology 4:673–684.
8. Denk H, Krepler R, Artlieb U, Gabbiani G, Rungger-Brandle E, Leoncini P, Franke WW (1983) Proteins of intermediate filaments. An immunohistochemical and biochemical approach to the classification of soft tissue tumors. Am J Pathol 110(2):193–208.

9. Gabbiani G, Kapanci Y, Barazzone P, Franke WW (1981) Immunochemical identification of intermediate-size filaments in human neoplastic cells. A diagnostic aid for the surgical pathologist. Am J Pathol 104(3):206–216.
10. Kahn HJ, Marks A, Thom H, Baumal R (1983) Role of antibody of S-100 protein in diagnostic pathology. Am J Clin Pathol 79(3):341–347.
11. Kurman RJ, Scardino PT, McIntire KR, Waldmann TA, Javadpour N (1977) Cellular localization of alpha fetoprotein and human chorionic gonadotropin in germ cell tumors of the testis using an indirect immunoperoxidase technique. A new approach to classification utilizing tumor markers. Cancer 40(5):2136–2151.
12. Motzer RJ, Rodriguez E, Reuter VE, Mazumdar M, Bosl GJ, Chaganti RSK (1995) Molecular and cytogenetic studies in the diagnosis of patients with midline carcinomas of unknown primary site. J Clin Oncol 13(1):274–282.
13. Motzer RJ, Rodriguez E, Reuter VE, Samaniego F, Dmitrovsky E, Bajorin DF et al. (1991) Genetic analysis as an aid in diagnosis for patients with midline carcinoma of uncertain histologies. J Natl Cancer Inst 83(5):341–346.
14. O'Connor DT, Burton D, Deftos LJ (1983) Immunoreactive human chromogranin A in diverse polypeptide hormone producing human tumors and normal endocrine tissues. J Clin Endocrinol Metab 57(5):1084–1086.
15. Osborn M, Weber K (1983) Biology of disease. Tumor diagnosis by intermediate filament type: a novel tool for surgical pathology. Lab Invest 48(4):372–394.
16. Tapia FJ, Polak J, Barbosa AJ, Bloom SR, Marangos PJ, Dermody C, Pearse AG (1981) Neuron-specific enolase is produced by neuroendocrine tumors. Lancet 1:808–811.
17. Whang-Peng J, Triche TJ, Knutsen T, Miser J, Douglass EC, Israel MA (1984) Chromosome translocation in peripheral neuroepithelioma. N Engl J Med 311(9): 584–585.
18. Shildt RA, Kennedy PS, Chen TT, Athens JW, O'Bryan RM, Balcerzak SP (1983) Management of patients with metastatic adenocarcinoma of unknown origin: a Southwest Oncology Group study. Cancer Treat Rep 67(1):77–79.
19. Nystrom JS, Weiner JM, Heffelfinger-Juttner J, Irwin LE, Bateman JR, Wolf RM (1977) Metastatic and histologic presentations in unknown primary cancer. Semin Oncol 4(1):53–58.
20. Karsell PR, Sheedy PF, O'Connell MJ (1982) Computerized tomography in search of cancer of unknown origin. J Am Med Assoc 248(3):340–343.
21. McMillan JH, Levine E, Stephens RH (1982) Computed tomography in the evaluation of metastatic adenocarcinoma from an unknown primary site. Radiology 143(1):143–146.
22. August CZ, Murad TM, Newton M (1985) Multiple focal extraovarian serous carcinoma. Int J Gynecol Pathol 4(1):11–23.
23. Chen KT, Flam MS (1986) Peritoneal papillary serous carcinoma with long-term survival. Cancer 58(6):1371–1373.
24. Dalrymple JC, Bannatyne P, Russell P, Solomon HJ, Tattersall MH, Atkinson K, Carter J, Duval P, Elliott P, Friedlander M, Murray J, Coppleson M (1989) Extraovarian peritoneal serous papillary carcinoma. A clinicopathologic study of 31 cases. Cancer 64(1):110–115.
25. Gooneratne S, Sassone M, Blaustein A, Talerman A (1982) Serous surface papillary carcinoma of the ovary: a clinicopathologic study of 26 cases. Int J Gynecol Pathol 1(3):258–269.
26. Hochster H, Wernz JC, Muggia FM (1984) Intra-abdominal carcinomatosis with histologically normal ovaries (Letter). Cancer Treat Rep 68(6):931–932.
27. Strnad CM, Grosh WW, Baxter J, Burnett LS, Jones HW 3rd, Greco FA, Hainsworth JD (1989) Peritoneal carcinomatosis of unknown primary site in women. Ann Intern Med 111(3):213–217.
28. Tobacman JK, Greene MH, Tucker MA, Costa J, Kase R, Fraumeni JF Jr (1982) Intra-abdominal carcinomatosis after prophylactic oophorectomy in ovarian cancer-prone families. Lancet 2:795–797.

29. Ransom DT, Patel SR, Keeney GL, Malkosian GD, Edmonson JH (1990) Papillary serous carcinoma of the peritoneum: a review of 33 cases treated with platin-based chemotherapy. Cancer 66(6):1091–1094.
30. Bhatia SK, Saclarides TJ, Witt TR, Bonomi PD, Anderson KM, Economou SG (1987) Hormone receptor studies in axillary metastases from occult breast cancers. Cancer 59(6):1170–1172.
31. Ashikari R, Rosen PP, Urban JA, Senoo T (1976) Breast cancer presenting as an axillary mass. Ann Surg 183(4):415–417.
32. Merson M, Andreola S, Galimberti V, Bufalino R, Marchini S, Veronesi U (1992) Breast carcinoma presenting as axillary metastases without evidence of a primary tumor. Cancer 70(2):504–508.
33. Patel J, Nemoto T, Rosner D, Dao TL, Pickren JW (1981) Axillary lymph node metastases from an occult breast cancer. Cancer 47(12):2923–2927.
34. Rosen PP (1980) Axillary lymph node metastases in patients with occult noninvasive breast carcinoma. Cancer 46(5):1298–1306.
35. Ellerbroek N, Holmes F, Singletary E, Evans H, Oswald M, McNeese M (1990) Treatment of patients with isolated axillary nodal metastases from an occult primary carcinoma consistent with breast origin. Cancer 66(7):1461–1467.
36. Gentile PS, Carloss HW, Huang T-Y, Yam LT, Lam WK (1988) Disseminated prostatic carcinoma simulating primary lung cancer. Cancer 62(4):711–715.
37. Tell DT, Khoury JM, Taylor HG, Veasey SP (1985) Atypical metastasis from prostate cancer: clinical utility of the immunoperoxidase technique for prostate specific antigen. J Am Med Assoc 253(24):3574–3575.
38. Johnson RO, Castro R, Ansfield FJ (1964) Response of primary unknown cancers to treatment wth 5-fluorouracil. Cancer Chemother Rep 38:63.
39. Moertel CG, Reitemeier RJ, Schutt AJ, Hahn RG (1972) Treatment of the patient with adenocarcinoma of unknown origin. Cancer 30(6):1469–1472.
40. Eagan RT, Therneau TM, Rubin J, Long HJ, Schutt AJ (1987) Lack of value for cisplatin added to mitomycin-doxorubicin combination chemotherapy for carcinoma of unknown primary site. Am J Clin Oncol 10(2):82–145.
41. Fiore JJ, Kelsen DP, Gralla RJ, Casper ES, Magill G, Cheng E, Ochoa M Jr (1985) Adenocarcinoma of unknown primary origin: treatment with vindesine and doxorubicin. Cancer Treat Rep 69(6):591–594.
42. Goldberg RM, Smith FP, Ueno W, Ahlgren JD, Schein PS (1986) 5-Fluorouracil, Adriamycin, and mitomycin in the treatment of adenocarcinoma of unknown primary. J Clin Oncol 4(3):395–399.
43. Kambhus SA, Kelsen D, Niedzwiecki D, Ochoa M Jr (1986) Phase II trial of mitomycin C, vindesine, and Adriamycin and predictive variables in the treatment of patients with adenocarcinoma of unknown primary sites (Abstract). Proc Am Assoc Cancer Res 27:185.
44. Milliken ST, Tattersall MH, Woods RL, Coates AS, Levi JA, Fox RM, Raghavan D (1987) Metastatic adenocarcinoma of unknown primary site. A randomized study of two combination chemotherapy regimens. Eur J Cancer Clin Oncol 23(11):1645–1648.
45. Treat J, Falchuk SC, Tremblay C, Spielman M, Woolley PV, Ronesse J (1989) Phase II trial of methotrexate-FAM (m-FAM) in adenocarcinoma of unknown primary. Eur J Cancer Clin Oncol 25(7):1053–1055.
46. van der Gaast A, Verweij J, Planting AS, Stoter G (1988) 5-Fluorouracil, doxorubicin, and mitomycin C (FAM) combination chemotherapy for metastatic adenocarcinoma of unknown primary. Eur J Cancer Clin Oncol 24(4):765–768.
47. Woods RL, Fox RM, Tattersall MHN, Levi JA, Brodie GN (1980) Metastatic adenocarcinomas of unknown primary: a randomized study of two combination-chemotherapy regimens. N Engl J Med 303(2):87–89.
48. de Campos ES, Menasce LP, Radford J, Harris M, Thatcher N (1994) Metastatic carcinoma of uncertain primary site: a retrospective review of 57 patients treated

with vincristine, doxorubicin, cyclophosphamide (VAC), or VAC alternating with cisplatin and etoposide (VAC/PE). Cancer 73(2):470–475.
49. Gill I, Guaglianone P, Grunberg SM, Scholz M, Muggia FM (1991) High dose intensity of cisplatin and etoposide in adenocarcinoma of unknown primary. Anticancer Res 11(3):1231–1235.
50. Lenzi R, Abbruzzese J, Amato R, Raber M, Frost P (1991) Cisplatin, 5-fluorouracil and folinic acid for the treatment of carcinoma of unknown primary: a phase II study. Proc Am Soc Clin Oncol (Abstract) 10:301.
51. Pasterz R, Savoraj N, Burgess M (1986) Prognostic factors in metastatic carcinoma of unknown primary. J Clin Oncol 4(11):1652–1657.
52. Raber MN, Faintuch J, Abbruzzese JL, Sumnull C, Frost P (1991) Continuous infusion of 5-fluorouracil, etoposide and cis-diamminedichloroplatinum in patients with metastatic carcinoma of unknown primary origin. Ann Oncol 2(7):519–520.
53. Jones AS, Cook JA, Phillips DE, Roland NR (1993) Squamous carcinoma presenting as an enlarged cervical lymph node. Cancer 72(5):1756–1761.
54. Barrie JR, Knapper WH, Strong EW (1970) Cervical nodal metastases of unknown origin. Am J Surg 120(4):466–470.
55. Bataini JP, Rodriguez J, Jaulerry C, Brugere J, Ghossein NA (1987) Treatment of metastatic neck nodes secondary to an occult epidermoid carcinoma of the head and neck. Laryngoscope 97(9):1080–1084.
56. Carlson LS, Fletcher GH, Oswald MJ (1986) Guidelines for the radiotherapeutic techniques for cervical metastases from an unknown primary. Int J Radiat Oncol Biol Phys 12(12):2101–2110.
57. Coker DD, Casterline PF, Chambers RG, Jacques DA (1977) Metastases to lymph nodes of the head and neck from an unknown primary site. Am J Surg 134(4):517–522.
58. de Braud F, Heilbrun LK, Admed K, Sakr W, Ensley JF, Kish JA, Tapazoglou E, al-Sarraf M (1989) Metastatic squamous cell carcinoma of an unknown primary localized to the neck. Advantages of an aggressive treatment. Cancer 64(5):510–515.
59. Fermont DC (1980) Malignant cervical lymphadenopathy due to an unknown primary. Clin Radiol 31(3):355–358.
60. Jesse RH, Perez CA, Fletcher GH (1973) Cervical lymph node metastasis: unknown primary cancer. Cancer 32(4):854–859.
61. Jose B, Bosch A, Caldwell WL, Frias Z (1979) Metastasis to neck from unknown primary tumor. Acta Radiol Oncol 18(3):161–170.
62. Leipzig B, Winter ML, Hokanson JA (1981) Cervical nodal metastases of unknown origin. Laryngoscope 91(4):593–598.
63. McCunniff AJ, Raben M (1986) Metastatic carcinoma of the neck from an unknown primary. Int J Radiat Oncol Biol Phys 12(10):1849–1852.
64. Mohit-Tabatabai MA, Dasmahapatra KS, Rush BF Jr, Ohanian M (1986) Management of squamous cell carcinoma of unknown origin in cervical lymph nodes. Am Surg 52(3):152–154.
65. Nordstrom DG, Tewfik HH, Latourette HB (1979) Cervical lymph node metastases from an unknown primary. Int J Radiat Oncol Biol Phys 5(1):73–76.
66. Pacini P, Olmi P, Cellai E, Chiavacci A (1981) Cervical lymph node metastases from an unknown primary tumour. Acta Radiol Oncol 20(5):311–314.
67. Spiro RH, DeRose G, Strong EW (1983) Cervical node metastasis of occult origin. Am J Surg 146(4):441–446.
68. Yang ZY, Hu YJ, Yan JH, Cai WM, Qin DX, Xu GZ, Wu XL (1983) Lymph node metastases in the neck from an unknown primary. Report on 113 patients. Acta Radiol Oncol 22(1):17–22.
69. Guarischi A, Keane TJ, Elhakim T (1987) Metastatic inguinal nodes from an unknown primary neoplasm. A review of 56 cases. Cancer 59(3):572–577.
70. Greco FA, Vaughn WK, Hainsworth JD (1986) Advanced poorly differentiated

carcinoma of unknown primary site: recognition of a treatable syndrome. Ann Intern Med 104(4):547–553.
71. Hainsworth JD, Wright EP, Gray GF Jr, Greco FA (1987) Poorly differentiated carcinoma of unknown primary site: correlation of light microscopic findings with response to cisplatin-based combination chemotherapy. J Clin Oncol 5(8):1275–1280.
72. Hainsworth JD, Wright EP, Johnson DH, Davis BW, Greco FA (1991) Poorly differentiated carcinoma of unknown primary site: clinical usefulness of immunoperoxidase staining. J Clin Oncol 9(11):1931–1938.
73. Fox RM, Woods RL, Tattersall MHN (1979) Undifferentiated carcinoma in young men: the atypical teratoma syndrome. Lancet 1:1316–1318.
74. Hainsworth JD, Greco FA (1986) Poorly differentiated carcinoma of unknown primary site. In: Fer MF, Greco FA, Oldham R (eds) Poorly differentiated neoplasms and tumors of unknown origin. Grune and Stratton, Orlando, pp189–202.
75. Richardson RL, Greco FA, Wolff S, Hande KR, Oldham RK (1979) Extragonadal germ cell malignancy: value of tumor markers in metastatic carcinoma in young males (Abstract). Proc Am Assoc Cancer Res 20:204.
76. Richardson RL, Schoumacher RA, Fer MF, Hande KR, Forbes JT, Oldham RK, Greco FA (1981) The unrecognized extragonadal germ cell cancer syndrome. Ann Intern Med 94(2):181–186.
77. Hainsworth JD, Johnson DH, Greco FA (1992) Cisplatin-based combination chemotherapy in the treatment of poorly differentiated carcinoma and poorly differentiated adenocarcinoma of unknown primary site: results of a 12-year experience. J Clin Oncol 10(6):912–922.
78. Pavlidis N, Kosmidis P, Skaros D, Briassoulis E, Beer M, Theoharis D, Bafaloukos D, Maraveyas A, Fountzilas G (1992) Subsets of tumors responsive to cisplatin or carboplatin combinations in patients with carcinoma of unknown primary site. Ann Oncol 3(8):631–634.
79. van der Gaast A, Verweij J, Henzen-Logmans SC, Rodenburg CJ, Stoter G (1990) Carcinoma of unknown primary: identification of a treatable subset. Ann Oncol 1(2):119–122.
80. Abbruzzese JL, Abbruzzese MC, Hess KR, Raber MN, Lenzi R, Frost P (1994) Unknown primary carcinoma: natural history and prognostic factors in 657 consecutive patients. J Clin Oncol 12(6):1272–1280.
81. Hainsworth JD, Johnson DH, Greco FA (1988) Poorly differentiated neuroendocrine carcinoma of unknown primary site: a newly recognized clinicopathologic entity. Ann Intern Med 109(5):364–371.

Index